Cash's Textbook of General Medical and Surgical Conditions for Physiotherapists

P

Cash's Textbook of General Medical and Surgical Conditions for Physiotherapists

edited by
PATRICIA A. DOWNIE FCSP

with Susan Boardman MCSP

Second edition

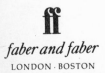

faber and faber
LONDON · BOSTON

First published under this title in 1984
by Faber and Faber Limited
3 Queen Square London WC1N 3AU

Second edition 1990

Photoset by Parker Typesetting Service, Leicester
Printed in Great Britain by
Richard Clay Ltd Bungay, Suffolk

Previously published as part of *Cash's Textbook of
Medical Conditions for Physiotherapists* 1951, 1957,
1965, 1971, 1976, 1979 and *Cash's Textbook of
Physiotherapy in Some Surgical Conditions* 1955, 1958,
1966, 1971, 1977, 1979

ISBN 0-571-14064-5

A CIP record for this book is
available from the British Library.

Contents

Contributors

Mary Anderson MB, ChB, FRCOG
Consultant Obstetrician and Gynaecologist
Lewisham Hospital
London SE13 6LH

Susan Boardman MCSP
Superintendent Physiotherapist, Mount Vernon Hospital
Northwood, Middlesex HA6 2RN

Mary W. Bromiley MCSP, SRP, RPT(USA)
Downs House, Baydon
Marlborough SN8 2JS

Christine V. Bungay MCSP
Superintendent Paediatric Physiotherapist
and Clinical Co-ordinator Child Development Centre
St George's Hospital, London SW17 0QT

Jane Burgess MCSP
Superintendent Physiotherapist, St John's Hospital for Diseases of
the Skin
London WC2H 7BJ

David Evans MD, FRCP, FRCPath
Consultant Pathologist, Llandough Hospital
Penarth CF6 1XX

Penelope A. Fenn Clark MCSP
Superintendent Physiotherapist, Dulwich Hospital (North)
London SE22 8DF

Sheila M. Harrison MCSP
Consultant Physiotherapist for Women's Health
Health Department of Western Australia, Perth

Margaret E. Jefferies SRP
formerly Senior Physiotherapist, Little Plumstead Hospital
Norwich NR6 5BE

Hilary Lawler BA, MCSP
Unit Head Physiotherapist for Mental Illness and Handicap
Hellesdon Hospital, Norwich NR6 5BE

Mary Lightbody MCSP
Superintendent Physiotherapist, Neurosurgical Unit
The Radcliffe Infirmary, Oxford OX2 6HE

D. B. McHutchison BPharm, MRPharmS
Principal Pharmacist, Addenbrookes Hospital
Cambridge CB2 2QQ

Julie McKenna MCSP
formerly Senior Obstetric Physiotherapist
The Royal Free Hospital, London NW3 2QG

Laura Mitchell MCSP, DipTP
8 Gainsborough Gardens
Well Walk, London NW3 1BJ

Brian Morgan MB, FRCS
Consultant Plastic Surgeon, University College Hospital, London
and Mount Vernon Hospital, Northwood, Middlesex

Jeanne M. Morgan MCSP
Senior Physiotherapist, Little Plumstead Hospital
Norwich NR13 5EW

James Partridge MA(Oxon), MSc
Maison de Bas
St Andrews, Guernsey CI

Stella Saywell MA, FCSP
Chairman, Avon Riding for the Disabled
Avon Riding Centre for the Disabled
Kingsweston Road, Henbury, Avon BS10 7QT

Paul J. Smith FRCS
Consultant Plastic Surgeon, Mount Vernon Hospital
Northwood, Middlesex HA6 2RN

David Stewart BA, ALA
Librarian, The Royal Society of Medicine
London WIM 8AE

Catherine M. C. Van de Ven MCSP
District Physiotherapist, Richmond, Twickenham and Roehampton
Health Authority
Queen Mary's University Hospital, Roehampton
London SWI5 5PR

Edward Welchew MB, ChB, FFARCS
Consultant Anaesthetist, Northern General Hospital, Sheffield
and Honorary Lecturer, Department of Anaesthetics, University of
Sheffield Medical School

Editor's Preface

There is a well-known quotation which is said to have originated in the ancient Greek school of medicine: its words set the theme for this new edition:

> 'To cure, occasionally,
> To relieve, often,
> To comfort, always.'

I asked all the contributors to highlight the practicalities of care for patients. I hope the resultant chapters do reflect this. I also asked that, where appropriate, they should comment upon wider issues which bear upon total patient care. This has certainly been achieved, and mention will be found of AIDS, child abuse, rape, abortion, infertility, euthanasia. I must thank particularly Mary Anderson who, despite a heavy professional timetable, has provided a most helpful chapter which includes a succinct section on the ethical and moral problems relative to obstetrics and gynaecology. I hope that physiotherapists will find such comments helpful to them in enabling them to formulate their own thoughts and opinions on these highly topical subjects.

James Partridge has brought up to date his doings and experiences after severe burns. As I said in the previous edition his chapter (16) should be compulsory reading for every physiotherapist whether student or trained, throughout the world, for it provides the *raison d'être* of so much of our work. His 'physio' is still remembered by him for her humanity, compassion and understanding.

'To comfort, always' – this is something which can never be quantified by research, yet it must ever remain the cornerstone of patient care. As medical science becomes increasingly sophisticated and technological so it also becomes less easy to remember the human aspect (within this book Figure 22/1, page 398, might well be captioned 'Find the baby'). Time to talk with, and listen to, patients is as much part of treatment as manipulation. Assuaging fears and worries, explanation of symptoms, encouragement to become independent, all should be seen within the context of total patient care. Currently, there is a great deal of talk and writing about holistic medicine, of wholeness and healing, but for many of us treatment of physical affliction has always meant care for the whole person, and his family. Cure a patient physically of his symptoms and leave mental anguish and you have failed; cure him physically and mentally and leave him bitter in spirit and you have failed; cure him physically and mentally and know he has peace of mind then you have probably succeeded.

Almost without exception each contributor has talked of team-work, of being part of a multidisciplinary team. If it is remembered that the most important person of any team is the patient then, through the varying skills of each team member, it should be pos-sible to provide that person with the necessary incentives to allow him to be cured, sometimes; relieved, often; and comforted, always.

I took heed of requests for certain additional subjects to be included and readers will now find new chapters on the elderly, adult mental handicap and psychiatric illness. To these authors I extend my thanks. To *all* the contributors, old and new, my grateful thanks for revising or re-writing existing chapters. As editor I am ultimately responsible for the overall content and this is reflected in my decision to include a chapter on veterinary physiotherapy. Mary Bromiley is a highly experienced physiotherapist working with animals and I am delighted that she is now able to share her knowledge with the wide readership of these textbooks.

My associate editor, Susan Boardman, has been a splendid assist-ant; Pauline Walker MCSP and Stella Saywell FCSP have both given invaluable help; to these three I really am indebted for much of the 'nitty-gritty' of putting together such a book, and I can only say thank you to them on behalf of the readership.

Yet again, Audrey Besterman has come up trumps – this time with equine and canine anatomical drawings. I thank her most warmly.

My final words go to the reader: do *enjoy* reading these chapters and may they help and encourage you all in the performing of your professional duties.

P.A.D. *Norwich, 1989*

Sadly, Paddy Downie died during the preparation of this volume. Thousands of physiotherapists will be grateful to Paddy Downie for her complete revision of Joan Cash's original physiotherapy textbooks. These books are now universally acknowledged as the best physiotherapy texts and this is due almost entirely to Paddy Downie's efforts. As well as editing and writing books she was also medical editor at Faber and Faber from 1977 to 1987.

Roger Osborne,
Medical Editor, Faber and Faber

Chapter 1

Using Medical Libraries

by D. W. C. STEWART BA, ALA

Medical libraries vary considerably in size and scope of coverage and run from what may be little more than a shelf of books to collections of hundreds of thousands of books, journals and other materials such as audiotapes and videos. Whatever their size and type they exist to provide relevant information to support education, training, research and the professional development of health care workers with the ultimate aim of improving the quality of patient care.

The average medical library forms part of an institution such as a hospital or research institute and as such will endeavour to identify a readership whose needs it can reasonably try to meet. A teaching hospital library, for example, will be concerned primarily with the needs of medical students, teaching staff, consultants and researchers. It will also cover the needs of other health professionals such as physiotherapists, radiographers and pharmacists and it may also aim to provide for administrative and technical staff not directly concerned with patient care. Provision of nursing literature may also be made but that often depends on whether there is a school of nursing in which case there will probably be a separate nursing library.

It is important to define which is your primary library, that is to say, the one to which you belong and on whose services you have a right to call. It may be the library of a hospital, an authority, a public library system or a professional society. The more libraries to which you can have access the better, as it can be more useful to visit another library if you are working on a subject in which it specializes rather than trying to gather a lot of material by inter-library loan. A visit will also give access to specialized material such as dictionaries and bibliographies which would not normally be made available on loan.

Most libraries produce some kind of printed guide; it may be a lavishly produced booklet or a single duplicated sheet. In addition to digesting this, try to make yourself known to the library staff and get an individual introduction to the library; explain also what you are working on so that the librarian can help you get the most out of the library. Larger libraries such as those of universities have formal introductory procedures for new readers while some have audio-visual presentations on how they work or on the use of some specific types of material such as government publications.

THE CATALOGUE

Make the acquaintance of the catalogue; this is all the more important if it seems daunting in its complexity. It is the key to the library and it is designed both to act as a list of what is held and to provide an alternative approach to the stock from that of the arrangement of books and journals on the shelves. Catalogues are constructed according to fairly elaborate rules to ensure conformity of entry; they deal with how one files a name such as Van Winkle (under 'Van' if he's American, under 'Winkle' if he's Dutch) and how the publications of organizations – as opposed to individuals – should be treated and so on. Unhappily not all libraries use the same rules and large older libraries may have rather old-fashioned styles of entry. Regular use of the catalogue should make the reader familiar with the peculiarities of the system.

Most library catalogues are on cards filed in cabinets but other forms are increasingly found such as microfilm or computer based. There is little difference in approach in using either card or microfilm catalogues but computerized catalogues, which permit the reader to sit at a terminal and make a search of the data-base which forms the catalogue, can give greatly improved and faster results though they may be less easy to browse through. It is important to know what is in a catalogue and what is not; for example, very few library catalogues aim to list individual articles in journals or chapters in books, though a highly specialized library may maintain such an index, possibly as a file separate from the catalogue itself.

Most libraries regard the author entry as the 'main entry' so that some catalogues may expect the reader to refer to the author card for the fullest details of the publication in question. While the author of a book is usually an individual the term 'author' is used to cover editors, compilers, sponsoring bodies, government departments and so forth. The name of a publisher is not normally used, so it is rarely any use going to a catalogue knowing that a report was published by the government and expecting to find it under Her Majesty's Stationery Office as it will have its entry under the name of the government department responsible for it. However, a publication such as the *Faber Medical Dictionary* would have an entry under publisher as the publisher's name is an integral part of the title. A good catalogue will try to cover some of the possible headings a reader might approach and there should be a good system of cross references. These consist of *'see'* references which direct from a heading not used, to one which is, such as 'Petrograd *see* Leningrad', and *'see also'* references which refer to a related heading, for example 'Music therapy *see also* Art Therapy'.

Dictionary catalogue

A subject approach may be provided by a separate subject catalogue but some libraries inter-file authors and subjects in a dictionary catalogue. Problems can arise here if a word can be used in different senses and a dictionary catalogue distinguishes between, say, 'Brain' as an individual's name (Lord Brain, the distinguished neurologist), the name of something (*Brain*, the neurology journal), the same word as the name of a place and the word as a common noun. A catalogue would file the entries in the order in which I have given them here. Dictionary catalogues should be used in rather the same way as one uses encyclopaedias.

Subject catalogue

Subject catalogues are usually arranged in the same order as the classification system used in the library with appropriate additional entries to bring together information on books which are not grouped together on the shelves. Classifications are based on analysing subjects and assigning numerical or alphabetical codes to identify groups and sub-groups of subjects and place the classified books, and the catalogue entries, in a logical relationship. The approach of classification systems varies and results in books being grouped in different ways.

National Library of Medicine Classification This is the most common classification system and is the scheme used in most British medical libraries. It is based on grouping all the material on a system (cardiovascular, nervous, digestive, etc.) in one place and sub-dividing by anatomy, physiology, pathology and so forth to produce a notation which looks like this:

WG	Cardiovascular System
WG 200	Heart, general works
WG 201	Cardiovascular Anatomy
WG 202	Cardiovascular Physiology

Physical Therapy is classified as:

WB 460 Physical medicine. Physical therapy
WB 469 Heat therapy
WB 480 Ultraviolet therapy. Sunlight. Light therapy
WB 510 Diathermy
WB 515 Ultrasonic therapy

Universal Decimal Classification (UDC) This scheme, and the related Dewey Classification usually found in public libraries, arranges medical material with anatomy, physiology and pathology as the main groupings sub-divided by parts of the body to produce a filing order like:

6 Applied Sciences. Medicine. Technology
61 Medicine
611 Anatomy
611.1 Cardiovascular Anatomy
612 Physiology
612.1 Cardiovascular Physiology
616 Pathology
616.1 Cardiovascular Disease

The Dewey and UDC class 615 covers treatment methods of all kinds, including pharmacology, with physiotherapy at 615.8. However, the treatment of a specific disorder is classified with material on the disorder so that books on physiotherapy may be located in other places if they deal with the treatment of a specific condition.

Thus in the one scheme you will find all physiological material together while in the other all cardiological material is in one place. However good a classification may be it is impossible always to keep related material together as many topics have quite complex relationships. Most classifications give librarians some latitude within the rules to suit the needs of the individual library so it is possible to find the same book classified in different ways in two libraries which use the same classification. It is useful to be in the habit of using the catalogue rather than relying on physiotherapy books being on the third shelf down inside the door.

Having found the entry for a book you want in the catalogue it should not be too difficult to find it on the shelves. The information on the catalogue card should include the author, the title and the subtitle, the 'collation' which indicates size, number of pages and other details of physical form, and perhaps an annotation which may provide additional information about the title, for example:

MORTON, L. T. and GODBOLT, S. (editors).

Information Sources in the Medical Sciences. 3rd edition.
London, Butterworths, 1984.

xviii,534p
(Butterworths Guides to Information Sources)

In addition the entry will include information such as an accession number which identifies the book for library administrative purposes and a classification number or other indicator of where the book is shelved.

A library may have more than one sequence of books depending perhaps on whether they are earlier than a specific date, available for reference only or of unusual size, so it is important to read the catalogue entry carefully for any indication of this. The libraries of medical schools often have a 'reserve' collection of course reading and standard texts which may be issued for limited periods only.

AUDIO-VISUAL MATERIAL

Audio-visual productions are important teaching and training media and all hospital libraries will have stocks and the appropriate equipment on which to use them. At the simplest they may be audiotapes which can be listened to on a car cassette player and they range through audiotapes with sets of slides, films and videos with accompanying training manuals to computer based video training systems which guide the user through a programme providing instruction and questions. Videos are particularly useful in illustrating conditions and procedures which cannot easily be described in print; there is a wide range available including examination techniques, the surgical management of hand injuries, knee joint arthroscopy, health worker – patient communication as well as programmes designed for use by patients.

A printed catalogue of audio-visual material is published by the Graves Medical Audio-visual Library, 220 New London Road, Chelmsford, Essex CM2 9BJ.

PERIODICALS

Medical libraries spend a fairly large proportion of their book grants on periodicals and give this kind of material special treatment. Periodicals may be listed in the catalogue but more often there is a separate list arranged by title which gives an indication of the holdings available. It may also be available as a printed handlist for distribution to readers. In addition the library will maintain a detailed stock record which gives precise details about dates of receipt of issues, what parts have not arrived and so on.

Indexing periodicals

While the library catalogue lists the book stock in some detail the contents of periodical issues are not normally indexed though special issues of importance may be. Instead, reliance is placed on what are known as 'secondary' publications (usually themselves journals) which index the contents of the 'primary' journals which publish original work. Some secondary publications are designed to keep practitioners and researchers aware of new material appearing while others provide a means of making searches of the literature for information on specific subjects. Occasionally a secondary journal may carry one or two original papers, usually reviews of the literature on some aspect of a subject, while some primary journals may have an abstracting section which draws attention to papers in other periodicals.

The Institute for Scientific Information (USA) publishes a series of weekly journals called *Current Contents* three of which relate to medicine and surgery and which slightly overlap: *Current Contents – Life Sciences*, *Current Contents – Clinical Medicine* and *Current Contents – Social and Behavioral Sciences*. Each issue reproduces the contents pages of the journals and books it covers and also provides a subject index and a list of authors' addresses. They are a useful means of keeping in touch with new articles in journals which your own library may not have.

Some other journals which have mainly original articles also have sections which review and abstract recent articles in other journals. *Physical Therapy* and *Surgery Gynecology & Obstetrics* have regular abstract sections of this kind.

The Index Medicus The *Index Medicus* (or the *Abridged Index Medicus*) is probably the most widely available of all medical indexing sources. It is a monthly index to the contents of some 2500 medical journals and to a small number of selected congresses, symposia, etc., which arranges the papers it indexes according to a carefully compiled list of index terms (Medical Subject Headings or 'MeSH') while also indexing by author. *Index Medicus* has been published almost continuously since 1879 and in its present form it cumulates annually for ease of retrospective searching. It is selective but it covers all aspects of medicine and a good range of journals world-wide though there is a slight bias in favour of US material. Some time spent getting familiar with *Index Medicus* is well worth while.

Index Medicus places physiotherapy in its subject category E2 – PROCEDURES AND TECHNICS – THERAPEUTICS. The main specific heading is PHYSICAL THERAPY; other specific headings of interest to physiotherapists include EXERCISE THERAPY, HYDRO-THERAPY, MAS-SAGE, and ULTRAVIOLET THERAPY. A useful broader heading is REHABILITATION.

Sub-headings are used to assist in arranging entries and include: anatomy, adverse effects, diagnosis, etiology, education, instru-mentation, methods, treatment, prevention and so on. An article will be indexed under three or so headings if appropriate and only under the most specific headings available. It is important to check the MeSH list before making a search to ensure that the most appropriate headings are being checked.

Excerpta Medica *Excerpta Medica* is an abstract journal in 42 different subject sections with Section 19 entitled 'Rehabilitation and Physical Medicine'. Papers are listed and abstracted in as many sections as are necessary so that an article on the physical rehabilita-tion of patients after mitral valve replacement will appear in the section on Rehabilitation and in the section covering Cardiovascular Disease and Surgery. All abstracts are in English and are full enough to make it unnecessary sometimes to read the original paper. There is an annual index for searching back-years and each issue is arranged so that it can be browsed with appropriate grouping of abstracts such as:

Diagnosis, Function Tests and Evaluation
Rehabilitation of Somatic Disorders (arranged by system, e.g. musculoskeletal, nervous, cardiovascular, respiratory, etc.)
Rehabilitation of Mental Disorders
Prostheses and Technical Aids

Most medical libraries will have the *Index Medicus* but only the largest will have many sections of *Excerpta Medica*, though sections important to a reasonable number of readers will be available.

Both of these important information sources and many other information files also exist as computerized information systems which can be searched on-line through computer terminals linked into national and international communications networks. A com-puter literature search can often be more precise than one made in the printed version of a file but because systems operate in different ways searches are usually done by librarians with the user of the information sitting-in to monitor progress so that the direction of the search can be changed as results appear on the screen. Among the files available are:

DHSS-DATA which covers medical equipment and supplies, primary health care, social services to the handicapped, occupational diseases and most of the topics which are the responsibility of the Departments of Health and Social Security.

HSELINE   is produced by the Health and Safety Executive and covers all aspects of industrial health and hygiene.

PSYCINFO   is a large file which aims to cover the world's literature in psychology and related literature.

The growth of computerized information files in recent years means that there is likely to be increasing availability of such facilities in libraries of all kinds.

Alternative versions of on-line files now becoming available are information systems in the form of a compact disc (CD ROM) similar to a compact audio disc but containing 'printed' information. *Index Medicus* is available in this form and is usually available in libraries for direct use, after appropriate instruction, by library readers.

The indexing sources mentioned above and the articles quoted in papers provide information on a wide range of possibly relevant material. When searching the *Index Medicus* or other sources it is important to make an accurate note of papers you would like to read. While the arrangement and layout will vary, the essential elements of a reference are: the title of the journal, the year, the volume and part number and the pages of the article. Useful are the authors and the title and it is best to note these also. If an article is a chapter in a book the name of the author or editor should also be noted as the chapter details are usually insufficient to identify the book of which it is part and make the obtaining of it from another library difficult.

INTER-LENDING SYSTEMS

No library can aim to provide everything its readers could want so libraries co-operate through various inter-lending systems locally, nationally and internationally. Within the National Health Service several regions have well-developed library systems which effectively make available to library users the resources of all the libraries in the region. A library will have available a range of listings of the periodical holdings of other libraries though it is rather more difficult to locate books and monographs. The University of London, for example, publishes a microform list of the periodical holdings of all the libraries of the University including the medical schools and the specialist institutes which is extremely useful. Some individual libraries publish their own lists and there are other listings such as *British Books in Print* which act as means of confirming that a publication actually exists or that the details are correct.

The British Library Document Supply Centre has a stock of publications which covers medicine and related subjects almost comprehensively and is often the main source of books and journals which a library cannot provide from its own stock. If necessary articles can be obtained from abroad. The BLDSC can only provide material in response to requests from libraries, not individuals, though there is a public reading room at the library in Boston Spa, Yorkshire.

The Science Reference and Information Service of the British Library is located in central London and can be used without formality. Medically related material is housed at the branch at Aldwych.

The *Directory of Medical and Health Care Libraries* (6th edition, London, The Library Association, 1986) lists all the significant medical libraries in Britain and Ireland by geographical location and is an invaluable guide to the resources in one's area. Copies are available in most medical libraries.

References for publication

Having found the material which you wish to consult you may then find yourself in the position of writing a paper for publication. There are many books on the writing of scientific papers and publishers will also have their own rules and recommendations on format and presentation. Most medical papers have to supply references to the work of other people which may have been quoted in the text; editors are very hard on the author who produces unsupported statements. Not only must references be provided but they must also be checked for accuracy both in content and presentation. Badly presented or inaccurate references reflect on the general accuracy and diligence of the author and a good paper can be spoiled by inadequate references. *Never* quote something which you have not read; at the time you read a paper make an accurate and complete note of it avoiding the shorthand like APM&R 3/77 48 which you may be unable to reconstruct accurately when you need to. Note the titles of papers and the last as well as the first page number as some publishers require it. If you have used a variety of libraries in your researches it may help to note where you saw something that took you a while to find as you may want to use it again. Five-by-three-inch index cards in a small file are still the best physical means of organizing reference lists.

The *Index Medicus* style of reference citation is increasingly being used as a standard and is known as the 'Vancouver' system (International Committee of Medical Journal Editors, 1988). Even if the project in hand is not intended for publication the system applied to reports and other documents greatly improves the appearance and usability of the finished work.

There are two other systems for citing references in papers; either by the quoting of the author's name with a superior numeral, e.g. Smith[3] or the author's name and the date of the paper, e.g. Smith (1976). The second system, generally and inexplicably known as the Harvard system, is still preferred by many journals. In the bibliography references are arranged numerically by the first system and alphabetically by the second system. Some publishers prefer that journal titles be given in full while others recommend abbreviations; a good standard abbreviation list appears in the first issue of *Index Medicus* each year.

When checking the references after typing your paper always check them from the original publication; do not take the short cut of looking them up in the *Index Medicus* for it can make mistakes and it may not give you all the information you need. One of the longest running wrong references appeared off and on in the literature from 1887 to 1938 and was only sorted out when someone took the trouble to read the original paper referred to!

REFERENCE

International Committee of Medical Journal Editors (1988). Uniform requirements for manuscripts submitted to biomedical journals. *British Medical Journal*, 296, 401–5.

BIBLIOGRAPHY

Jenkins, S. (1987). *Medical Libraries: A User Guide*. British Medical Association, London.

Morton, L. T. (1980). *How to Use a Medical Library*, 6th edition. William Heinemann Medical Books Limited, London.

Morton, L. T. and Godbolt, S. (eds) (1984). *Information Sources in Medical Sciences*, 3rd edition. Butterworths, London.

Chapter 2

Inflammation and Healing

by D. M. D. EVANS MD, FRCP, FRCPath

In Shakespeare's time most disease was ascribed to the four 'humours', used as a cloak to hide the almost complete ignorance of disease processes. Sometimes the relationship between a disease and its cause was dimly appreciated, as between the 'ague' (malaria) and marshland districts, but several hundred years elapsed before the relationship between marshland, the breeding of mosquitoes and their role in the transmission of malarial parasites to man was discovered.

Before its disorders could be understood, the normal human body had to be studied. This required international co-operation. An Englishman, William Harvey (1578–1657) paved the way by his work on the circulation of blood. A Dutchman, Anton Van Leuwenhoek (1632–1723) developed microscopes with which he discovered the existence of red blood cells and the capillary circulation. With the aid of the microscope an Italian, Marcello Malpighi (1628–1694) investigated the cellular structure of normal organs, earning the title 'Father of Histology'. A German, Rudolph Virchow (1821–1901) used the microscope to study diseased tissues and became the founder of cellular pathology. A Frenchman, Louis Pasteur (1822–1895) demonstrated the existence of bacteria and their importance in causing disease. A Russian, Ilya Metchnikoff (1845–1916) elucidated the process of inflammation in living tissues. Workers from many other countries have advanced our knowledge to its present stage.

INFLAMMATION (Latin, *inflammare*, to burn)

Inflammation is the sequence of changes which take place in living tissue in response to damage. The termination '-itis' as in meningitis indicates inflammation of the relevant tissue, in this case the meninges.

Causes

The main causes of inflammation are injury, infection, infarction and immune reactions.

Injury This may be physical, thermal, radiational, electrical or chemical.

1. *Physical* injury (trauma) includes bruises, wounds, surgical intervention, fractures and crush injuries.
2. *Thermal* injury is produced by excessive heat or cold. Heat injury includes scalds from hot water bottles, wax baths and various types of burn. Cold injuries include chilblains and frostbite.
3. *Radiational* injury includes sunburn, ultraviolet irradiation burns and flash burns from nuclear explosions.
4. *Electrical* injury is the result of an electric current passing through the tissues, of sufficient power to damage them. Short wave diathermy may produce a similar type of burn injury.
5. *Chemical* injury includes burns from acids, alkalis and corrosive metal salts. There are other poisons which can damage various organs, such as cantharides (Spanish fly) which produces its aphrodisiac effect by causing inflammation of the urinary tract.

Infection This may be due to viruses, rickettsiae, bacteria, fungi, protozoa and metazoa.

1. *Viruses* are organisms too small to be visible with the light microscope, but with the electron microscope they have been found to have a wide range of size and shape. Many of the infectious diseases are caused by viruses, including colds, influenza, measles, mumps, poliomyelitis, hepatitis and AIDS. They can only multiply inside living cells which are often killed in the process, but the resting stage of many viruses is able to survive outside the body for long periods.
2. *Rickettsiae* are slightly larger than viruses and are just visible with the highest magnification of the light microscope. They cause a number of severe diseases such as typhus and psittacosis. Like viruses they can survive for long periods outside the body and may be transmitted by mosquitoes, lice and, in the case of psittacosis, by birds.
3. *Bacteria* are larger than the viruses and rickettsiae: using the light microscope different groups of bacteria can be recognized by their shapes (Fig. 2/1) and staining properties. Organisms that stain with methyl violet (Gram's stain) and are not decolourized

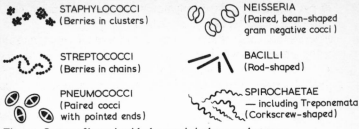

Fig. 2.1 Groups of bacteria with characteristic shapes and patterns

by alcohol are called Gram positive, and those which are decolourized are called Gram negative. Small round organisms are called cocci (Latin, berries). Gram positive cocci include: staphylococci, causing boils, pustules and abscesses; streptococci, causing tonsillitis, cellulitis and septicaemia; and pneumococci, causing pneumonia and meningitis. Gram negative cocci (Neisseria) include *N. gonorrhoeae* causing gonorrhoea; and *N. meningitidis* causing meningitis. Rod-shaped organisms are called bacilli of which there are numerous different Gram positive and negative types, causing many varieties of infection, for example tetanus, gas gangrene and Legionnaire's disease from Gram positive bacilli; gastroenteritis and typhoid from Gram negative bacilli. Some organisms are corkscrew-shaped, the best known probably being *Treponema pallidum*, causing syphilis.

Mycoplasmae have many of the characteristics of bacteria but have no definite shape. This is because they have no capsule and their outer skin is so thin that they can bend into any shape. An example is *Mycoplasma pneumoniae* which produces primary atypical pneumonia.

Actinomyces are generally considered as bacteria but they have branching threads, like fungi. Fortunately actinomycosis, the disease which they cause, is fairly rare. It has recently been found that contraceptive devices left in the uterus for a year or two may be associated with actinomyces or actinomyces-like organisms. Only occasionally are they involved in pelvic infections such as tubo-ovarian abscess.

4. *Fungi* are rather larger than bacteria. They have branching threads or hyphae and produce spores by which infection is spread. They cause superficial infections such as athlete's foot or ringworm. In debilitated patients they can cause internal infections such as aspergillosis of the lung or torulosis of the brain.

INFLAMMATION AND HEALING 15

Fungi can also produce inflammation as an immune reaction in sensitized subjects, e.g. farmer's lung.

5. *Protozoa* are small animals composed of a single cell. An example is the amoeba of which one variety, *Entamoeba histolytica*, causes a particularly unpleasant form of dysentery which can give rise to liver abscesses. Protozoa include malarial parasites: *Trichomonas vaginalis* causing sexually transmitted vaginal infection; and trypanosomes causing sleeping sickness. Many protozoal infections are tropical diseases and are spread by mosquitoes or other insects.

6. *Metazoa* are larger multicellular animals. A major group causing human disease are the parasitic worms or helminths. They are encountered most frequently in hot countries. They include roundworms, tapeworms and flukes.

Many of these parasites also infect animals which usually act as an 'intermediate host'. In the case of hydatid disease man and sheep are the intermediate hosts, being infected by eggs from a tiny tapeworm, *Echinococcus granulosus*, which lives in the intestine of the dog (Cheesebrough, 1987).

Infarction This is produced by blockage of the blood supply to an organ. An example is a heart attack due to a coronary artery being blocked by a blood clot. Deprivation of a blood supply causes tissue death which then gives rise to an inflammatory response. Infarction is considered in more detail on page 45. Tissue death from other causes, e.g. hormonal effects on the endometrium at the onset of menstruation, produces an inflammatory reaction which is visible in histological sections of endometrial curettings taken before and during menstruation.

Immune Reactions These are reactions which give rise to inflammation resulting from hypersensitivity either to a foreign protein or to one or more of the body's own proteins (autoimmunity).

A. *Foreign protein hypersensitivity* may be immediate, episodic (reaginic) or delayed.
(i) *Immediate hypersensitivity* follows the injection of antisera, foreign proteins, e.g. insulin (usually obtained from pigs), or substances, e.g. penicillin, that combine with body protein to produce what is in effect a foreign protein to which the patient has become sensitized.
(ii) *Episodic (reaginic) hypersensitivity* includes hay fever and asthma which usually occur after exposure to certain pollens, also various

skin allergies and gastro-intestinal allergies (e.g. to shellfish) with vomiting and diarrhoea.

(iii) *Delayed hypersensitivity* occurs after infection with certain viruses, bacteria or fungi. The patient's lymphocytes become sensitized to the organism. It occurs in tuberculous infection or after immunization with BCG (Bacille Calmette-Guérin, a modified tubercle bacillus) and accounts for a positive Mantoux test. In this test, a small quantity of the extract from tubercle bacilli is injected into the skin. A positive reaction is a red, slightly raised area at the site of injection reaching its maximum 48 hours after injection.

B. *Autoimmunity* is an immune reaction produced by the body against its own tissues. Examples are thyroiditis, atrophic gastritis, rheumatoid arthritis and chronic active hepatitis. They may be considered as examples of a misdirected protective mechanism which reacts against the body's own cells, destroying them and producing inflammation.

ACUTE INFLAMMATION

A mild form of acute inflammatory reaction is produced by making a firm stroke across the skin with a metal spatula. This produces a transient pallor followed by a dull red line (the *flush*), with an irregular surrounding zone of redness (the *flare*); if the stroke is sufficiently firm a linear swelling (the *wheal*) is produced. The sequence of flush, flare and wheal formation was described by Lewis and Grant (1924) and is known as the *triple response* which they considered to be mainly due to histamine or histamine-like substances. There is evidence that the flare is also mediated through a local axon reflex (Walter and Israel, 1987a). These changes gradually subside.

With more severe inflammation, as with an acutely infected finger, the four cardinal signs of inflammation develop, originally described by Celsus in the first century AD (Walter and Israel, 1987a). They are redness (*rubor*), swelling (*tumor*), heat (*calor*) and pain (*dolor*). These changes persist until the cause of the inflammation, e.g. infection, is controlled. If sufficiently severe, the inflammatory changes cause loss of function (*functio laesa*) of the affected part, sometimes incorrectly included as Galen's fifth cardinal sign (Rather, 1971).

The inflammatory reactions described above are related to a sequence of changes in which the small blood vessels supplying the area play a crucial part. They have been studied in living tissues which are sufficiently transparent for the blood vessels and cells to be seen, as in the web of a frog's foot.

Initially there is a momentary arteriolar constriction producing the transient pallor. This is followed by arteriolar dilatation, with increased blood flow, dilatation of capillaries and venules and resultant redness (*rubor*) and heat (*calor*). The walls of the vessels become more permeable, allowing the escape of protein-rich fluid. This causes the swelling (*tumor*) and the resulting pressure on the nerves is the main cause of the pain (*dolor*). With the loss of fluid the blood cells become more densely packed together (haemoconcentration) and the blood flow slows. The leucocytes, mainly polymorphs, leave the centre of the capillaries and move to the margins of the vessels. There they stick to the altered surface of damaged endothelial cells. They then pass through the walls of the capillaries by squeezing between the endothelial cells. Having left the vessels the leucocytes actively move towards the site of infection. At this stage virtually all the leucocytes are polymorphs. They have the ability to engulf bacteria and dead tissue cells, a process known as phagocytosis (Greek, *phago*, I eat), described by Allison et al (1955) and Florey (1979) and outlined on page 20.

To summarize, the acute inflammatory process has four major components which will be described in detail:

Blood flow changes
Exudation of protein-rich fluid
Leucocyte emigration
Lymphatic drainage.

Blood Flow Changes The blood supply to a part is controlled very largely by the muscle tone in its arterioles. Increasing the muscle tone constricts the arterioles so that less blood can flow through, producing the transient pallor which precedes the triple response. This is followed by a relaxation of the muscle tone in the arterioles which is a major factor in the inflammatory process. The lumen of the vessels becomes wider. This reduces the resistance to blood flow and allows a larger volume of blood to flow more rapidly through the arterioles (hyperaemia). This increased blood flow reaches the capillaries under a higher pressure than previously. As a result many capillaries which were partially or completely shut down are opened up and so the affected part becomes engorged with blood (Fig. 2/2(1)). There is a phase of rapid blood flow which may persist for an hour or so. It is followed by a gradual slowing of the rate of flow.

There are a number of factors which cause this slowing. The loss of fluid causes the cells to become concentrated (haemoconcentra-

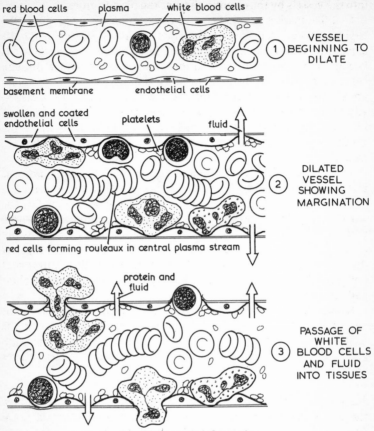

red blood cells   plasma   white blood cells

basement membrane   endothelial cells

① VESSEL BEGINNING TO DILATE

swollen and coated endothelial cells   platelets   fluid

red cells forming rouleaux in central plasma stream

② DILATED VESSEL SHOWING MARGINATION

protein and fluid

③ PASSAGE OF WHITE BLOOD CELLS AND FLUID INTO TISSUES

Fig. 2.2 The vascular changes which occur in inflammation

tion); water and other small molecules are lost more rapidly than larger ones, leading to increased protein in the plasma which makes it more viscous. The increased protein causes the red cells to come together in rouleaux, like heaps of pennies (Fig. 2/2(2)).

The leucocytes attached to the walls of the vessels, sometimes in several layers, reduce the effective size of the lumen.

Exudation of Protein Rich Fluid   In normal tissue there is some fluid in the spaces between the cells (tissue fluid) which contains little protein. The blood pressure at the arterial end of capillaries is sufficient to filter this fluid out through the vessel walls. By the time blood has reached the venous end of the capillaries the blood pressure has fallen sufficiently for the tissue fluid to be absorbed back into the vessels by the osmotic effect of the plasma proteins.

In inflammation the dilatation of the arterioles causes a rise in the capillary blood pressure so that more fluid is exuded from the capillaries and little is reabsorbed. In addition the vessel walls become more leaky so that plasma proteins can pass out through small holes between the endothelial cells (Fig. 2/2(3)). These holes are visible with the electron microscope. They open very occasionally in the absence of inflammation to release a molecule of protein into the tissue spaces. In the early stage of inflammation, lasting about 30 minutes, protein exudation occurs from the venules but not from the capillaries.

There is evidence that histamine is involved in producing this effect. Local injection of histamine has been shown to produce gaps between endothelial cells (Fox et al, 1980). In mild inflammation the changes may then gradually subside. In more severe inflammation protein exudation then occurs from the capillaries as well. It is not certain which substance produces this effect. It may be at least partly due to direct damage to the capillaries (with death and disruption of endothelial cells) by whatever is causing the inflammation (Robbins and Kumar, 1987).

In addition to histamine there are other substances, such as kinins and prostaglandins, which probably act as chemical mediators in the inflammatory process, but until more reliable information is available the role of individual substances remains ambiguous (Walter and Israel, 1987a).

Leucocyte Emigration   During the early stage of rapid blood flow the leucocytes are mainly in the centre of the bloodstream (axial flow) (Fig. 2/2(1)). As the blood flow slows the leucocytes move towards the margin of the vessels (margination) (Fig. 2/2(2)). There they stick to the endothelial cells which have become swollen and appear to be covered by a gelatinous layer (Wilkinson and Lackie, 1979). The fact that leucocytes also stick to each other and that red cells and platelets become more sticky suggests the presence of a plasma factor (Allison et al, 1955). These changes occur mainly in the venules and nearly all the leucocytes are polymorphs. They extend pseudopodia into the junctions between endothelial cells actively forcing a gap through which they squeeze (Fig. 2/2(3)) (Marchesi, 1961). One or more cells may follow through, including occasional red cells passively ejected from the blood vessel (diapedesis). The gap then closes behind them and the leucocytes are guided chemically towards the site of tissue damage (chemotaxis or leucotaxis (Ward, 1974)). In pyogenic infections, such as pneumonia, chemotactic agents released from the affected tissue or from bacteria not only cause them to move to the infected site but also stimulate the bone marrow to produce large numbers of polymorphs. In other types of infection, such as typhoid, there is little stimulus to polymorphs and instead the main cell to respond is the monocyte, which emigrates into the tissue to become a macrophage (Greek, large eater).

Phagocytosis A phagocyte is a cell which ingests bacteria and other particulate matter. Both macrophages and polymorphs are phagocytes, the latter sometimes being termed microphages (Greek, small eaters). Macrophages have a long life-span but polymorphs only live for three to four days (Walter and Israel, 1987a). It has been shown by *in vitro* studies that no phagocytosis takes place unless serum is present; the relevant factors in serum are proteins called opsonins (Stossel, 1974). An opsonin is a substance which coats the surface of bacteria. It may be likened to butter, making the bacteria palatable.

Opsonins may be non-specific or specific (Stossel, 1974). The non-specific type or 'natural antibody' is effective against a number of different bacteria but often not against the more virulent organisms with capsules. For these a specific 'immune opsonin' is needed which is an antibody against the particular strain of organism causing the infection, e.g. pneumococcus type 2. It takes time for the body's immune system to produce sufficient specific antibody. Once such immunity has developed phagocytosis becomes a major feature of the inflammation.

It has also been shown that phagocytosis of such organisms can take place even in the absence of immune opsonin, provided the physical conditions are right (Smith and Wood, 1958). If the bacteria are trapped on surfaces, as on a fibrin clot, alveolar wall or even between two leucocytes the phagocyte can ingest them without the aid of opsonin (surface phagocytosis).

Lymphatic Drainage The lymphatics are thin-walled vessels which assist in the drainage of tissue fluid. In resting tissue many of these channels are collapsed and inactive. During inflammation these collapsed lymphatics open up and assist in the removal of excess fluid, protein and breakdown products of inflammation. The promotion of lymphatic drainage, e.g. by raising the affected limb to allow gravity to assist, will often relieve excess swelling and so reduce pain and discomfort.

Outcome of inflammation

The interaction between the infection and the body's defence now enters a critical phase. The outcome is determined by the number and virulence of the infecting organisms balanced against the effectiveness of the body's resistance. The balance may be tipped in favour of the patient by appropriate treatment such as the administration of an antibiotic to which the organism is sensitive. The most favourable outcome is complete resolution (see p.23). Other possibilities are incomplete resolution (see p.24), suppuration, chronic inflammation, spread of inflammation and death.

Suppuration

If there is much tissue destruction a hole or cavity is produced – an abscess. The cavity is filled with semi-liquid material called pus which is composed of dying or dead polymorphs, known as pus cells, dead tissue cells and bacteria, both living and dead. The process of pus formation is known as suppuration. When it occurs in the skin it is called a boil or carbuncle. Although this may appear very unsightly it has the effect of walling off the infection instead of allowing it to spread through the body. Before the days of antibiotics abscesses were frequent and it was often necessary to drain them surgically. Even today it is occasionally necessary.

CHRONIC INFLAMMATION (Greek, *chronos*, time)

A chronic inflammation is one which persists for a long time, e.g. months or years. It is a process in which destruction and inflammation are proceeding at the same time as attempts at healing (Walter and Israel, 1987b); an example is tuberculosis. As the infection continues the cells at the site of infection change. The short-lived polymorphs disappear and are replaced by macrophages. These larger cells live longer than polymorphs and are able to phagocytose larger particles, including tubercle bacilli which can remain alive inside them.

The macrophages come from the blood where they initially circulate for a day or two as monocytes and then leave the vessels to become histiocytes (Greek, *histos*, tissue and *cytos*, cell). They form the epithelioid cells and giant cells which are characteristic of tuberculous infection. They also give rise to the fibroblasts, cells which form collagen and produce fibrous tissue, a feature of chronic inflammation.

Lymphocytes, too, migrate to the site of chronic inflammation, often in large numbers. Some lymphocytes of the type called T cells are sensitized to kill specific organisms such as the tubercle bacillus. Lymphocytes of T-cell type can even become sensitized against tissue cells as in a heart transplant rejection or kidney rejection and also in autoimmune inflammations such as thyroiditis, causing myxoedema, or atrophic gastritis, sometimes causing pernicious anaemia.

In many inflammations which persist for more than about a week a number of lymphocytes of the type called B cells turn into plasma cells and produce specific antibodies against an organism or its toxin. They are produced in viral infections, sub-acute bacterial infections, syphilis and also in rheumatoid disease and other autoimmune inflammations.

The various patterns of immune response are considered in Chapter 3, pages 34–8, under the heading 'Defence Mechanisms against Infection'.

Persistence and Progression of Inflammation   Sub-acute inflammation occurs with an intermediate type of infection, halfway between acute and chronic inflammation. It is characterized by infiltration of the affected tissue by plasma cells. Thus an acute inflammation of the Fallopian tubes may persist and become sub-acute salpingitis.

An example of progression of infection is the entry of bacteria or viruses into the bloodstream (bacteraemia or viraemia), multiplication of organisms in the bloodstream (septicaemia) and the production of further abscesses as a result of organisms spreading in the bloodstream (pyaemia). Some degree of bacteraemia or viraemia occurs in a number of infections and contributes to fever and malaise.

The more severe conditions of septicaemia and pyaemia give rise to rigors. These are attacks of uncontrollable shivering in which the patient feels cold while at the same time the body temperature is rising rapidly. He may then suddenly feel very hot and sweat profusely with resultant fall in temperature. With uncontrolled infection, e.g. of the urinary tract, a patient may suffer bout after bout of rigors and become extremely debilitated. Rigors are a typical feature of untreated malaria, occurring regularly (at two- or three-day intervals depending on the type), each time that malarial parasites are released from the red cells into the bloodstream.

Sometimes rigors may persist until the temperature reaches a dangerously high level called hyperpyrexia (over 41°C) which may damage the temperature control centre so that the temperature continues to rise. Unless steps are taken to bring down the temperature artificially, e.g. by tepid sponging, the patient will die.

Types of chronic inflammation

Inflammation persisting for a year or more may be due either to recurrent attacks of acute inflammation or to inflammation which is essentially chronic from its onset.

Recurrent acute inflammation can affect the bronchus, gall bladder, kidney, bladder, cervix and large intestine. Each attack of acute inflammation produces local and general symptoms similar in nature to those already described, modified by the anatomical site involved. In the bronchus, for example, it causes cough and expectoration of purulent sputum, the persistent state being known as chronic bronchitis.

Essentially chronic inflammation includes many major diseases. Tuberculosis, leprosy and syphilis are examples in which the bacterial cause is known. The dust diseases such as silicosis characterized by fibrosis of the lung also have a clearly recognized cause. Rheumatoid disease, Crohn's disease and sarcoidosis are chronic inflammatory conditions whose cause is unknown and whose nature is only partially understood. Each of these conditions tends to cause progressive damage to the affected organs. As a result there is scarring and impairment of function which if untreated may become progressively worse, as with the grossly deformed joints which can occur in rheumatoid arthritis. Physiotherapy can play an important part in the prevention of such deformities and in encouraging the maximum mobility in affected joints.

HEALING

Tissue repair may take place by *resolution, organization* or *regeneration*. When tissue damage is slight, healing takes place by *first intention*. When damage is more extensive or the healing process is complicated by infection, it takes place by *second intention*.

Resolution

The inflammatory process resolves and the tissue returns to its original state. This may occur in lobar pneumonia: the pneumococci are phagocytosed by the polymorphs, the polymorphs are liquefied by their own enzymes, the fibrin undergoes lysis and the liquefied exudate is re-absorbed to leave an intact lung which can function normally again. Not all cases of pneumonia will resolve so completely. Where there is tissue damage and abscess formation, healing occurs at the affected sites by organization, resulting in a scarred lung.

Organization

If resolution is incomplete, organization of residual fibrin occurs. Fibroblasts and capillary loops grow into the fibrin from the margin. New capillaries grow out from existing capillaries, initially in the form of solid buds. They link up with adjacent new capillaries to form loops and arcades. Within hours of their appearance blood starts to flow through them. Red cells, leucocytes and proteinaceous fluid escapes from these new capillaries. Excess fluid is removed from the site by newly formed lymphatics which bud out from adjacent pre-existing lymphatics, linking up with each other to form a lymphatic drainage system (and apparently never linking up with a blood capillary by mistake). This vascularized tissue is called granulation tissue. While this blood supply and lymph drainage is developing, the fibroblasts multiply and start to lay down collagen, at first of primitive and later of more mature type. The blood supply is remodelled and eventually greatly reduced to form relatively bloodless scar tissue. This restores the continuity of the organ but never replaces the function of the tissue it replaces, e.g. lung or skeletal muscle.

Regeneration

In some organs damaged tissue can be replaced by functioning normal tissue. In addition to fractured bone and torn fibrous ligaments, thyroid, liver, pancreas and salivary glands are all capable of regeneration, provided the general alignment of the supporting tissues is retained. Peripheral nerves are able to regenerate provided the severed proximal end of the nerve is in continuity with the distal end which dies, leaving a neural tube up which the regenerating nerve grows at the rate of one millimetre a day. It has always been considered that there is no possibility of regeneration if the brain or spinal cord is damaged. Recent work, however, suggests that some regeneration is possible by reproducing the conditions present in the fetus. Fetal brain tissue has been used in the treatment of adult brains damaged by Parkinson's disease (Madrazo et al, 1988).

Healing by first intention (Fig. 2/3)

The healing of a clean operation wound with the edges in close apposition is a typical example of healing by first intention. Slight haemorrhage occurs into the narrow space between the wound margins and so the gap becomes filled with blood clot (first day). The clot is composed mainly of fibrin which undergoes organization as already described. At the same time epithelial cells spread over the surface from the adjacent epidermis (second to third days).

After covering the surface with a single layer they multiply to form the stratified squamous epithelium of which epidermis is composed (fourth to fifth days). This is the first tissue in which continuity of all its components is restored (14th day). Meanwhile fibroblasts lay down collagen in the granulation tissue which eventually becomes converted into a narrow band of scar tissue.

Healing by second intention

When the gap between the wound margins is wide or when the occurrence of infection interferes with the healing process a large amount of granulation tissue is formed. If the surface of the wound is large the spread of epithelial cells over the surface and eventual formation of stratified squamous epithelium may take a long time.

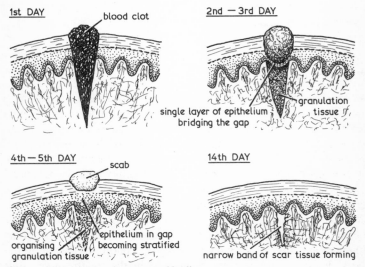

Fig. 2.3 The stages in primary wound healing

The delicate epithelium may even be stripped off if care is not taken when changing dressings. The large amount of granulation tissue results in the formation of a large amount of scar tissue. The scar tissue may later contract and produce distortion, interfering with function, as in an infected wound of the hand.

Factors influencing tissue repair

The factors affecting the repair of tissue damage are its site, size, supply and support, also sepsis, sinuses, sutures and other foreign bodies, to which may be added age and temperature.

Site   The site of tissue damage determines whether it can regenerate. Under favourable conditions full regeneration in bone marrow, fibrous tissue, mesothelium (peritoneum, pleura, synovium), intestinal and bladder mucosae, liver, pancreas and peripheral nerves is possible, whereas scar tissue replacement often occurs in heart muscle and lung. *Joint cartilage* is a halfway tissue, small defects being made good by regeneration but larger injuries, which produce a haematoma, being converted either into fibrous tissue or bone (Walter and Israel, 1987c). *Tendon* regeneration is good although slow, provided the tendon ends are accurately united and under some tension (Matthews and Richards, 1974). Otherwise union is by scar tissue. Some adhesions usually occur but may not limit movement significantly.

Skeletal muscle and, possibly, cardiac muscle are capable of significantly more regeneration than used to be considered possible (Hay, 1971). In a surgical wound regenerating muscle cells on either side of the incision may unite so that eventually the continuity of the muscle is restored (Gay and Hunt, 1954). Damage to muscle with obstruction to the blood supply results in much fibrosis, as in Volkmann's ischaemic contracture (Seddon, 1964; *BMJ*, 1980).

Skin and other squamous epithelia show good regeneration but hair follicles, sweat and sebaceous glands and rete ridges are not replaced. *Gastric mucosa* shows good regeneration after acute ulceration with intact underlying connective tissue. With chronic peptic ulcers fibrosis occurs and healing is inhibited. When healing does occur the new epithelium may be of intestinal type (Walter and Israel, 1987c).

Size   Where the size of tissue damage is small repair can take place with the minimum of scarring. Extensive tissue damage may lead to extensive scarring. In the case of skin this may be overcome by skin grafting. Extensively damaged kidneys may require to be replaced by a kidney transplant from a donor of the right tissue type.

Supply *Blood supply* to the site of tissue damage is a crucial factor in its repair. A good blood supply promotes rapid healing. The scalp is well supplied and sutures in scalp wounds may be removed after only five to six days. A part which has been irradiated may have a poor blood supply so that tissue repair is slow.

Poor venous and lymphatic drainage may also lead to slow healing as in the case of varicose ulcers in the region of the ankle where gravity and incompetent valves in the leg veins produce venous stasis. Physiotherapy may improve circulation by means of ultra-violet light, ultrasound, moderate exercise and appropriate posture (raising leg).

Nerve supply to the damaged part apparently needs to be intact for healing to occur. If the nerve supply is impaired, as in syringomyelia or tabes dorsalis, trophic ulcers occur. The exact mechanism is not fully understood, but loss of pain sense allows tissue to be damaged more readily.

Food supply to the part by the bloodstream is dependent on adequate nutrition of the body. Adequate proteins and vitamins in the diet, particularly vitamin C, are essential.

Hormone supply is again provided by the bloodstream, particularly thyroxin. Deficiency of thyroxin, as in myxoedema and cretinism, impairs healing.

Support Fractures require firm support and alignment if bone union is to take place. The support may be by internal fixation or external splintage. It has been found that union is more rapid if support is not too rigid. Internal fixation by carbon fibre plates, which allows a very slight flexing, induces firmer and more rapid union than metal plates which allow no movement at the fracture site.

Protection from injury and infection by the use of petroleum jelly gauze, sterile dressings and bandages promotes wound healing. Good management requires sufficient immobilization for repair to proceed, yet allowing sufficient movement to assist circulation and reduce muscular wasting to a minimum.

Sepsis Sepsis delays healing. *Asepsis* is the avoidance of infection by using sterile instruments, sheets, gowns, gloves and swabs and a non-touch technique in the changing of dressings. *Antisepsis* is the removal of infection by appropriate chemical agents. Because of their effects on living tissue some of these agents may impair healing, e.g. carbolic acid (phenol).

Sinuses and Fistulae A sinus is a blind tract leading to an epithelial surface, e.g. to the skin from a foreign body embedded in a wound. A fistula is a tract leading from one epithelial surface to another, e.g. a rectovaginal fistula (from rectum to vagina) which occasionally complicates Crohn's disease. Surgical removal of the lesion and its cause (if removable) is indicated.

Sutures and Other Foreign Bodies Initially sutures promote healing by bringing tissue surfaces together. Sutures which are left in too long (unless they are absorbable (catgut)) act as foreign bodies. Surgical swabs, pieces of clothing, dead tissue or any other foreign material left in a wound prevent healing and may give rise to sinus formation.

Age Healing tends to be more rapid in childhood than old age.

Temperature Healing is impaired by excessive heat or cold.

Summary

From the above it can be seen that healing is promoted by:

1. Control of infection.
2. Removal of any foreign material, dead tissues, sinuses or fistulae.
3. Facilitation of repair with the minimum of scar tissue (first intention) by suturing together clean cut un-infected wound tissues and where appropriate by skin grafting.
4. Rest and protection of the affected part and, if necessary, immobilization, e.g. for a fracture.
5. The maintenance of good general health with adequate protein and vitamins (especially C) in the diet.
6. Encouraging a good circulation and ensuring venous and lymphatic drainage by appropriate posture.
7. Where appropriate, physiotherapy to hasten the healing process, e.g. by the use of ultraviolet irradiation, infrared irradiation, short wave diathermy, local massage in the case of varicose ulcers; and graded exercise(s) to maintain and/or restore muscle tone.

REFERENCES

Allison, F., Smith, M.R. and Wood, W.B. (1955). Studies on the pathogenesis of acute inflammation. *Journal of Experimental Medicine*, **102**, 655–75.

Cheesebrough, M. (1987). *Medical Laboratory Manual for Tropical Countries*, 2nd edition, vol. 1, pp. 296–8. Butterworths, London.

Florey, H.W. (ed.) (1979). Inflammation: microscopical observations. In *General Pathology*, pp. 40–123. Lloyd-Luke, London.

Fox, J., Galey, F. and Wayland, H. (1980). Action of histamine on the mesenteric microvasculature. *Microvascular Research*, **19**, 108–26.

Gay, A.J. and Hunt, T.E. (1954). Reuniting of skeletal muscle fibres after transection. *Anatomical Record*, **120**, 853–71.

Hay, E.D. (1971). Skeletal muscle regeneration. *New England Journal of Medicine*, **284**, 1033–4.

Leading Article (1980). Volkmann's ischaemic contracture. *British Medical Journal*, **1**, 430.

Lewis, T. and Grant, R.T. (1924). Vascular reactions of the skin to injury. *Heart*, **11**, 209–65.

Madrazo, I. et al (1988). Transplantation of fetal substantia nigra and adrenal medulla to the caudate nucleus in two patients with Parkinson's disease. *New England Journal of Medicine*, **318**, 51.

Marchesi, V.T. (1961). The site of leucocyte migration during inflammation. *Queensland Journal of Experimental Physiology*, **46**, 115–33.

Matthews, P. and Richards, H. (1974). The repair potential of digital flexor tendons. *Journal of Bone and Joint Surgery*, **56B**, 618–25.

Rather, L.J. (1971). Disturbance of function (*functio laesa*): the legendary fifth cardinal sign of inflammation, added by Galen to the four cardinal signs of Celsus. *Bulletin of the New York Academy of Medicine*, **47**, 303–22.

Robbins, S.L. and Kumar, V. (1987). *Basic Pathology*, 4th edition, p. 31. Saunders, Philadelphia.

Seddon, H. (1964). Volkmann's ischaemia. *British Medical Journal*, **1**, 1587–92.

Smith, M.R. and Wood, W.B. (1958). Surface phagocytosis. *Journal of Experimental Medicine*, **107**, 1–13.

Stossel, T.P. (1974). Phagocytosis. *New England Journal of Medicine*, **290**, 717, 774, 883.

Walter J.B. and Israel, M.S. (1987a). *General Pathology*, 6th edition, pp. 82–96. Churchill Livingstone, Edinburgh.

Walter J.B. and Israel, M.S. (1987b). *ibid*, p. 142.

Walter J.B. and Israel, M.S. (1987c). *ibid*, pp. 130–41.

Ward, P.A. (1974). Leukotaxis and leukotactic disorders. A review. *American Journal of Pathology*, **77**, 520–38.

Wilkinson, P.C. and Lackie, J.M. (1979). The adhesion, migration and chemotaxis of leucocytes in inflammation. *Current Topics in Pathology*, **68**, 47–88.

BIBLIOGRAPHY

See end of Chapter 5, page 65.

Chapter 3

Infection

by D. M. D. EVANS MD, FRCP, FRCPath

The types of organism which cause infection are described on page 13. All such organisms are called pathogens (Greek, *pathos-gen*, disease producer). There are also many organisms present on the surface of skin, hair, nasal cavity, mouth, intestines and vagina of healthy people. They are called commensals (Latin, *con-mensa*, sharing the same table) and live in peaceful co-existence with their host.

Whether or not infection is produced depends partly on the organism (the 'seed') and partly on the relevant tissue (the 'soil'). The nature of the 'soil' often determines whether the 'seed' multiplies and produces an infection. *Staphylococcus aureus* is an organism which is quite often present on the skin or in the nose of healthy people without producing any ill effect. But if it gains access to an open wound it will probably cause sepsis. Preventing such access by using aseptic techniques is a major factor in the control of cross-infection.

MODES OF INFECTION

Transmission by direct contact, droplets, water, food and fomites are the main ways in which infection is spread.

Direct contact

There is a danger that infection may be spread by direct contact from the skin of the hand to an open wound in hospital. It is prevented by scrubbing the hands adequately, putting on sterile gloves and using sterile instruments to avoid direct contact. A physiotherapist with a boil (*Staphylococcus aureus* folliculitis) or other skin infection, particularly if it is on the hand, should avoid handling patients. Long hair which may infect a wound should be controlled by a cap.

The sexually transmitted diseases are spread by direct contact. These include AIDS and hepatitis, where transmission of infection can occur during heterosexual intercourse but also occurs commonly between male homosexuals through the rectal mucosa which is readily susceptible to damage and haemorrhage. Blood is the main vehicle of transmission, e.g. in drug addicts by needle sharing (see fomites). When handling AIDS and hepatitis patients with skin lesions, including simple scratches, rubber gloves should be worn. Similarly a physiotherapist with a cut or desquamating skin lesion should wear gloves when handling AIDS and hepatitis patients. It should however be emphasized that the infectivity of AIDS is extremely low, except by needle inoculation of infected blood, sexual intercourse and, possibly, by intimate kissing. Excessive isolation procedures, e.g. gowns and masks, are inappropriate (Gordon et al, 1987).

Droplets

It is well known that coughs and sneezes spread diseases. It is not so generally appreciated that talking also spreads fine droplets for a distance of three metres or so. The use of an adequate face mask cuts down the risk of such spread. A plain gauze mask which does not include a cellophane barrier is inadequate to prevent the spread of fine droplets. Diseases spread by droplet infection include measles, mumps, chickenpox, rubella, influenza, the common cold (coryza) and many other viral infections of the upper and lower respiratory tract. A patient with a dangerous respiratory infection, such as open tuberculosis, should be isolated. There is no evidence that AIDS is spread by droplets (Gordon et al, 1987).

Water

In developed communities tap water is generally considered safe, particularly if it has been chlorinated. Cholera and typhoid have been transmitted by water in the past and have not yet been eliminated. Recently there have been occasional cases of Legionnaire's disease, even in hospitals, from infection of the water in air-conditioning systems or from showers, by fine droplets (aerosols). Taps and water filters may themselves become infected. When dressing wounds, infection is avoided by the use of sterile saline, etc.

Food

Contaminated food can cause food poisoning (Salmonella infections and botulism), dysentery, typhoid and other diseases. A boil on the hand can infect food or milk with *Staph. aureus*. If this is then given a chance to multiply, particularly in warm conditions, it can cause severe gastroenteritis. Food can also be contaminated by 'healthy carriers' – persons with typhoid bacilli in their gall bladders which can persist for many years, as observed by the author in the head waiter of a large hotel. Selection of clean food, cleanliness in food handling, 'non-carrier' food handlers and refrigerated storage help to prevent food-borne infection.

Fomites (Latin, *fomites*, tinder)

A fomite is the term used for any material which is infected and can then spread infection. Dirty dressings, swabs and utensils may all transmit infection. Care in the disposal of used dressings and the cleansing of utensils prevents such transmission. Clothing can act as a fomite. Where appropriate this is prevented by the use of sterile gowns.

The practice of sharing needles by intravenous drug users provides ready transmission of infections such as AIDS, hepatitis and syphilis. The risk is particularly high in 'shooting galleries' where drug addicts rent injection equipment which is then rented to the next customer (Des Jarlais and Friedmann, 1987). Infected blood products for haemophiliacs have been responsible for many cases of AIDS. Safe products are now available. The risk of transmission by blood transfusion has been reduced by AIDS antibody testing but not eliminated.

PREVENTION OF CROSS-INFECTION

Once the modes of infection are understood, the prevention of cross-infection is essentially applied common sense, as outlined above. The strictness with which precautions need to be applied depends very much on the circumstances. In dealing with open wounds strict asepsis is indicated. When deciding whether a patient with a given infection should be isolated the guiding factors are its *infectivity* and the *virulence* of the infecting organism.

Infectivity

The infectious diseases, many of which are due to viruses, such as chickenpox, measles, mumps and rubella ('baby blight'), have a high degree of infectivity. Leprosy is often thought to be highly infectious but in fact has a low degree of infectivity. When assessing the infectivity of an individual case it is helpful to consider the mode(s) of spread of the infection concerned, the stage of the disease and whether the infection is still active.

Virulence

Virulence is the term used of an organism to indicate the severity of infection which it produces. The smallpox virus is an example of a highly virulent organism which produced a high mortality rate. By giving it to a cow its virulence was greatly reduced and the modified virus so produced was used for vaccination which gave its recipients immunity against smallpox. Rubella is an infection which can prove highly virulent for the unborn human fetus but causes only a mild infection during postnatal life. The virulence of an organism is related to its *invasiveness, toxin production* and *immunologically mediated damage*.

Invasiveness An example of a highly invasive organism is the *Streptococcus pyogenes* which is a common cause of tonsillitis. If it infects an open wound it spreads readily through the tissue, digesting away barriers which might obstruct its progress by enzymes. It spreads along the lymphatics to produce a lymphangitis, reaching lymph nodes to cause a lymphadenitis, and penetrates the bloodstream (bacteraemia) where it multiplies (septicaemia), and can then settle in various tissues, producing multiple abscesses (pyaemia).

Invasion of tissues by an organism is assisted by its having a protective capsule or sheath. The tubercle bacillus has a lipid sheath which resists digestion by macrophages. So the macrophage transports living tubercle bacilli and actually assists the spread of infection. The same occurs with lepra bacilli (causing leprosy) which, like many viruses and rickettsiae, spread widely in the body without leaving any trace at the site of entry (Walter and Israel, 1987a).

Toxin Production A toxin is a poisonous substance. If a toxin is released by living organisms it is called an *exotoxin* (Greek, *exo-toxin*, external poison). A toxin present within the organism such as the tubercle bacillus which does not escape into the host's tissues until the organism dies is called an *endotoxin* (Greek, *endon-toxin*, internal poison).

Exotoxins produce damage at the site of infection or in distant tissues or both. In gas gangrene the toxic damage is in tissues at the site of infection. In tetanus the toxin produces an effect on the nervous system, making it unduly sensitive to any stimulus, such as a noise, which causes uncontrollable and painful muscle spasm, often including spasm of the masseter muscles (lockjaw). In diphtheria the toxin causes both local tissue damage and a distant effect on nerve tissue and heart muscle. The gastroenteritis caused by *Staph. aureus* is also due to an exotoxin called enterotoxin. In general, exotoxins are extremely potent, that of botulism being a million times more toxic than strychnine (van Heyningen, 1970). They are simple proteins, often having specific enzyme activity and acting on specific tissues, and they are neutralized by a specific antibody (Govan et al, 1986a).

Endotoxins are much less potent, weight for weight, although they can be equally lethal if present in sufficient amount. They form an integral part of the bacterial wall, e.g. in typhoid, dysentery and food poisoning organisms, and are lipid–polysaccharide complexes (Govan et al, 1986a). They are not specific for each organism and they do not stimulate antitoxin production. They cause fever, shock, intravascular coagulation, often neutropenia followed by neutrophilia, and destruction of platelets causing thrombocytopenia and a bleeding tendency. Macrophages are activated so that they not only become more phagocytic but also release a variety of active substances, some of which cause further damage (Walter and Israel, 1987a).

Immunologically Mediated Damage Organisms may produce damage by reacting with sensitizing antibodies (Webb, 1968). The development of hypersensitivity in tuberculosis not only signals immunity and resistance to the infection; it is also accompanied by the caseating destructive response to the tubercle bacillus (Robbins and Kumar, 1987a). A fatal but fortunately rare complication of measles is sub-acute sclerosing panencephalitis in which a high level of antibodies is present in both blood and cerebrospinal fluid (Walter and Israel, 1987b).

DEFENCE MECHANISMS AGAINST INFECTION

The natural defence mechanisms against the infection are: (1) intact skin and mucous membranes; (2) the acute and chronic inflammatory reactions; and (3) the immune responses. To this may be added (4) the artificial defences provided by immunization, antiseptics, antibiotics and the preventive measures of aseptic techniques and isolation.

Skin and mucous membranes

The skin provides mechanical protection against many infections. A small cut is sufficient to allow organisms to enter and *Staph. aureus* is able to infect an intact hair follicle to produce a boil. The eyes are protected by secretion from the tear glands which contain lysozyme, capable of killing many bacteria and fungi. The respiratory tract is protected by the secretion of mucus which forms a protective blanket, continually moved along by cilia. The stomach secretes hydrochloric acid which is strong enough to kill many organisms. The urethral sphincter is normally sufficient to prevent organisms from entering the urinary tract, although the shorter urethra in the female urinary tract makes it more susceptible to infection than the male tract.

Inflammatory reactions

The acute and chronic inflammatory reactions described in Chapter 2 are important defence mechanisms. Phagocytosis of organisms by polymorphs and macrophages is often successful in killing them although some organisms, such as the tubercle bacillus, are resistant. Further protection is provided by the immune responses which are closely linked with the inflammatory reactions.

The immune responses

Immunological responsiveness is dependent on lymphocytes. They provide immunity in two ways: cellular immunity in which T cells participate and humoral antibodies which are derived from B cells.

Cellular Immunity The lymphocytes which provide cellular immunity are derived from bone marrow but at about the third month of intra-uterine life they migrate to the thymus (Halloran, 1987a) where they differentiate into T cells (T for thymus). The differentiated T cells leave the thymus, most of them settling in the paracortical areas of lymph nodes and the peri-arteriolar sheaths of the spleen but some continuing to circulate in the blood and thoracic duct lymph (Robbins and Kumar, 1987b).

Cellular immune reactions are triggered off by the presence of an antigen to which particular T cells are sensitive. Macrophages assist in the reaction by presenting the antigen to the T cells in a form to which they can respond. The relevant T cells then undergo *transformation* into large 'blast' cells with subsequent division to provide an army of effector cells capable of reacting to that particular antigen.

An example of such a cell is the cytolytic (*killer*) T cell capable of non-phagocytic destruction of target cells, e.g. a virus infected cell (Robbins and Kumar, 1987b).

Some T cells become *helper cells* and assist B cells or other T cells in providing the optimal immune response, e.g. against infection. Other T cells become *suppressor cells* and regulate or suppress an immune response. There is evidence that helper and suppressor cells are produced from different clones (Robbins and Kumar, 1987b). Transformed T cells can act both as stimulators and inhibitors of the chemotactic migration of polymorphs and the phagocytic activity of macrophages. T cells are also involved in stimulating the bone marrow to produce a leucocytosis and in the production of interferon and other factors (Halloran, 1987a).

Humoral Immunity Antibody production is the function of a distinct set of lymphocytes. These are also formed in the bone marrow but do not migrate to the thymus. In birds they migrate to an organ associated with the hind gut called the bursa of Fabricius, whence the term B cells (B for bursa). Mammals, including humans, do not have such an organ. It is possible that lymphoid tissue in the alimentary tract such as Peyer's patches may perform a similar function (Robbins et al, 1987b). When differentiation is complete the B cells migrate to the primary and secondary follicles of the lymph nodes and spleen (Halloran, 1987a).

Stimulation of an appropriate B cell by an antigen requires the assistance of a macrophage, as with cellular immunity, and in addition a T-helper cell is often needed. The B cell then undergoes *transformation* into a large 'blast' cell and then proceeds to division and produces plasma cells (Govan et al, 1986b). It is from the plasma cells that the various antibodies (immunoglobulins) are produced, e.g. antitoxins and bacterial agglutinins. Typically the first antibody produced against an antigen is a large immunoglobulin (macroglobulin or IgM). Later the corresponding antibody is a smaller immunoglobulin (gamma globulin or IgG). Other recognized types of antibody are IgA, IgD and IgE. IgE is the antibody involved in allergic reaction of *immediate hypersensitivity* type, e.g. hay fever and asthma (Halloran, 1987a). The role of immunoglobulins IgA and IgD is less certain.

Patterns of immunity

Immunity may be *passive* or *active*. Each type of immunity may occur *naturally* or be induced *artificially*. In addition there is a *species* immunity. Thus man as a species has a high degree of immunity against foot and mouth disease, whereas animals with cloven feet such as cattle are very susceptible. There is also some degree of *racial* immunity. Jews tend to have a higher degree of immunity to tuberculosis than the Irish. Eskimos tend to have a lower degree of immunity to infectious diseases than most town dwellers. Immunity to infections can be greatly reduced by diseases affecting the immune system (see p.38).

Passive Immunity

Natural: A baby receives passive immunity in the form of antibodies from its mother. These are immunoglobulins whose molecules are small enough to cross the placenta or be transmitted in breast milk. This gives temporary immunity to the baby, lasting three to six months, against infections to which the mother had herself developed immunity.

Artificial: The giving of antitoxin against diphtheria or tetanus toxin are examples of passive immunization which in the past have been used successfully in the treatment of these infections. The antisera were often made by immunization of horses. Unfortunately a number of patients became sensitive to the horse serum and suffered anaphylactic shock or serum sickness, sometimes with a fatal outcome; tetanus antitoxin made from horse serum is now no longer used. Purified human gamma globulin however can now be used against hepatitis B and in the treatment of tetanus and other infections.

Active Immunity

Natural: The recovery phase of many infections is associated with the formation of antibodies against the relevant organism and its toxins. This provides an immunity which in the case of infections like measles and diphtheria is normally long lasting, although it may wane in later life. The cells which produce the antibodies are lymphocytes and plasma cells of B-cell type. In other types of infection, such as tuberculosis, immunity is mainly of the cellular type provided by lymphocytes of T-cell type. Sometimes both types of immunity are involved, as in syphilitic infection: the detection of the syphilitic antibody produced provides the basis of diagnosis in all but very early cases.

Artificial: The body's defences against an infection such as tetanus are greatly enhanced by previous artificial immunization through the injection of tetanus toxoid. It results in production of antitoxin by B cells at a very early stage of the infection so that tetanus toxin is immediately neutralized, thus preventing the painful muscle spasms and lockjaw. Artificial active immunization against poliomyelitis, measles and whooping cough either protects against these infections completely or greatly reduces their severity and is strongly recommended in early childhood. Immunization against rubella is also strongly recommended for children aged 1–12 years, especially girls. It should not be given to pregnant women, nor to girls if there is a risk of their becoming pregnant (Downham, 1976).

DISEASES AFFECTING IMMUNITY

Diseases causing deficiency of immunity against infection may be primary (congenital) or acquired.

Primary immune deficiency

Bruton (1952) reported the absence of antibodies (agamma-globulinaemia) in a boy who for more than four years suffered repeated pneumococcal infections. These stopped when he was injected with immune human gammaglobulin. This form of immune deficiency is linked to the X chromosome and occurs only in males. Many different types of primary immune deficiency have since been described (Rosen et al, 1984). There are three main groups: (1) with defects mainly affecting antibodies (humoral immunity); (2) with defects mainly affecting T cells (cellular immunity); and (3) with other defects together with (1) and/or (2) above.

Acquired immune deficiency syndrome (AIDS)

This condition results from infection by the human immuno-deficiency virus (HIV) of which there are two or more sub-types, most infections being due to HIV 1. Transmission of infection can occur (1) during homosexual or heterosexual intercourse; (2) by intravenous drug abuse with infected needles; (3) by the injection of infected blood products in the treatment of haemophilia or by blood transfusion (see p.32); or (4) by accidental puncture of the skin by a needle contaminated by blood from an AIDS victim. There has been an occasional case when infection has occurred from infected blood splashing into the normal eye or on to the skin of a nurse with dermatitis. Apart from such rare exceptions, the disease has not spread to laboratory workers, physiotherapists or other health care professionals working with AIDS victims or their blood (Halloran, 1987b).

The disease is probably now worldwide, with geographical hot spots associated with homosexual promiscuity and intravenous drug usage. There is a danger that overcrowding, drug abuse and homosexuality in prisons (Conacher, 1988) could be followed by heterosexual spread into the community when prisoners are released. After infection has occurred there is an incubation period of between six weeks and 12 months before the HIV antibody test becomes positive. There is a further incubation period of one to two years, or sometimes considerably more, before symptoms develop.

The prodromal phase with diarrhoea, wasting, lymphadenopathy and fever is followed by the immunodeficiency syndrome characterized by opportunistic infection, e.g. by *Pneumocystis carinii*, viruses, fungi and protozoa, and also Kaposi's sarcoma and malignant lymphoma of B-cell type. In the late stages the central nervous system is often seriously affected by the HIV infection.

The immunodeficiency is due to a T-cell lymphopenia with practically no killer cells or helper cells but with normal numbers of suppressor cells (Govan et al, 1986c). Immunoglobulins are increased, but although antibody reaction to previously experienced infections is normal, no antibody to new infections can be produced in the absence of helper cells. The absence of an effective immune system makes the victims vulnerable to overwhelming infection by organisms which would normally have little pathogenic effect. *Children* with AIDS have, initially, B-cell defects rather than T-cell defects although the latter develop later (Bernstein et al, 1985). The number of affected children may be expected to increase as the number of affected women increases. In 1986 only 7 per cent of all AIDS patients were women but heterosexual transmission is anticipated to cause this figure to rise significantly (Novick and Rubinstein, 1987).

The main treatment for AIDS is antibiotics for infections as they arise. The use of antiviral agents, especially zidovudine (Retrovir), previously known as AZT (Azidothymidine), appears to have a life-prolonging effect (Yarchoan et al, 1986). It also produces a considerable improvement in the patient's general condition. In children with AIDS, whose main immunological deficiency initially is humoral due to B-cell defects, periodic intravenous gamma-globulin can extend life expectancy and prevent recurrent bacterial infections (Cavelli and Rubinstein, 1986). The best prophylaxis is the avoidance of risk of exposure to infection. Condoms provide some degree of protection but cannot be considered 100 per cent safe.

Provided care is taken to avoid inoculation by infected blood there is no evidence that a physiotherapist is at risk when involved in the care of patients with AIDS. A physiotherapist whose skin is abraded, cut or scaling should take appropriate protective measures, e.g. by covering a cut with adhesive plaster and/or wearing gloves.

Other acquired conditions affecting immunity

Cellular immunity is suppressed during measles, rubella and lepromatous leprosy and also following measles vaccination (Halloran, 1987b), leading to an increased susceptibility to other infections which is of limited duration and generally returns to normal. Hodgkin's disease and its treatment cause more prolonged suppression of cellular immunity, resulting in increased susceptibility to infection by tubercle bacilli, viruses and fungi (Halloran, 1987b). Lymphocytic lymphoma and chronic lymphatic leukaemia cause deficiency of both cellular and humoral immunity.

Organ transplantation: In the management of kidney, heart, lung and liver transplant cases, immunity has to be suppressed by cytotoxic and other drugs to prevent the transplanted organs from being rejected. As a result such patients are very susceptible to infection (Halloran, 1987b) and need special consideration and protection.

Artificial Antibacterial Defences

Antiseptics: The chances of a wound becoming infected may be greatly reduced by debridement. This involves cleaning the wound surface and the surrounding skin. Any foreign material is removed and an appropriate antiseptic such as hydrogen peroxide is used to kill organisms which may have entered the wound. In general, antiseptics are applied to the site of possible infection. Their effect is purely local and they have no effect on organisms which have penetrated more deeply into the body. Many antiseptics are poisonous if swallowed. Suitable antiseptics may, however, be used for sterilizing instruments which have been previously cleaned.

Antibiotics: Antibiotics, like antiseptics, can kill susceptible organisms. Unlike antiseptics they can reach organisms that have penetrated deeply into the body tissues. They are given either by mouth or by injection, reaching the tissues via the bloodstream. They can also be applied locally when appropriate. Some antibiotics have a narrow range of organisms against which they act: thus penicillin is effective against much *S. pyogenes* but useless against Gram negative bacilli.

Some antibiotics (broad spectrum) have a wide range of organisms against which they act. This apparent advantage has the drawback that they cause diarrhoea by removing the bacteria normally present in the gut and allowing the proliferation of fungi. Before any antibiotic is given to a patient, a swab or specimen should be sent to the bacteriology laboratory to culture the organism concerned and test its sensitivity against an appropriate range of antibiotics.

Asepsis: Prevention is better than cure. It is better to avoid the introduction of organisms than to treat the resultant infection by antiseptics which may damage the tissues or antibiotics which may have harmful side-effects. Modern surgery has only been made possible by the use of rigid aseptic techniques. These include scrubbing up to remove excess organisms from the hands, the wearing of sterile gowns, caps, masks and gloves, the use of sterilized instruments, swabs, dressings and towels and the practice of a non-touch technique. The latter is the use of sterile instruments, rather than hands, for holding swabs, dressings and tissues, and carefully discarding any potentially contaminated materials or instruments. A similar technique is used in the dressing of wounds or changing dressings postoperatively.

An important adjunct to aseptic techniques is the cleansing of skin adjacent to a wound or pre-operatively by skin antiseptics.

An extension of the aseptic technique is the early skin grafting of extensive burns which would otherwise become infected, producing scarring and deformity. This is a great advance, both cosmetically and functionally. It is particularly important for the physiotherapist who has to ensure that as much mobility as possible is retained, especially following burns of the hand.

REFERENCES

Bernstein, L.J., Ochs, H.D., Wedgwood, R.J. and Rubinstein, A. (1985). Defective humoral immunity in paediatric acquired immune deficiency syndrome. *Journal of Pediatrics*, **107**, 352–7.

Bruton, O.C. (1952). Agammaglobulinemia. *Pediatrics*, **9**, 722–7.

Cavelli, T.A. and Rubinstein, A. (1986). Intravenous gammaglobulin in infant acquired immunodeficiency syndrome. *Pediatric Infectious Disease*, **5**, 5207–10.

Conacher, G.N. (1988). AIDS, condoms and prisons. *Lancet*, **2**, 41–2.

Des Jarlais, D.C. and Friedmann, S.R. (1987). Editorial review: HIV infection among intravenous drug users: epidemiology and risk reduction. *AIDS*, **1**, 67–76.

Downham, M.A.P.S. (1976). Immunisations. *British Medical Journal*, **1**, 1063–6.

Gordon, F.M., Willoughby, A.D., Levine, L.A., Gurel, L. and Neill, K.M. (1987). Knowledge of AIDS among hospital workers: behavioral correlates and consequences. *AIDS*, **1**, 183–8.

Govan, A.D.T., Macfarlane, P.S. and Callander, R. (1986a). *Pathology Illustrated*, 2nd edition, p. 53. Churchill Livingstone, Edinburgh.

Govan, A.D.T., Macfarlane, P.S. and Callander, R. (1986b). *ibid*, p. 111.

Govan, A.D.T., Macfarlane, P.S. and Callander, R. (1986c). *ibid*, p. 120.

Halloran, P.F. (1987a). The immune system. In *General Pathology*, 6th edition (ed. Walter, J.B. and Israel, M.S.), pp. 155–67. Churchill Livingstone, Edinburgh.

Halloran, P.F. (1987b). Immunity to infection. *ibid*, pp. 187–99.

van Heyningen, W.E. (1970). Pathogenicity and virulence of micro-organisms. In *General Pathology* (ed. Lord Florey), p. 882, Lloyd-Luke, London.

Novick, B.E. and Rubinstein, A. (1987). The paediatric perspective. *AIDS*, 1, 3–7.

Robbins, S.L. and Kumar, V. (1987a). *Basic Pathology*, 4th edition, pp. 437–43. Saunders, Philadelphia.

Robbins, S.L. and Kumar, V. (1987b). *ibid*, pp. 129–31.

Rosen, F.S., Cooper, M.D. and Wedgwood, R.J.P. (1984). The primary immunodeficiencies. *New England Journal of Medicine*, 311, 235–42, 300–10.

Walter, J.B. and Israel, M.S. (1987a). *General Pathology*, 6th edition, pp. 106–7. Churchill Livingstone, Edinburgh.

Walter, J.B. and Israel, M.S. (1987b). *ibid*, p. 316.

Webb, H.E. (1968). Factors in the host-virus relationship which may affect the course of an infection. *British Medical Journal*, 4, 684–6.

Yarchoan, R. et al (1986). Administration 3-Azido-3 deoxythymidine, an inhibitor of HTLV-3/LAV replication, to patients with AIDS or AIDS-related complex. *Lancet*, 1, 575–80.

BIBLIOGRAPHY

See end of Chapter 5, page 65.

Chapter 4

Circulatory Disturbances

by D. M. D. EVANS MD, FRCP, FRCPath

Circulatory disturbances may be divided into general and local.

The most important *general* disturbance of the circulation is cardiac failure. Its main causes are excessive load, damaged heart muscle and conduction system, and inefficient heart valves. Excessive load is most commonly due to high blood pressure, the immediate cause being increased tone in the muscular arteries and arterioles. Damaged heart muscle and conduction system are most commonly due to obstruction of the coronary arteries which supply the heart, by atheroma and thrombosis. Inefficient valves may be due to congenital defects or to damage resulting from infection. Rheumatic fever was a common cause but has now become rare as a result of treating streptococcal infections by antibiotics. Whatever the cause of cardiac failure one effect is slowing of the circulation. This in turn can contribute to local circulatory disturbance such as thrombosis. Another common effect of cardiac failure is oedema due to the increased venous pressure.

The most important *local* disturbance of circulation is obstruction of the blood supply. This is usually due to thrombosis or embolism but may also be due to disease of the vessel wall, compression, invasion by a growth or vascular spasm.

THROMBOSIS

Thrombosis is the formation of a thrombus (Greek, *thrombos*, a clot). Normally blood does not clot when it flows through healthy blood vessels. Factors which promote thrombosis are stasis (slowing of the bloodstream) and injury or disease of the vessel wall. Stasis may be part of general slowing of the bloodstream, as from cardiac failure or from prolonged recumbency without the benefit of physiotherapy.

Local factors include the compression of veins by tight clothing, the bar of a deckchair, a pregnant uterus or a tumour, and the narrowing of the lumen of coronary arteries by atheroma. Damage to a vessel wall, usually a vein, may be due to a fracture or an operation in its close vicinity. An adjacent inflammatory process may precipitate thrombosis, e.g. of uterine veins in pelvic sepsis (French and Macfarlane, 1970). Following an operation there may be a period of recumbency with a consequent slowing of the circulation, although nowadays this is kept as short as possible with early mobilization. Following childbirth and surgical procedures, particularly splenectomy, there is a rise in platelet count which increases the patient's susceptibility to thrombosis temporarily.

Platelets have the property of adhering to a variety of surfaces, particularly collagen which is exposed when a vessel is damaged. Blood vessels constantly suffer minor damage. The integrity of the vessel wall is restored by a layer of platelets laid down soon after the damage occurs, together with a small amount of fibrin. The fibrin and platelets are rapidly covered by endothelial cells so that the smooth lining is restored and no further platelets are laid down (Walter and Israel, 1987).

The formation of a blood clot results from conversion of the soluble blood protein fibrinogen into insoluble fibrin which forms a web of fine threads in which the blood cells become enmeshed. This conversion is brought about by thrombin. Normally circulating blood contains no thrombin, otherwise it would clot. Instead it contains an inactive substance called prothrombin which, in the presence of calcium, is converted into thrombin by thromboplastin (also called thrombokinase). Normally circulating blood contains no thromboplastin, otherwise it would clot. Instead it contains a number of factors, platelets being one of these factors. If there is any damage to the blood vessel wall platelets tend to stick to the damaged vessel wall and the clotting process may be triggered off by the production of thromboplastin. This clotting tendency is increased if the circulation is slowed. Oral contraceptive hormones may predispose to such thrombosis (Vessey and Doll, 1968).

The tendency to clot is diminished by regular physiotherapy with exercise. It is also diminished by anticoagulant therapy, a treatment not without hazards (*Lancet*, 1988).

Once a thrombus has formed in a vein the stasis resulting from the blockage of the lumen causes further clotting (propagated thrombus) which usually extends to the point at which the next tributary joins the vein. However, since blood flow may not have stopped completely in the early stage of thrombosis the pattern of fibrin deposition in the first formed thrombus follows the direction of blood flow and is laid down in broad bands (Jorgensen, 1964). Initially such thrombus may be only loosely attached to the vessel wall and there is a danger that part of it may become detached. Later an inflammatory reaction develops. Capillary buds and fibroblasts grow into the clot so that it becomes organized and firmly attached to the vessel wall. Eventually the thrombus may become re-canalized, with one or more channels extending through the length of the clot so that circulation is re-established (Akrawi and Wilson, 1950). Alternatively the vein may end up as a fibrous cord.

EMBOLISM

When a clot occurs in a leg vein there is a danger that part of the clot may break away and form an embolus (Greek, *embolos*, a wedge or stopper). This is carried off in the bloodstream until it becomes wedged, usually in the pulmonary artery or one of its branches. The process is then referred to as pulmonary embolism (French and Macfarlane, 1970). A large pulmonary embolus is often fatal.

Another example of embolism is when a portion of thrombus breaks away from the left atrium, a not uncommon complication of atrial fibrillation. The embolic thrombus is ejected into the aorta from which it may escape into a carotid artery and then become wedged in a cerebral artery, blocking the blood supply to part of the brain. Alternatively it may travel the whole length of the aorta and become wedged astride its bifurcation into the two common iliac arteries (saddle embolus) blocking the blood supply to one or both legs. A smaller embolus may pass straight down into one of the leg arteries and cause a block at almost any level (author's observations).

INFARCTION

Infarction is tissue death due to a blocked vessel. The extent of the tissue death reflects the distribution of the vessel. In the case of a blocked artery in an organ such as the kidney it is often cone-shaped, as is the tissue supplied by the artery. It is called an infarct (Latin, *infarctum*, stuffed) because in the early stages it is stuffed with blood, at least in soft tissues such as the lung. Infarcts in firmer tissues are only haemorrhagic at the edges due to seepage of blood into the dead tissue from vessels at the margin of the infarct. The blood gradually becomes absorbed and it changes from a red into a white infarct. It also becomes fibrotic and shrinks in size.

Infarction only occurs in tissues which do not have an adequate collateral (secondary) blood supply. Thus, in addition to pulmonary vessels, the lung has a secondary supply from bronchial vessels. So a small pulmonary embolism may not produce an infarct unless there is also cardiac failure, making the bronchial supply inadequate. It is patients who have poor circulation, as in cardiac failure, who are more likely to get leg vein thrombosis with the possibility of pulmonary embolism and resultant pulmonary infarction.

Infarction may occur from a blocked vein such as a mesenteric vein undergoing thrombosis or from blockage of both artery and vein, as from torsion of an ovarian cyst when the whole cyst becomes infarcted. A common cause of death is infarction of heart muscle due to blockage of a coronary artery by atheroma and thrombosis. The brain may undergo infarction either from embolism due to a clot released from a damaged heart or from thrombosis of a cerebral artery. Gangrene of an extremity due to arteriosclerosis is another example of infarction.

Signs: symptoms: management

Thrombosis, embolism and infarction are closely related conditions, any one of which may give rise to signs and symptoms. Leg vein thrombosis may give rise to pain and tenderness at the site of thrombosis with swelling of the affected limb. Management is a compromise between resting the limb to avoid dislodging an embolus and sufficient movement of the rest of the body to discourage further thrombosis, assisted by anticoagulant administration. Prevention is by adequate movement and physiotherapy for recumbent patients, particularly postoperatively and especially if they are obese.

Not uncommonly leg vein thrombosis may be symptomless and the first indication of its existence may be the effects of pulmonary embolism. A large embolus causes extreme distress, shock and breathlessness and may be fatal within minutes.

A smaller embolus may give rise to transient pleuritic pain which may be associated with signs and symptoms resembling pneumonia. Sometimes there is little clinical evidence that pulmonary embolism has occurred and a puzzling shadow on the radiograph may be the first clue to what has happened. Pulmonary infarction may be complicated by chest infection which will then require treatment as for pneumonia. Otherwise management is mainly directed to the prevention of further pulmonary embolism by anticoagulants and physiotherapy.

Thrombosis of a coronary artery may give rise to a typical heart attack, with chest pain and shock, often with breathlessness and cyanosis. Quite often the pain is described as indigestion or back pain; it may radiate down the arm or into the neck. Management depends on severity and available facilities. It varies from intensive care with cardiac monitoring in a coronary care unit, possibly with dramatic resuscitation procedures, to bed rest at home. Once the acute phase is over, graduated exercise plays an important part in the recovery phase.

Embolism from the heart to the brain or thrombosis of a cerebral artery can cause cerebral infarction, i.e. a stroke. A small infarct may cause slight weakness on one side (hemiparesis), sometimes involving only one limb. A larger infarct may cause complete paralysis of one side (hemiplegia). Physiotherapy and occupational therapy play an important part in regaining maximum movement and control. This may include training the left hand to undertake functions previously performed by the right hand.

Embolism from the heart to a leg artery causes pain and discoloration of the leg. Immediate operation to remove the embolus (embolectomy) is sometimes successful. If this cannot be done, keeping the limb cool with minimal movement (to reduce metabolism) may keep gangrene at bay, allowing a collateral circulation to develop and re-canalization to occur (Akrawi and Wilson, 1950). If gangrene develops, amputation may be necessary; the rehabilitation and training in the use of the prosthesis is described in Chapter 17.

If a leg artery becomes progressively blocked by atheroma a point is reached when the patient suffers pain after walking a certain distance, a condition known as intermittent claudication (Latin *claudicare*, to limp). It is now possible to restore the circulation by introducing a catheter into the artery carrying a rotating cutter which literally cuts away the obstructing atheroma (Höfling et al, 1988).

OEDEMA

There is normally a small amount of tissue fluid in the intercellular spaces. Oedema occurs when tissue fluid is formed more rapidly than it is re-absorbed. This commonly presents clinically as swelling of the feet and ankles. A finger pressed on the swollen tissues produces an indentation which persists for a while after the finger is removed (pitting oedema).

Tissue fluid is formed by filtration from the blood as it flows through the capillaries. The capillary lining acts as a semi-permeable membrane. It allows water and electrolytes to pass through but holds back the cells and virtually all the proteins. At the arterial end of the capillaries the blood pressure is higher than the osmotic pressure of the plasma proteins and so fluid passes through the capillary wall into the tissue spaces. By the time blood reaches the venous end of

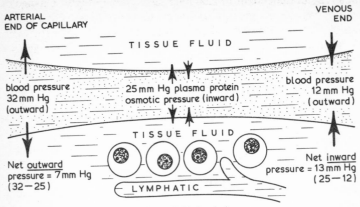

Fig. 4.1 The factors controlling tissue fluid circulation

the capillary the blood pressure has normally fallen sufficiently for the osmotic pressure of the plasma proteins to draw the tissue fluid back into the vessels (Fig. 4/1). Tissue fluid drainage is also provided by re-absorption into the lymphatics. This tissue fluid circulation enables the cells to be provided with food and oxygen and also removes waste products. Oedema occurs when the reabsorption of tissue fluid cannot keep pace with its formation (Roberts, 1970). There are five main causes: (1) increased venous blood pressure; (2) reduced plasma protein osmotic pressure; (3) increased permeability of the capillary wall, allowing more protein to pass through; (4) increased osmotic pressure of the tissue fluid; and (5) obstruction of lymphatic drainage (Thomson and Cotton, 1983).

Increased venous pressure

General   The venous pressure is increased in cardiac failure. The causes for this have already been outlined at the beginning of this chapter. The raised pressure at the venous end of the capillary counteracts the osmotic pressure of the plasma proteins, thus impeding the re-absorption of tissue fluid. Oedema results. Its treatment involves the appropriate management of cardiac failure, including the use of drugs such as digoxin and diuretics.

Local

Gravity: An important factor in determining the site of oedema. Even in healthy people oedema of the feet and legs can occur if the limbs remain dependent for too long, as on a long flight. Change of posture can be of great importance in controlling oedema. An example is the prevention of oedema of the lungs in a patient with left ventricular failure by sleeping propped-up in bed against pillows.

Inactivity: The venous return, especially from the legs, depends on compression of the veins by muscular activity in conjunction with competent valves in the veins which prevent reverse flow. If the muscles are inactive the venous return is poor, the venous capillary pressure is raised and so oedema occurs. An extreme example is paralytic oedema. A less extreme example is the oedema due to poor muscle tone. In the latter instance the physiotherapist can help to restore the strength and tone of the muscles by teaching graded exercises. If there is also laxity of the fascia the limb is elevated and a firm (but not tight) elastic bandage may be used. In the case of paralytic oedema passive measures to promote venous return will be required. These include: (1) elevation of the affected limb; (2) passive movement of joints; (3) artificial exercise of the paralysed muscles by interrupted direct current (now rare); or (4) light massage which is sometimes effective in dispersing the fluid into regions not affected by the paralysis. Care must be taken neither to increase the paralytic vasodilation nor to bruise or stretch the atonic muscle fibres.

Varicose veins: These greatly impair venous return from the legs. The dilatation of the veins causes valves to become incompetent so that even with muscular activity the venous return is poor. Venous return can be improved by raising the legs or by providing support, e.g. with an elastic stocking. Surgical treatment of varicose veins is often effective.

Pressure: Tight clothing, e.g. garters and elasticated hosiery, may obstruct both veins and lymphatics. Pressure may also be produced by the pregnant uterus, tumours or by inflammation. Treatment is to educate the patient about clothing, and investigate the medical causes of pressure.

Venous Thrombosis Factors involved in venous thrombosis have been described already. When thrombosis occurs in the deep veins of the leg it obstructs the venous capillary pressure behind the obstruction so that tissue fluid cannot be re-absorbed and oedema results. The leg becomes swollen and painful (white leg (phlegmasia alba dolens)).

In the initial stages the leg has to be rested to avoid provoking embolism and anticoagulant therapy given to prevent extension of the thrombosis. By elevating the leg the severity of the oedema can be reduced. Not until the danger of embolism is past is it possible to introduce more active measures to promote re-absorption of oedema, e.g. alternating muscle contraction and relaxation.

Traumatic Oedema The swelling which occurs after minor trauma is usually due mainly to oedema. The discomfort may be alleviated by simple measures such as cold compresses. Re-absorption of the oedema fluid is often quite rapid. With more severe trauma including fractures much of the swelling is due to haemorrhage (a bruise or haematoma) which takes considerably longer to re-absorb. The swelling associated with extensive burns is usually mainly oedema; it will be considered further under increased capillary permeability.

Reduced plasma proteins

The plasma proteins may be reduced by inadequate intake as in starvation, or excessive loss as in protein-losing nephritis. Proteins may also be lost in large amounts into the alimentary tract, e.g. from the surface of a colonic carcinoma; a number of gastro-intestinal conditions with hypoproteinaemia have been grouped together as 'protein-losing gastro-enteropathy' (Jarnum, 1963). Management includes raising the level of plasma proteins, particularly albumin, by intravenous infusion, and treatment of the cause.

Increased capillary permeability

The sluggish circulation associated with raised venous pressure tends to cause anoxia of the endothelial cells. The resulting increased capillary permeability is thus a factor in circulatory oedema. Damage to the capillary endothelium is also a factor in the oedema occurring in nephritis, e.g. peri-orbital oedema. Allergy, e.g. wasp sting may also damage the endothelium of capillaries and produce local oedema which can be a hazard to life if the sting involves the tongue. The oedema of nettle-rash is similar and may be controlled by anti-histamine drugs, histamine being one of the main substances causing damage to the capillary endothelium in allergic states.

Burns are an important cause of increased capillary permeability. The resulting oedema fluid has a high protein content so that it clots and organizes readily. This may result in permanent disfiguration if appropriate steps are not taken to promote its re-absorption (see Chapter 15). The underlying principles and practical measures have already been described but unfortunately their application may be impeded by the extent of injury caused by the burns. An over-riding consideration is the maintenance of blood pressure by the infusion of plasma or plasma substitute to replace the fluid and protein lost from the circulation into the tissue spaces as oedema fluid.

Increased osmotic pressure of the tissue fluid

Excess sodium ions in the tissue fluid increases its osmotic pressure, thus preventing fluid re-absorption and causing oedema. This occurs in cardiac failure and in any conditions where sodium excretion is impaired, e.g. in renal failure and in adrenal steroid oversecretion or overtreatment. Excess salt in the diet can produce a similar effect (Thomson and Cotton, 1983).

Obstruction to lymphatic drainage

In addition to the factors already mentioned under raised venous pressure, which obstruct both veins and lymphatics, there may also be selective lymphatic obstruction. This occurs after repeated attacks of lymphadenitis and lymphangitis; following radical surgery, e.g. for carcinoma of the breast; and as a long-term effect of filarial infection (elephantiasis). The oedema produced by lymphatic obstruction is usually of the non-pitting variety due to fibrosis. Unless treated early it rarely responds significantly to physiotherapy.

Important precaution

In all forms of oedema the vessels in the oedematous region should not be encouraged to dilate since this exacerbates the oedema. The application of heat to the affected part is therefore to be avoided.

REFERENCES

Akrawi, Y. Y. and Wilson, G. M. (1950). Observations on the development and function of elastic-coated vascular channels in occluded arteries. *Journal of Pathology and Bacteriology*, **62**, 69–73.

French, J. E. and Macfarlane, R. G. (1970). Haemostasis and thrombosis. In *General Pathology* (ed. Lord Florey), pp. 273–317. Lloyd-Luke, London.

Höfling, B., Polnitz, A. V., Backa, D., Arnim, Th. v., Lauterjung, L., Jauch, K. W. and Simpson, J. B. (1988). Percutaneous removal of atheromatous plaques in peripheral arteries. *Lancet*, **1**, 384–6.

Jarnum, S. (1963). *Protein-Losing Gastro-Enteropathy*, pp. 1–232. Blackwell Scientific Publications Limited, Oxford.

Jorgensen, L. (1964). Experimental platelet and coagulation thrombi. *Acta Pathologica et Microbiologica Scandinavica*, 62, 189–223.

Leading Article (1988). Management of venous thromboembolism. *Lancet*, 1, 275–7.

Roberts, K. B. (1970). Oedema. In *General Pathology* (ed. Lord Florey), pp. 370–93. Lloyd-Luke, London.

Thomson, A. D. and Cotton, R. E. (1983). *Lecture Notes on Pathology*, pp. 122–3. Blackwell Scientific Publications Limited, Oxford.

Vessey, M. P. and Doll, R. (1968). Investigation of relation between oral contraceptives and thrombo-embolic disease. *British Medical Journal*, 2, 199–205.

Walter, J. B. and Israel, M. S. (1987). *General Pathology*, 6th edition, pp. 522–3. Churchill Livingstone, Edinburgh.

BIBLIOGRAPHY

See end of Chapter 5, page 65.

Cellular Pathology

by D. M. D. EVANS MD, FRCP, FRCPath

The human body is a complex organization of cells. If cellular function in any part of the body is impaired the whole body may suffer. Cell death is called necrosis. Lesser degrees of cell damage from which recovery is possible are called degenerations.

NECROSIS (Greek, *nekrosis*, a killing)

Necrosis means death of cells while they still form part of a living body. It implies permanent cessation of function of the affected cells (Dixon, 1967). Anything which damages cells can cause necrosis. This includes all the factors described in Chapter 2 as causes of inflammation, especially infection, infarction and injury. One example of necrosis is the pressure sore which may occur over a bony point in a bedridden patient.

Gangrene

When necrosis affects a mass of tissue such as a digit or limb it is called gangrene. An example is the gangrene of a toe resulting from an obstructed blood supply. The toe becomes purplish and may eventually go black. This blackening is probably due to the slow drying and oxidation of haemoglobin in the tissues (Walter and Israel, 1987a). The main cause of the necrosis is lack of oxygen (tissue anoxia). Two types of gangrene are recognized, dry and moist.

Dry Gangrene This occurs when there is no oedema or infection. The affected digit or limb mummifies and there is a clear line of demarcation due to an inflammatory reaction in the living tissue next to the blackened dead tissue (Thomson and Cotton, 1983a).

Moist Gangrene This occurs when oedema and infection are present. The affected part undergoes swelling and putrefaction. It is seen in infarction of a loop of bowel as in a strangulated hernia. Moist gangrene may also complicate dry gangrene of a digit or limb if it becomes infected (Thomson and Cotton, 1983a). This is particularly likely to happen if the patient has diabetes mellitus.

ATROPHY (Greek, a-trophē, without nourishment)

Atrophy is a wasting away of part of the body. It may simply be a reduction in the size of the affected cells but if severe may also involve a reduction in the number of cells, called apoptosis (Greek, dropping off) (Walter and Israel, 1987b). Atrophy may be generalized or local.

Generalized

This occurs in starvation and in protein deprivation (kwashiorkor). In starvation, body fat and protein are mobilized to provide the essential energy requirements for life. Practically all the soft tissues and organs of the body become reduced in size. In kwashiorkor there is insufficient protein for the growth and replacement of tissues which normally take place. It is characterized by wasting and weakness of the muscles which is in marked contrast to the associated swelling of the abdomen. The term kwashiorkor is from the Ghanaian language and means 'the sickness which the old one gets when the next baby is born', i.e. the older child is deprived of breast feeding and weaned on a diet consisting mainly of carbohydrates (Robbins and Kumar, 1987).

Generalized muscular wasting also occurs in patients who are confined to bed for any length of time. Muscular inactivity is the main cause and the legs, being relatively more immobile than the arms, tend to be more severely affected. Appropriate physiotherapy can prevent or greatly reduce such muscular wasting.

Other causes of generalized atrophy include toxaemia due to prolonged infection such as tuberculosis; systemic conditions such as rheumatoid disease; endocrine deficiency such as myxoedema; ulcer or carcinoma of the oesophagus or stomach; and cardiac failure. The latter has been known to cause cachexia (severe wasting) leading to a diagnosis of a carcinoma when in fact none was present (author's observation).

Senile atrophy is of importance to physiotherapists because not only is there atrophy of the soft tissues but also the skeleton undergoes atrophic change known as osteoporosis in which the amount of bone tissue per unit volume of bone is reduced (*BMJ*, 1971). Elderly women, and sometimes younger postmenopausal women, are particularly susceptible. Their bones may become so fragile that they fracture spontaneously; the neck of the femur is a common site. Vertebrae are also affected; vertebral bodies can collapse causing compression of nerve roots with considerable pain. It is important to recognize this condition. Handling frail elderly women requires special care. The progression of the bone fragility may be controlled by replacement hormone therapy.

Osteoporosis can also affect anyone who is immobilized, including healthy male volunteers placed in plaster casts from the waist to the toes, 1–2 per cent of the total body calcium being lost in 6–7 weeks (Deitrick et al, 1948). This is probably due to increased reabsorption of bone by osteoclasts (*Lancet*, 1963). Other causes of osteoporosis include starvation, intestinal malabsorption, adult scurvy, acromegaly, thyrotoxicosis, Cushing's disease and rheumatoid disease treated by steroids (Walter and Israel, 1987b). To this may be added prolonged weightlessness in space. Conditions which may be mistaken for osteoporosis include osteogenesis imperfecta (Smith, 1984) and hyperparathyroidism.

Local

Local atrophy results from a number of conditions which interfere with the nourishment or health of the affected part. They include impaired blood supply, disuse, pressure, impaired nerve supply and primary muscle disease.

Impaired Blood Supply Partial loss of blood supply to a group of muscles causes them to waste and, if severe, results in replacement fibrosis. Its most serious form is seen in the heart as myocardial ischaemia. It can cause progressive cardiac failure or a heart attack which may be mild, severe or fatal. Carefully controlled exercise under medical supervision may improve the blood supply to the affected part by encouraging the development of an alternative blood supply by collateral vessels. This applies to the heart as well as to skeletal muscles.

Disuse Disuse atrophy of muscles is one of the most important conditions that a physiotherapist may be called upon to treat or, infinitely better, to prevent. Untreated it can progress with remarkable speed. Active exercises provide the most effective treatment; but in the case of paralysis, passive measures, including electrical stimulation of muscles, may have to be used. This is particularly important where the paralysis is temporary and eventual recovery is anticipated.

Atrophy may occur in bone adjacent to an inflammatory process. Atrophy also occurs round an ankylosed or inflamed joint, particularly around rheumatoid or tuberculous arthritis (Walter and Israel, 1987b).

Pressure Pressure atrophy is produced when there is prolonged pressure, probably as a result of reducing the blood supply to the affected cells (Thomson and Cotton, 1983b). The more serious condition of pressure sores has already been mentioned under necrosis. Lesser degrees of pressure cause atrophy of the compressed tissues. Constant awareness of the danger, particularly in elderly bedridden patients, is the key to its prevention.

Impaired Nerve Supply In addition to the disuse atrophy already described, the absence of a nerve supply can, in itself, lead to tissue atrophy. It is minimized by taking steps to restore the nerve supply as quickly as possible. This may require surgical intervention to suture a severed nerve together, so that nerve axons may grow down the tube provided by the dead distal part of the nerve at the rate of about one millimetre a day.

Primary Muscle Disease Primary muscular dystrophies are a group of diseases of skeletal muscle, many of which are due to an inherited defect, possibly an enzyme deficiency. They are often present in early childhood with progressive muscular weakness. The affected muscles may not appear wasted but instead may appear enlarged, particularly the calf muscles, due to the presence of fat. It is important to recognize muscular dystrophies because misapplied physiotherapy may be harmful.

The term myopathy is used to denote conditions such as the muscle weakness and wasting which may occur in association with certain tumours, e.g. carcinoma of lung (oat cell), breast or colon (Walters and Israel, 1987c). There are also a number of congenital myopathies (Dubowitz, 1978). They all present with muscle weakness which may date from birth, early infancy (the 'floppy infant syndrome') or later in life. The various types are distinguished by muscle biopsy with histochemistry and electron microscopy.

DEGENERATIONS

Cell degeneration results from damage which is insufficient to cause cellular necrosis and from which recovery is possible. Two of the commoner forms of degeneration are cloudy swelling and fatty degeneration.

Cloudy swelling

This occurs in many febrile conditions, e.g. acute specific fevers such as measles and whooping cough. It also occurs in anaemia, anoxia, malnutrition and minor grades of poisoning by chemical substances. If the kidney is examined the cut surface is seen to pout. Under the microscope the kidney cells appear swollen with a hazy, granular cytoplasm; the granules are protein from damaged cell organelles. Alterations in the mitochondria can be seen by electron microscopy (Trump et al, 1965). Normally it is a transient condition and complete recovery is the rule.

Fatty change

This form of degeneration indicates more severe cellular damage. It is a change commonly seen in the liver of alcoholics. The liver is large and pale and the cut surface is greasy. Under the microscope the liver cells are seen to contain fatty droplets. In the early stages the cytoplasm of the cells contains a number of small droplets. These coalesce to form one large droplet which may push the nucleus to one side resembling the appearance of a fat cell in adipose tissue. When many liver cells are affected the tissue section appears to be full of holes like a sieve, an appearance seen only too frequently in liver biopsy specimens. If the alcoholic gives up drinking the fatty liver cells return to normal. Often, however, the condition is complicated by cirrhosis of the liver, a condition with nodules of liver surrounded by fibrosis, which does not revert to normal. The heart and kidneys may also be affected by fatty degeneration. In Western society alcohol is probably the most important cause of fatty degeneration, the liver being the main target. Other causes include infections, anaemia, anoxia and kwashiorkor. In the latter the liver is greatly enlarged, in marked contrast to the wasting of the limbs (Robbins and Kumar, 1987).

NEOPLASIA (Greek, *neos*, new and *plasso*, to form)

Neoplasia means new growth, i.e. tumour formation. It includes both benign and malignant forms of tumour. When a benign tumour grows it may compress surrounding tissue but does not invade it. Malignant tumours (cancers) not only invade surrounding tissues but may also spread to more distant tissues either along lymphatic channels to produce lymph node deposits; or through the bloodstream to produce deposits in liver, lungs, brain or bone; or else across spaces such as the peritoneal cavity to implant at other sites and on other organs in the cavity.

The term cervical intra-epithelial neoplasia (CIN) is used to describe the changes that occur in the lining of the uterine cervix before an invasive growth or cancer develops (Coleman and Evans, 1988a). The term CIN 1 is used when the inner third or less of the epithelial thickness consists of neoplastic cells; CIN 2 when the inner one- to two-thirds of the thickness is so affected; and CIN 3 for more severe lesions. If left untreated a significant proportion (possibly 40 per cent) of the more severe lesions will eventually develop into the invasive cancer (Fidler et al, 1968). Although invasion usually develops from CIN 3 it can occasionally develop from less severe lesions (Coleman and Evans, 1988b).

The recognition that such changes may be detected and treated before the neoplasia becomes invasive is an important step in the control of malignant growth.

Tumours may be divided broadly into two groups, those which arise from epithelial cells and those arising from connective tissue. Tumours in each group can be either *benign*, *malignant* or *intermediate*. Benign tumours do not invade but can damage surrounding tissues by pressure atrophy. Malignant tumours always invade the surrounding tissues; they can also spread by vascular channels and metastasize to distant parts of the body (Walters and Israel, 1987d). The term *intermediate tumour* was introduced by Morehead (1965) to include a lesion which is locally invasive but shows little or no tendency to metastasize, e.g. basal cell carcinoma of skin (rodent ulcer); such tumours are also described as being *locally malignant*.

Epithelial tumours

Benign The benign epithelial tumours are papillomata and adenomata. A *papilloma* is a protuberant tumour arising from an epithelium such as skin. A *pedunculated* papilloma is one with a stalk. A *sessile* papilloma is one without a stalk which appears to sit on the epithelium from which it is arising.

An *adenoma* is a benign tumour arising from glandular tissue such as salivary gland or gastro-intestinal tract. An adenoma arising in the gut usually protrudes into the lumen as a polyp. Although an adenoma is a benign tumour it is likely to recur if it is not completely removed, particularly one arising from the salivary gland.

Malignant Malignant epithelial tumours are all called carcinomas (Greek, *karkinos*, a crab). If the epithelium from which they arise is glandular and the tumour is of glandular type the term adeno-carcinoma is appropriate, being the malignant version of an adenoma; this more clearly defines the type of carcinoma. Other types of carcinoma are defined by their component cells such as squamous cell carcinoma or oat cell carcinoma. They are also defined by their site of origin, e.g. squamous cell carcinoma of lung. From experience it is known that a squamous cell carcinoma grows more slowly and is more likely to be cured by surgery than an oat cell carcinoma of lung.

The term cancer (Latin, *cancrum*, a crab) includes *all* forms of malignant tumour.

Connective tissue tumours

Benign connective tissue tumours are designated by the ending *-oma* following a prefix indicating the tissue involved. This fibroma arises from fibrous tissue, lipoma from fatty tissue, myoma from muscle and osteoma from bone. *Malignant* connective tissue tumours are all called sarcomas. One arising from fibrous tissues is a fibrosarcoma, one from bone is an osteosarcoma and from skeletal muscle a rhab-domyosarcoma. Like carcinomas, sarcomas infiltrate surrounding tissues; they have a much greater tendency to spread by the blood-stream, particularly to lungs, than carcinomas which more fre-quently spread by lymphatics to the related lymph nodes.

Patterns of tumour growth

There is a group of malignant connective tissue tumours arising in the central nervous system called gliomas. They infiltrate the sur-rounding nervous tissue of brain or spinal cord but do not spread outside the nervous system.

Another important group of tumours arise from the pigment-forming cells (melanocytes) of the skin or eye. The benign form is called a pigmented naevus, commonly known as a mole. The malignant form is a malignant melanoma. Any pigmented tumour which starts to grow, itch or bleed should be looked upon with suspicion and excised with a wide margin of clearance. Malignant melanomas can spread both by lymphatics, like carcinomas, and by the blood-stream, like sarcomas. Sometimes there is an interval of several years between the initial tumour, thought to have been removed completely, and the appearance of metastases. Breast cancer may have a similar latent interval.

The tissues of which benign tumours are composed are similar to the normal tissue from which they are formed. Malignant tumours are variable. If they are well differentiated they closely resemble their tissue of origin but if they are poorly differentiated their tissue type may be difficult to recognize. In general, poorly differentiated cancers invade and spread more rapidly than well-differentiated cancers.

The term benign suggests that such tumours are not harmful. This is not always true. A meningioma is a benign tumour arising from the meninges, the membranes enclosing the brain and spinal cord. As a meningioma grows it compresses the adjacent nervous tissue, causing progressive damage to the brain or spinal cord. If diagnosed early it can be removed before irreparable harm is caused. A benign thyroid adenoma may suddenly enlarge due to haemorrhage into its substance and compress the trachea, causing asphyxia unless prompt action is taken.

Conversely the diagnosis of malignancy does not imply a sentence of death if it is diagnosed at an early stage. Cancer of the cervix can cause death by infiltrating the ureters which run nearby, producing uraemia. Yet many cases of cervical cancer are now being prevented or cured by early recognition and treatment. Other malignant tumours such as Hodgkin's disease of lymph nodes and even the highly malignant Ewing's sarcoma of bone have been successfully treated by surgery, radiotherapy and chemotherapy.

Spontaneous regression of a malignant tumour is a rare but now well-recognized phenomenon. A malignant tumour may undergo maturation into its related benign tumour, e.g. neuroblastoma into a ganglioneuroma (Smithers, 1969). Very occasionally incomplete resection of an inoperable tumour such as oat cell carcinoma of lung may result in a complete cure (Smith, 1971).

Cancer causation

In recent years there has been considerable advance in the understanding of the nature of cancer. It is now known that there is no single cause, but many causes. A number of cancers are due to factors in the environment – these factors are known as carcinogens and in certain cases are controllable, the most notable factor being tobacco smoke.

There are also intrinsic and extrinsic factors concerned with the development of tumours.

Intrinsic Factors There is at present little evidence of a hereditary factor for most of the common tumours. Occasional 'cancer families' have been described in which there is a relatively high frequency of certain tumours, usually carcinoma of the breast, ovary or large intestine (Mulvihill, 1985). Polyposis coli and xeroderma pigmentosum are inherited conditions which predispose to the development of cancer. Genetic factors are also involved in the development of certain rare tumours such as retinoblastoma. People with high risk factors should be screened regularly.

Malignant disease occurs in all races but the types of cancers vary. Carcinoma of the liver is rare in Europeans but common in Bantus. People whose skins are pale and who do not tan easily are more likely to develop skin cancer if they live in a hot climate where their skin is exposed to the sun.

Carcinoma of the testis is almost unknown in black Africans. Carcinoma of the prostate and chronic lymphatic leukaemia are very rare in the Japanese and Chinese (Doll, 1972).

There is also a different incidence of certain cancers according to the sex of the person. Carcinoma of the bronchus has been more common in the male than the female. At present, the numbers occurring in the female population are increasing which suggests that it was related to smoking habits rather than the sex of the individual. Age is significant in relation to the development of tumours. The majority develop or become apparent over the age of 50 although some types can occur at any age. Sarcomas tend to develop in younger people and likewise some types of leukaemia develop in children.

Alterations in the level of hormone secretions which cause hyperplasia of tissue may promote the formation of a malignant growth. There is certainly a connection between oestrogen levels and the development of endometrial and breast cancer, and in the male a connection between hormones and prostatic carcinoma.

Chronic inflammation such as ulcerative colitis can increase the risk of a cancer developing.

Extrinsic Factors Substances which are known to contribute to the formation of malignant tumours are known as carcinogens. There is an enormous variety of ways in which these carcinogens work and the production of a tumour depends on their concentration and the length of exposure or the interaction of various substances which are not carcinogenic on their own but are when combined. The following are examples of carcinogens:

1. *Chemical:* Hydrocarbons such as benzpyrene (active compound of soot and tar); fine fibres such as asbestos (*BMJ*, 1976).
2. *Physical:* Radiant energy – x-rays, alpha, beta and gamma rays.
3. *Viral:* Oncogenic viruses, e.g. leukaemia – sarcoma virus of cats, rats, guinea pigs and hamsters.

A number of virally produced tumours have been found in animals. Over many years researchers have hoped that a virus would be found to be responsible for cancer in humans as it might then be possible to protect people by vaccination. There is growing evidence of viral infection being a factor in the causation of some tumours, e.g. Burkitt's lymphoma and also cervical, breast and naso-pharyngeal carcinomas (Walter and Israel, 1987d).

Development and control of early cancer

There is growing evidence that the development of cancer is preceded by cellular changes occurring in a series of steps, usually extending over a long period of time. Some of these steps are reversible. Smoking produces squamous metaplasia in the bronchial epithelium. Giving up smoking before irreversible change has occurred allows the bronchial epithelium to revert towards normality, with a corresponding reduction in the risk of developing cancer.

There is strong evidence that the uterine cervix usually undergoes intra-epithelial neoplasia (CIN) before it reaches the stage of invasive cancer. As the degree of CIN becomes more severe so the chances of invasive cancer developing are found to increase (Coleman and Evans, 1988b); but even at the stage of CIN 3 spontaneous regression can occur. However, since it is not possible to distinguish between cases which will regress and those that will progress, the usual procedure is to remove the more severe lesions by cone biopsy. Less severe cases are now being treated more conservatively, e.g. evaporation of the abnormal epithelium by laser beam, or treatment by cautery, including large loop excision of the transitional zone (Coleman and Evans, 1988c).

Just as the early stages of cervical cancer can be detected by cervical cytology so the early stages of urinary tract cancer can be detected by urine cytology. This is of particular value in detecting early cancer in industrial or laboratory workers who have been exposed to carcinogens such as aromatic amines, perhaps many years previously. Multiple biopsies have shown that atypia, hyperplasia, dysplasia and early cancer may be present simultaneously in the same bladder. If detected early, bladder cancer can be treated successfully.

Treatment

Some cancers may be prevented by the removal of the relevant carcinogen from the environment. There is considerable evidence about the effect of carcinogens as seen by the dramatic rise of deaths from lung cancer which relates to the smoking habits of man. Great efforts are being made to reduce smoking by advertising the health risks. Similarly, preventive measures are being taken where carcinogens are involved in work situations. Protective clothing and masks are compulsory for workers in asbestos industries, and similar rules apply in furniture-making factories where wood dust has been found to be a cause of cancers of the nasal sinuses. These known industrial carcinogens are now listed and Acts of Parliament embody preventive measures as well as procedures for compensation should it be proved that a cancer has been caused through working with a specific substance.

It is of note that if two carcinogens are present in the environment their effect may be multiplicative. Thus if smoking increases the lung cancer risk by 10 times and asbestos by five times, the two together increase it by 50 times (Selikoff et al, 1968).

The main forms of treatment are surgical excision, radiotherapy and chemotherapy. Successful treatment depends on early diagnosis so that the malignant tumour may be removed before it spreads. This is not easy as many tumours do not have significant effects on health until they have spread. Early diagnosis is itself dependent on tests such as regular chest radiographs (in situations where there is a known hazard) or through early diagnostic units to which 'well persons' may be referred for preventive check-ups and instruction in, for example, breast self-examination.

Physiotherapy This is largely related to patients undergoing surgery and the treatment will depend on the particular surgical procedure. The physiotherapist may also be concerned with helping a patient who is terminally ill with cancer (see p. 526). This may involve help and advice on maintaining independence for as long as possible – provision of walking aids or helping to remove secretions from the chest to improve respiration.

REFERENCES

Coleman, D. V. and Evans, D. M. D. (1988a). *Biopsy Pathology and Cytology of the Uterine Cervix*, pp. 197–239. Chapman and Hall, London.

Coleman, D. V. and Evans, D. M. D. (1988b). *ibid*, p. 240.

Coleman, D. V. and Evans, D. M. D. (1988c). *ibid*, pp. 29–33.

Deitrick, J. E., Whedon, G. D. and Shore, E. (1948). Effects of immobilization upon various metabolic and physiologic functions of normal men. *American Journal of Medicine*, **4**, 3–36.

Dixon, K. C. (1967). Events in dying cells. *Proceedings of the Royal Society of Medicine*, **60**, 271–5.

Doll, R. (1972). Cancer in five continents. *Proceedings of the Royal Society of Medicine*, **65**, 49–55.

Dubowitz, V. (1978). *Muscle Disorders in Childhood*, pp. 70–107; 223–31. W. B. Saunders, London.

Fidler, H. K., Boyes, D. A. and Worth, A. J. (1968). Cervical cancer detection in British Columbia. *Journal Obstetrics and Gynaecology of the British Commonwealth*, **75**, 302–404.

Lancet Annotation (1963). Disuse osteoporosis. *Lancet*, **1**, 150.

Leading Article (1971). Osteoporosis. *British Medical Journal*, **1**, 566–7.

Leading Article (1976). Exposure to asbestos dust. *British Medical Journal*, **1**, 1361–2.

Morehead, R. P. (1965). *Human Pathology*, p. 181. McGraw-Hill, New York.

Mulvihill, J. J. (1985). Clinical ecogenetics: cancer in families. *New England Journal of Medicine*, **312**, 1569–70.

Robbins, S. L. and Kumar, V. (1987). *Basic Pathology*, 4th edition, pp. 235–7. W. B. Saunders, Philadelphia.

Selikoff, I., Hammond, E. C. and Churg, J. (1968). Asbestos exposure, smoking and neoplasia. *Journal of the American Medical Association*, **204**, 106–12.

Smith, R. (1984). Osteogenesis imperfecta. *British Medical Journal*, **289**, 394–6.

Smith, R. A. (1971). Cure of lung cancer from incomplete surgical resection. *British Medical Journal*, **2**, 563–5.

Smithers, D. W. (1969). Maturation in human tumours. *Lancet*, **2**, 949–52.

Thomson, A. D. and Cotton, R. E. (1983a). *Lecture Notes on Pathology*, p. 130, 3rd edition. Blackwell Scientific Publications Limited, Oxford.

Thomson, A. D. and Cotton, R. E. (1983b). *ibid*, p. 135.

Trump, B. F., Goldblatt, P. J. and Stowell, R. E. (1965). Studies on necrosis of mouse liver *in vitro*; ultrastructural alterations in the mitochondria of hepatic parenchymal cells. *Laboratory Investigations*, **14**, 343–71.

Walter, J. B. and Israel, M. S. (1987a). *General Pathology*, 6th edition, p. 67. Churchill Livingstone, Edinburgh.

Walter, J. B. and Israel, M. S. (1987b). *ibid*, pp. 325–9.

Walter, J. B. and Israel, M. S. (1987c), *ibid*, p. 367.

Walter, J. B. and Israel, M. S. (1987d). *ibid*, p. 339.

BIBLIOGRAPHY

Anderson, J. R. (ed.) (1985). *Muir's Textbook of Pathology*, 12th edition. Edward Arnold Limited, London.

Robbins, S. L. and Kumar, V. (1987). *Basic Pathology*, 4th edition. Saunders, Philadelphia.

Spector, W. G. (1980). *An Introduction to General Pathology*, 2nd edition. Churchill Livingstone, Edinburgh.

Thomson, A. D. and Cotton, R. E. (1983). *Lecture Notes on Pathology*, 3rd edition. Blackwell Scientific Publications Limited, Oxford.

Tiffany, Robert (ed.) (1988). *Oncology for Nurses and Health Care Professionals*, 2nd edition, vol. 1 *Pathology, Diagnosis and Treatment*. George Allen and Unwin, London.

Walter, J. B. and Israel, M. S. (1987). *General Pathology*, 6th edition. Churchill Livingstone, Edinburgh.

Chapter 6

Drugs

by D. B. McHUTCHISON B Pharm, M R Pharm S

A drug may be broadly defined as a substance which modifies the activity of living tissues. The study of this activity in relation to the diagnosis, treatment or prevention of disease is termed *pharmacology*, while the application of the principles of pharmacology in clinical practice is known as *therapeutics*. A very large number of substances known to exert a pharmacological action have been studied, but only a small number of these are suitable for therapeutic use.

ADMINISTRATION AND ABSORPTION

In order to exert its therapeutic action a drug must first be absorbed by the body and transported to the tissues where its activity is required. Administration of drugs may be by one or more of the following routes.

Gastro-intestinal tract

The majority of drugs are absorbed into the bloodstream from the gastro-intestinal tract, and may be given as a solution, suspension or solid dose form, i.e. tablet or capsule. The rate at which a drug is absorbed after oral administration is dependent on a complex set of factors such as the chemical nature of the drug, the rate at which it dissolves, the pharmaceutical form used, and the contents of the gut at the time the dose is given. When more than one drug is given at the same time their rates of absorption may be further modified. Some preparations are designed specifically to delay absorption, to prevent gastric disturbance, or to prevent chemical change during passage through the gut. Enteric-coated tablets pass through the stomach unchanged and release their active ingredients in the small intestine. Slow-acting, or sustained-release, tablets or capsules prolong absorption by delaying the release of the drug from an insoluble matrix during passage through the gut. This allows a single dose to exert action for much longer, perhaps all day or all night.

A small number of drugs are absorbed from the buccal cavity, and in these cases absorption is often very rapid. This effect is exploited by the use of sub-lingual tablets which dissolve quickly under the tongue, for example glyceryl trinitrate used for the rapid relief of anginal pain.

Some drugs are also absorbed from the rectum when given as suppositories or as a retention enema. Aspirin, indomethacin and aminophylline are examples of drugs which may be given success-fully by this route. (Suppositories are also widely used where purely local action on the rectum is required.)

The lungs

Administration via the lungs is a long-established practice. Tradi-tionally inhalations were used, but modern pharmaceutical tech-niques have refined this and aerosol therapy is now common, particularly in the treatment of asthma. Solutions may be given by nebulizer, or dry powders by metred pressurized aerosols which can deliver exact doses of highly active drugs such as salbutamol.

By injection

The use of drugs by injection is widespread in hospital practice and, though generally a more expensive therapy, has many advantages over the oral route. The possibility of erratic absorption or chemical breakdown in the gut is avoided; this is particularly important in the use of antibiotics to treat severe infections. The intravenous (IV) route ensures total absorption and achieves desired tissue levels rapidly, and can be used even with drugs which would cause necrosis if concentrated in muscle tissue, e.g. some cytotoxic agents. Intra-muscular (IM) and subcutaneous (SC) routes also ensure total absorption, but distribution to the tissues is slower than the IV route. Depot injections can be given by the IM route, with the drug in an oily solution or as a suspension, allowing slow absorption from the injection site over a period of days or even weeks. Special techniques of injection such as intrathecal (IT) into the cerebro-spinal fluid, and intra-articular (IA) into joints allow adequate doses to be delivered directly to the tissues where the action is required.

Topically

In a suitable formulation many drugs will be absorbed through the skin and the mucous membranes. This method of administration is normally used where drug action is desired at the site of application, for example creams and ointments to treat skin conditions, or treatment of the eye with drops or ointment.

DISTRIBUTION

As a general principle, drugs, once they are absorbed into the bloodstream, will be distributed to all tissues in the body; the object of therapeutics is to give a dose such that a sufficient concentration of the drug is present in the particular tissue where action is required. Several factors control the rate at which this distribution takes place, and thus the time needed to achieve adequate tissue levels. Blood flow varies in different parts of the body, and in disease may change significantly in specific tissues, for example the liver or the kidneys. When in the bloodstream a drug may exist freely in solution or be chemically bound to plasma proteins, and the stronger the protein binding the slower the rate of distribution. Different drugs may bind to different proteins, but complications can occur when two drugs given together bind to the same protein. One will usually be bound preferentially and thus the other will be distributed more rapidly, achieve higher than expected tissue levels and hence exert a greater therapeutic effect than anticipated. For example, the anticoagulant warfarin is more active in the presence of aspirin because the latter displaces the warfarin from its binding sites. Transfer through membranes occurs in the capillaries, when the drug passes into the interstitial fluid, and at the cell wall where the drug diffuses from the interstitial fluid into the cell itself. The rate at which this transfer takes place may depend on the chemical nature of the drug, physical properties such as the size of the molecule (its molecular weight) and its degree of protein binding.

METABOLISM AND EXCRETION

During the course of their distribution many drugs will undergo biochemical changes, i.e. will be metabolized. These changes may reduce or even eliminate the pharmacological activity of the drug by producing inactive metabolites, or may convert the administered drug into pharmacologically active compounds which exert the actual therapeutic effect. A few of these changes may occur in the gut during absorption and in some cases in particular organs such as the kidney, but the vast majority of metabolic changes take place in the liver. Breakdown of the drug may be by reduction, oxidation or hydrolysis in the first phase of metabolism. In the second phase the drug, or the phase one breakdown product, may combine (be conjugated) with other molecules such as glucuronic acid or amino acids such as glycine.

Reference will often be seen to *hepatic first-pass metabolism*, a factor of importance in deciding the best route of administration. When absorbed from the gut drugs enter the hepatic portal system and thus all the dose goes through the liver. If the drug is rapidly metabolized by the liver the amount reaching the systemic circulation may be significantly reduced. This is known as the first-pass effect. In such cases it is often desirable to give the drug by injection, which allows passage around the systemic circulation before entering the liver.

When two or more drugs are given at the same time interactions may result from their effect on liver enzymes. Some drugs are known to enhance the activity of liver enzymes, either by stimulating their production or delaying their breakdown. If the affected enzyme is involved in the metabolism of a second drug being used at the same time the rate of metabolism of the latter drug may be increased and its therapeutic effect therefore reduced. For example, barbiturates inhibit the action of the anticoagulant warfarin and phenytoin reduces the efficacy of oral contraceptives by this mechanism.

After metabolism, and having exerted their pharmacological action, drugs and their metabolites will be eliminated from the body. The most important route of excretion is via the kidney. As with their absorption, the mechanism and the rate at which drugs and their metabolites are excreted by the kidneys are dependent on their chemical composition, molecular weight, and degree of protein binding. Some drugs are excreted by this pathway unchanged and this may be of considerable importance if the desired site of action is in fact the kidney itself, for example, antibiotics used to treat urinary tract infections. Some drugs are excreted by the liver, usually as metabolites which are passed into the bile and thus to the small intestine. Excretion is then via the faeces, though in some cases the drug or metabolites may be re-absorbed and return to the liver again. This may have the effect of prolonging the activity of the drug since some will continue to pass around the entero-hepatic circulation until all has been metabolized. Examples of drugs which undergo entero-hepatic re-cycling are phenytoin and rifampicin.

In a few cases drugs may be excreted by other routes such as in the sweat, via the lungs if the drug is a gas, e.g. anaesthetics, or in breast milk. The latter is particularly important in breast-feeding mothers when the baby could receive doses of unwanted drugs.

PHARMACOKINETICS

This is the mathematical treatment of the progress of a drug along its pathway through the body. It is concerned with measuring such factors as the rate of absorption and distribution; peak plasma levels and time of onset of action; duration of action; path and rate of metabolism and excretion; the half-life (time taken for the measured drug concentration to fall by 50 per cent). These studies are used, in the first instance, with new drugs, to determine the best route of administration, the strength of tablet, injection, etc., and the frequency at which doses are best given. The concepts are very broad and with some drugs individual patient variation is considerable. In such cases the principles can be applied to the individual patient, by use of the procedure known as therapeutic drug monitoring (TDM). Blood samples are taken to measure the actual concentration of active drug at a known time after administration. The results can then be analysed, usually by computer program, to decide the dose and dose-interval which will give the optimum therapeutic effect, while avoiding side-effects. TDM services will be found increasingly in major hospitals, and in some areas may be available to general practitioners as well.

MECHANISM OF ACTION AND DRUG RECEPTORS

In the body the functions of the tissues and organs are controlled by a variety of substances produced in the body itself and usually known as messengers or endogenous regulators. Some examples are acetylcholine, histamine, insulin and the catecholamines, e.g. noradrenaline. Many drugs act in a similar way to these endogenous substances. The basic concept is that once the drug or messenger has reached its site of action it will react in some way with a group of molecules forming a receptor site in the tissue. Drugs or messengers which by their action at the receptor sites stimulate the activity of the tissues are referred to as agonists, while those which inhibit activity are known as antagonists or blockers.

Many types of receptor are now recognized and an important consideration is that the same type of receptor may influence different tissues in different ways; receptors are also now divided into sub-types. Histamine receptors are divided into types H_1 and H_2. At

H_1 receptors histamine causes constriction of smooth muscle, e.g. in the bronchioles, tissue oedema, inflammation, and pain. These effects are antagonized by H_1 receptor blocker drugs, usually known as antihistamines. At H_2 receptors histamine causes an increase in gastric acid secretion, and this effect is not controlled at all by antihistamines, but is antagonized by the H_2-receptor antagonists such as cimetidine or ranitidine.

Adrenergic receptors (those at which the catecholamines act) are divided into α and β sub-types. α-receptor stimulation causes, for example, inhibition of intestinal or bladder movements, vaso-constriction of the arterioles and dilation of the pupils. Stimulation of β_1 receptors increases the rate and force of heart movements, while β_2-receptor stimulation leads to decreased bronchial secretions, relaxation of bronchial muscle and dilation of the cor-onary and peripheral arterioles.

The search for new pharmacologically active compounds seeks to produce substances in which parts of the molecule are structurally similar to parts of the molecule of known endogenous regulators. The hope is that such substances will be pharmacologically active in either mimicking or inhibiting the action of the natural regulator. The term *structure activity relationship* is often used in this context.

If a drug acts at receptors that are common to many tissues, or on more than one sub-type of receptor, it may produce undesirable side-effects as well as effects of therapeutic benefit. The ideal there-fore is to use a drug which is selective and will act only at receptors of a specific sub-type or in a specific tissue. Selectivity can sometimes be improved by chemical modification of an existing drug or by pharmaceutical formulation.

While most drugs are thought to act at tissue receptor sites a few are known which act by comparatively simple chemical or physical means. For example, chelating agents used to treat heavy metal poisoning, such as by lead, combine chemically with the poison allowing it to be excreted. Mannitol, a carbohydrate used to reduce intracranial pressure or to promote diuresis, acts physically by changing the osmolarity of body fluids.

ADVERSE REACTIONS AND INTERACTIONS

Any substance used to interfere with a biological process in a desir-able way is also likely to produce unwanted effects as well, usually referred to as side-effects or adverse reactions. In drug treatment it is usually necessary to consider a balance of advantage. In treating life-threatening conditions a quite high incidence of side-effects may be accepted. These effects may be many and varied, some minor and a nuisance, such as skin rash or gastric disturbance, others more serious and even potentially fatal, such as liver damage or suppression of the bone marrow. New drugs in particular are closely monitored to attempt to detect all adverse effects, though where the incidence is low it may be many years before the effect is recognized. For example, the β blocker, practolol, was found, after many years' successful use in cardiovascular treatment, to cause eye and intestinal damage in a very small number of patients.

DRUG GROUPS

Drugs are usually considered in groups relating to their effect on a particular organ or body system. It is not possible here to more than outline some groups which will be of particular relevance to the physiotherapist's practice.

DRUGS ACTING ON THE RESPIRATORY SYSTEM

Mucolytics

These are agents which reduce the viscosity of sputum and therefore make expectoration easier. Traditionally, inhalations were used, such as menthol and eucalyptus or compound benzoin tincture in hot water. The volatile ingredients help to clear the nasal passages, while the inhaled steam reduces the viscosity of the sputum, and expectoration can be facilitated by postural drainage. Drugs, such as tyloxapol, were developed in an attempt to achieve a similar effect when administered by nebulizer, and are thought to act by breaking down sputum proteins.

Acetylcysteine, carbocisteine, methylcysteine, and bromhexine are thought to act systemically by altering the composition and increasing the flow of bronchial secretions. They may be given orally, as tablets, syrups or granules and, in addition, bromhexine may also be given by IM or IV injection.

Antitussives

Many cough medicines are prescribed and sold, some of which may increase bronchial secretions, but there is no good evidence that any will stimulate the cough centre to increase expectoration. Cough suppressants are drugs used for the opposite effect, that is to depress the cough centre in the brain and relieve dry unproductive coughs which may be painful and distressing. Examples are codeine, diamorphine and pholcodine, all administered as linctus. Such preparations are not recommended in patients where expectoration is necessary, as retention of sputum and inhibition of ventilation may result.

Respiratory stimulants

Where inhibition of respiration occurs in patients with chronic obstructive airway disease, respiratory stimulants may be used as an adjunct to physiotherapy. Such drugs are usually given by IV injection or infusion and their use requires careful medical supervision. They are often used for short-term treatment in association with oxygen therapy. Examples are nikethamide and doxapram, both of which act on the respiratory centre in the brain to increase the rate and depth of respiration.

Drugs in asthma

In an asthma attack the bronchi contain thickened mucus, their walls are oedematous and the bronchial muscle is constricted. Asthma may be inherent or intrinsic and treatable with corticosteroids; or triggered by some outside stimulus (antigen) and known as extrinsic asthma, and treatable, for example, with β_2 stimulants.

Corticosteroids The anti-inflammatory glucocorticosteroids are used in asthma for their action of reduction of capillary permeability, bronchial congestion and oedema. In severe cases they may be given by injection, for example as hydrocortisone, or as short courses of oral treatment, for example as prednisone tablets. When given orally steroids may exert other effects, some undesirable; as an alternative, inhalation therapy has been developed. Beclomethasone and betamethasone are examples of potent steroids administered either from pressure-metered aerosols or powder inhalers. By this technique a small controlled dose is given, sufficient only to act in the lung and avoid undesirable systemic effects. In many cases sufficient control can be achieved to avoid the use of oral steroids entirely.

Bronchodilators The bronchodilator drugs play the major role in the treatment of asthma, bronchitis and other diseases causing bronchospasm. Drugs once widely used, and still in limited use today, such as adrenaline, isoprenaline or ephedrine are non-specific, having both α- and β-agonist properties. Thus while they do produce bronchodilation they also give rise to unwanted side-effects by their action on the heart, gastro-intestinal tract and bladder. The drugs now most widely used are the more selective β_2 stimulants: fenoterol, pirbuterol, reproterol, rimiterol, salbutamol and terbutaline. These are available in a variety of formulations for administration orally as tablets or syrup, by injection, by metered aerosol, powder inhaler or by nebulizer.

Salbutamol is probably the most widely used. Given by aerosol or powder inhaler it produces prompt bronchodilation, relieves bronchospasm and reduces bronchial secretions. It may also be given orally or by injection, but the inhaled route is considered to have the advantage of rarely producing side-effects, and the bronchodilation is more prolonged. The side-effects of oral or injected doses result from the limited β_1-agonist activity that salbutamol also exhibits. Tachycardia and tremor are the most noted, though night cramps and increased insulin and free fatty acid levels have been observed also. The other drugs listed above have broadly similar effects to salbutamol, though with some variation in their rates of absorption and duration of action. Though some would hold that to have several different drugs of similar type available is unnecessary it can often help the prescribing physician, as if one becomes ineffective another in the group may enable the patient's treatment to continue.

Patients with chronic bronchitis may not respond to the β_2 stimulants, and here the alternative anticholinergic bronchodilator, ipratropium, may be effective, administered by aerosol or nebulizer solution.

An alternative treatment in some forms of asthma is a prophylactic one using sodium cromoglycate or nedocromil sodium. These act by preventing the release of histamine, and other substances which cause bronchospasm, from sensitized cell membranes. Treatment, which is by aerosol, needs to be regular since the drug is of no value in treating an attack. Ketotifen has similar effects and is active orally, given as tablets or capsules.

Respirator solutions: In hospital, and occasionally in the home, respirator solutions of salbutamol or terbutaline are often used in the treatment of severe acute asthma (status asthmaticus), severe bronchospasm resulting from acute episodes of bronchial asthma and bronchitis, or in bronchial infections. The undiluted solutions, 2ml of salbutamol 5mg/ml, or 1ml of terbutaline 10mg/ml, may be given up to four times daily in oxygen-enriched air over a period of about three minutes. A suitable intermittent positive pressure ventilator such as the Bird respirator is used. Alternatively these solutions may be administered continuously with equipment such as the De Vilbiss or Wright's nebulizer and the Ventimask. In these cases the solutions are diluted with sterile water or saline to a concentration of 100 micrograms per ml and are given at the rate of 1 to 2mg per hour. To avoid contamination and infection such solutions in nebulizers should be replaced with fresh material at least every 24 hours. It is important to remember that these drugs are Prescription Only Medicines (see p.80) and may therefore *only* be administered by the physiotherapist *when prescribed by a physician*. On completion of the treatment the details, such as dose and time given, must be recorded by the physiotherapist in the appropriate section of the patient's treatment card or case notes.

DRUGS IN RHEUMATIC DISEASE

Patients suffering from the rheumatic diseases will form a significant portion of the physiotherapist's workload. Drugs are used extensively, but none have to date effected a cure. They may be considered in two groups; those affecting the course of the disease, and those relieving the symptoms of pain and inflammation.

The actions of those drugs affecting the course of the rheumatic diseases are not well understood. Those used are penicillamine, auranofin, sodium aurothiomalate, chloroquine, hydroxychloroquine and the immunosuppressant azathioprine. They are effective only when the disease is active and their benefits may take many months to appear. Side-effects are common and may be severe, requiring withdrawal of the treatment. All are given orally, as tablets, except sodium aurothiomalate which can only be given by IM injection. Close medical supervision, blood and urine tests are all necessary when therapy is undertaken with any of these agents.

Non-steroidal anti-inflammatory agents are widely used to relieve the symptoms of pain and inflammation, but these drugs have no effect on the course of the disease.

The relief of pain is probably the most widely used therapy. In theory it can be achieved in one of several ways, for example by suppressing the perception of pain in the brain or by overcoming the stimulus at the actual site of pain. An important modifying factor is the significant emotional content and individual variation in the perception of pain. Possibly for this latter reason the choice of analgesic/anti-inflammatory drug for a particular patient can often be a matter of trial and error. It is therefore fortunate that a wide range of such drugs are at the physician's disposal. Most of these drugs are administered by mouth as tablets, capsules or syrup and a few are also available as suppositories which can be a useful adjuvant to treatment in that they help to reduce morning stiffness by their long action.

Non-steroidal anti-inflammatory agents are all considered to exert their action at the site of pain production. To a greater or lesser degree they all inhibit the production in the tissues of prostaglandins, the endogenous regulators responsible for the production of fever, pain and oedema in inflammatory disease. In addition to relieving pain and inflammation some of these drugs, notably aspirin and its derivatives, also exert a significant antipyretic action. This is also thought to result from suppression of prostaglandin release, in this case in the temperature regulating centre in the brain. The latest edition of the *British National Formulary (BNF)* should be consulted for details of the dosage of those drugs currently in use in the United Kingdom.

Corticosteroids have a significant part to play in the treatment of rheumatic disease. They have a powerful anti-inflammatory action, but are only used systemically where the non-steroidal agents have been unsuccessful. Prednisolone in tablet form is usually used, at the lowest dose which will control the symptoms. If treatment is prolonged, tolerance may lead to the need to increase the dose with the consequent danger of side-effects. Steroids exert their anti-inflammatory action locally if given by intra-articular injection, when relief of pain and improved joint movement can be quite spectacular. They act by reducing fluid production and cellular exudates in the joint. To maintain the effect repeated injections are necessary every few weeks, but this is approached with caution as joint damage can ultimately result. Aseptic technique is essential with intra-articular injections, since infection introduced into a joint will increase the inflammatory process and may prove very difficult to treat. Table I lists those steroids available as intra-articular injections in the United Kingdom.

TABLE I   CORTICOSTEROIDS FOR INTRA-ARTICULAR INJECTION

Approved name	Dose range	Proprietary name
dexamethasone sodium phosphate	0.8 to 4mg	Decadron
hydrocortisone acetate	5 to 50mg	Hydrocortistab
methylprednisolone acetate	4 to 80mg	Depo Medrone
prednisolone acetate	5 to 25mg	Deltastab
triamcinolone acetonide	2.5 to 40mg	Kenalog
triamcinolone hexacetonide	2 to 30mg	Lederspan

NOTE: The dose required depends primarily on the size of the joint involved

Although not often used in rheumatic disease the rubifacients or counter-irritants are popular for symptomatic relief of musculo-skeletal pain, for example in sports injuries. They act by producing irritation of the skin itself and this has the effect of relieving pain deeper in the tissues. Poultices such as kaolin, and liniments or ointments containing methyl salicylate are widely used.

DRUGS IN EPILEPSY AND RAISED INTRACRANIAL PRESSURE

The drug treatment of epilepsy is a good example of an area where pharmacokinetic principles may be applied to determine optimum treatment schedules for individual patients. Measurements of plasma drug concentrations are used to enable the physician to adjust both dose and frequency to each patient's needs. A drug with a long half-life may only need to be given once a day, while dosage two or three times a day may be needed with shorter half-life products, or in cases where a high total daily dose is needed which would produce side-effects if given more frequently.

Phenytoin is still widely used, and to a lesser extent pheno-barbitone, though newer products are now more favoured by clinicians, because of their more predictable response. Sodium val-proate is the drug of choice in absence and myoclonic seizures, and carbamazepine in tonic-clonic and partial seizures. Current thinking is to control the condition with a single drug whenever possible, rather than with the multiple regimes which have been favoured in the past.

Raised intracranial pressure may result from trauma, stroke, or brain tumour, and may be treated with osmotic diuretics such as mannitol or urea, or by use of glucocorticoids such as dexa-methasone. The mode of action of the latter is unclear, but it may act by stabilizing the vascular system. In acute cases treatment is started by a large IV dose, followed by a reducing IV regime over about a week. Subsequently control may be maintained orally by the use of tablets.

CANCER CHEMOTHERAPY

The drug treatment of cancers involves the use of substances which will interfere with cell multiplication or will stop the synthesis of DNA or RNA. Unfortunately these agents, usually known as cyto-toxic drugs, cannot be confined in their actions to the malignant tissues and will therefore adversely affect the normal cells of the body as well. This is particularly a problem in tissues where the cells are normally dividing rapidly, such as the ovaries, testes, gut or bone marrow.

Different groups of these drugs act at different points in the dividing cell cycle and it is common therapeutic practice to use several agents in a regime designed to attack the malignant cells at several points at the same time. The cytotoxic agents currently in use may be divided into the following groups.

Antimetabolites: These act by interfering with the synthesis of essential cell constituents such as folic acid and pyrimidine. Examples of such drugs include methotrexate and cytarabine.

Alkylating agents: These interfere with the synthesis of DNA and include such drugs as busulphan, cyclophosphamide and melphalan.

Cytotoxic antibiotics: Antibiotics are substances produced by micro-organisms which interfere in some way with the growth of other cells. The majority in therapeutic use act against bacterial cells and are therefore used to treat infections. A few however act against human tissue cells by inhibiting formation of nucleic acids and proteins, for example actinomycin, bleomycin and doxorubicin.

Vinca alkaloids: These alkaloids are extracted from the periwinkle plant and are thought to act by interfering with the synthesis of micro-tubular protein, thus preventing cell division. Three drugs have been isolated, vincristine, vinblastine and vindesine. They are widely used and exhibit a particular side-effect which is of significance to the physiotherapist, in that they give rise to peripheral neuropathy. This probably arises from their mode of action in that they also interfere with micro-tubular protein in nerve tissue. The incidence of neuropathy is usually dose-related, and patients treated for lymphoma are generally much more susceptible than others. The symptoms may present in various forms including autonomic, e.g. constipation; motor, e.g. muscle weakness and loss of tendon reflexes; or sensory, e.g. jaw pain and paraesthesia. The symptoms normally disappear on withdrawal of the drug, and of the three agents vincristine is the most often implicated.

In addition to the main groups there are several other agents with varying uses and modes of action. A few examples are procarbazine used in Hodgkin's disease; tamoxifen, an anti-oestrogen used in breast cancer; and cis-platin used in testicular and ovarian cancers. The latter drug is notable as the first platinum salt used therapeutically, and like the vinca alkaloids may also give rise to peripheral neuropathy.

PAIN RELIEF

In patients under terminal care (Chapter 28) pain control is often a major factor in maintaining their remaining quality of life, and, similarly, in acute postoperative pain adequate relief is of significant psychological importance in the patient's recovery. In the first mentioned, weaker analgesics may be used initially but it is usually necessary to progress to the stronger drugs of the opioid group as tolerance develops. There should never be any hesitation by the physician in prescribing the strongest drug needed in each case. Pain can be of several different types, and the opioids, morphine and diamorphine, are particularly useful in visceral pain, soft tissue pain, and bone pain. Both drugs can be administered by mouth or by injection, and morphine by suppository. Diamorphine is generally preferred for injection as its higher solubility enables larger doses to be given in smaller volumes. Morphine is preferred orally, given as a simple solution or as sustained-release tablets.

In any form of pain control, and particularly in terminal care, analgesics should always be given regularly, never 'when necessary'. The object of good therapy is to determine the dose which given regularly, usually 4-hourly for injections and simple solutions, or 12-hourly for sustained-release tablets, will produce continuous pain relief, while avoiding side-effects such as respiratory depression. The therapist should always bear in mind that pain is totally subjective. Only the patient can judge the control achieved, and should never be asked to 'try to wait a little longer'. If the patient complains of inadequate control the physician should always be informed immediately so that the necessary dosage adjustment can be made.

PHOTOSENSITIZERS

Some drugs have the effect of increasing the sensitivity of the skin to ultraviolet light. This reaction may be an unwanted side-effect but in some cases can be of therapeutic use.

Methoxypsoralen is an example of a drug used for its photosensitizer effect. It may be given orally as tablets or capsules or applied topically as a lotion, and subsequent exposure to ultraviolet light or sunlight results in increased melanin formation in the skin. It has therefore been used to treat idiopathic vitiligo. In addition exposure to long wavelength ultraviolet light following topical or oral methoxypsoralen results in an inflammatory phototoxic reaction in the skin and this effect is utilized in the treatment of resistant psoriasis.

LEGAL ASPECTS

In the United Kingdom all drugs for human use are controlled at all stages of their development, import, manufacture or use by the Medicines Act 1968. Drugs may only be licensed for use after they have satisfied stringent safety requirements; they must be manufactured in approved premises by approved procedures; and they may only be promoted for treatment of conditions for which successful clinical trials have been completed.

For supply to the patient the Act divides medicines into three categories:

General Sales List: A very small group of materials which may be sold by the retailer, e.g. small packs of analgesics such as aspirin or paracetamol.

Pharmacy Only Medicines: These are drugs which may be sold without prescription, but only from a registered pharmacy.

Prescription Only Medicines: These are drugs which may be sold or supplied only against a prescription from a medical or dental practitioner. The majority of drugs fall into this category. In hospital practice this differentiation does not normally apply, as all drugs are administered only in accordance with a prescription.

In addition more stringent controls are applied to the small group of drugs which are liable to cause addiction, for example the amphetamines and narcotic analgesics such as morphine and diamorphine (heroin). These controls are contained in the Misuse of Drugs Act 1972.

FURTHER INFORMATION

Succinct information on the majority of drugs in current use in the United Kingdom will be found in the *British National Formulary* (*BNF*) which is now published every six months.

The pharmacies in most large hospitals have a drug information section capable of answering the majority of queries for information on drugs which may arise in day to day practice. Links are also established with regional and national centres where more detailed information is needed.

BIBLIOGRAPHY

Davies, D. M. (ed.) (1985). *Textbook of Adverse Drug Reactions*, 3rd edition. Oxford University Press, Oxford.

Gillies, H. C., Rogers, H. J., Spector, R. G. and Trouncer, J. R. (1986). *A Textbook of Clinical Pharmacology*, 2nd edition. Hodder and Stoughton, London.

Gilman, A. G., Goodman, L. S., Rall, T. W. and Murad, F. (eds) (1985). *The Pharmacological Basis of Therapeutics*, 7th edition. Macmillan Publishing Company, New York.

Hopkins, S. J. (1989). *Drugs and Pharmacology for Nurses*, 10th edition. Churchill Livingstone, Edinburgh.

Hopkins, S. J. (1988). *Principal Drugs: An Alphabetical Guide to Modern Therapeutic Agents*, 9th edition. Faber and Faber, London.

Martindale: The Extra Pharmacopoeia, 29th edition (1989). The Pharmaceutical Press, London.

British National Formulary is published six-monthly by the British Medical Association and the Pharmaceutical Society of Great Britain. It is available through book shops. All pharmacy departments receive a supply to be distributed free to specific personnel in the hospital.

MIMS (Monthly Index of Medical Specialties). Only lists proprietary products, and is distributed free to GPs, pharmacy departments and selected medical personnel. It may be supplied on subscription to others who write to the publishers: Haymarket Publishing, 38/42 Hampton Road, Teddington TWII OJE.

ABPI Data Sheet Compendium is published annually by the Association of the British Pharmaceutical Industry, and reproduces in full the data sheets of proprietary products currently marketed by the Association's members. It is distributed to all pharmacies and other hospital staff.

Chapter 7

Cardiac Arrest and Resuscitation

by E. WELCHEW MB, ChB, FFARCS

INTRODUCTION

The leading causes of sudden death before old age, in people over the age of 44, are ventricular fibrillation from asymptomatic ischaemic heart disease or non-traumatic accidents such as drowning and poisoning. In people under the age of 38, the commonest causes are traumatic, due to accident or violence. In such instances death may be prevented if airway obstruction can be reversed, apnoea or hypoventilation avoided, blood loss prevented or corrected and the person not allowed to be pulseless or hypoxic for more than two or three minutes. If, however, there is circulatory arrest for more than a few minutes, or if blood loss or severe hypoxia remain uncorrected, irreversible brain damage may result.

Immediate resuscitation is capable of preventing death and brain damage. The techniques required may be used anywhere, with or without equipment, and by anyone, from the lay public to medical specialists, provided they have been appropriately trained.

Resuscitation may be divided into three phases:

1. *Basic Life Support* using little or no equipment.
2. When equipment and drugs become available *Advanced Life Support* may start, in which a spontaneous circulation is restored.
3. *Prolonged Life Support* which is usually conducted in an intensive therapy unit and is directed towards salvaging cerebral function in the comatose patient, maintaining a stable circulation, restoring oxygenation to normal and other aspects of intensive care.

When confronted by an apparently unconscious patient, first establish that they are unconscious by *shaking* him and *shouting* at him. Then *call for help without leaving the patient*. Immediately check that he has a patent airway, and, if not, provide one. If the patient is unconscious but is breathing through a patent airway, then he should be rolled into a stable position on his side with the face

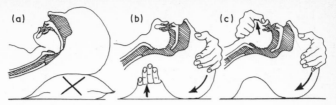

Fig. 7.1 Head positioning to prevent airways obstruction. (a) *Wrong*: on a pillow the head is flexed forward causing pharyngeal obstruction by the tongue. (b) *Correct*: tilting the head backward and lifting the back of the neck upward stretches the anterior neck structure bringing the base of the tongue off the pharyngeal wall. (c) *Correct*: tilting the head backward and pulling the chin upward also prevents the tongue obstructing the pharynx

pointing slightly downwards. The head should be tilted backwards and the jaw supported to keep the airway patent (Fig. 7/1). In this position, it will be less likely that the tongue will fall backwards to obstruct the pharynx, and saliva, blood and vomitus will be able to drain forwards out of the mouth instead of being aspirated into the lungs. If the patient is not breathing then, while keeping the airway patent, he should be put on to his back and artificial ventilation started. Finally, his pulse should be palpated – preferably at the carotid artery in the neck. If no pulse can be felt and the patient is unconscious, it must be assumed that he is in cardiac arrest. While continuing to provide artificial ventilation, external cardiac massage should also be given to maintain the patient's circulation (Fig. 7/2).

Where a patient is already in hospital having his ECG monitored when he has a cardiac arrest, and it is known that he went into witnessed ventricular fibrillation during the last 30 seconds, then the treatment of choice would be to first attempt to defibrillate him using 200 joules (J). If this did not succeed, then one should immediately proceed to Basic Life Support with the maintenance of a patent airway and ventilation as well as keeping the patient's circulation going with external cardiac massage as described below.

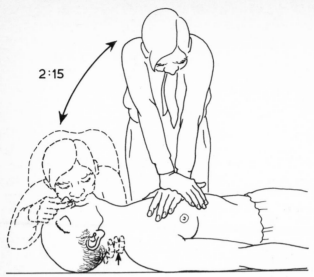

2:15

Fig. 7.2 Artificial ventilation and external cardiac massage with one operator only. 15 sternal compressions are alternated with 2 inflations of the lungs. The chest should be compressed at a rate of about 80 per minute; the return of a spontaneous pulse should be checked every 2 minutes or so

THE ABC OF RESUSCITATION

Basic Life Support

A. *Airway*
1. Ensure that the patient has a patent airway (Fig. 7/1).
2. Remove fluid and debris from the mouth using fingers and suction as necessary.
3. Insert a pharyngeal airway if necessary and available.

B. *Breathing*
1. Maintain a *patent airway.*
2. If the patient is breathing *roll him on to his side* into a stable position with the head tilted back. Maintain a patent airway and *check that breathing does not stop.* Check his pulse.
3. If the patient is not breathing leave him on his back; and
4. *Inflate the patient's lungs* rapidly 3 to 5 times using one of the

following methods:
(a) Use mouth to mouth or mouth to nose ventilation.
(b) Insert a Brook airway, give mouth to airway ventilation.
(c) Ventilate the patient using a bag and mask.

5. *Look for the rise of the patient's chest* with each ventilation. If this is not seen there may be (a) an obstruction in the airway, (b) a poor seal with the patient's airways during inflation, or (c) simply not enough air being blown into the patient.
6. Feel for the carotid pulse.
7. If the pulse is present, but no spontaneous ventilation, then continue 12 lung inflations per minute.

C. Circulation

1. If the pulse is present and there is obvious external haemorrhage, control bleeding by applying pressure to the bleeding point and elevating it if appropriate.
2. If the pulse is absent, and
3. If there is no spontaneous breathing or gasping, then
4. Transfer the patient to the floor, if he is not already on a hard surface, and start external cardiac massage:

Single operator: Alternate 2 quick lung inflations with 15 sternal compressions (Fig. 7/2). Compress the sternum at a rate of 80/min (Fig. 7/3).

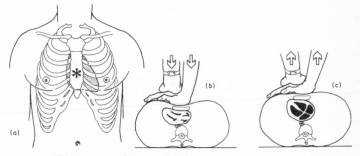

Fig. 7.3 (a) The correct position to place the hands when giving external cardiac massage. (b) Compression of the chest with the heel of the hand on the sternum and the second hand on the first. The heart and major vessels in the chest are compressed between the sternum and the vertebral body. (c) Without losing contact with the patient's chest, the pressure on the chest should be released for 50% of each cycle to allow the heart and blood vessels to fill with blood

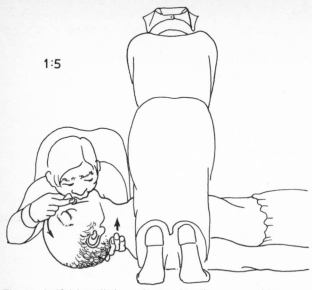

1:5

Fig. 7.4 Artificial ventilation and external cardiac massage with two operators. The first operator compresses the chest at one per second, the second operator inflates the lungs once every fifth compression

Two operators: Alternate 1 lung inflation with 5 sternal compressions (Fig. 7/4). Compress at a rate of 60/min.

The lower third of the sternum should be compressed about 5cm (2in) each time.

Resuscitation should be continued until a spontaneous pulse returns.

Advanced Life Support (The restoration of a spontaneous circulation)

D. Drugs
1. Cardiac compression and ventilation of the lungs should not be interrupted.
2. A central or peripheral intravenous catheter or needle should be inserted if not already in place.
3. The trachea should be intubated (when possible this should be done by someone appropriately skilled in the procedure). Not only will this make maintenance of the patency of the airway

much easier, it will also protect the airway to some extent from contamination by fluid or vomitus, and make artificial ventilation much easier to perform effectively.

4. The following drugs may be used:
   (a) adrenaline 0.5–1mg, repeated every 3–5 minutes as necessary.
   (b) sodium bicarbonate 1mEq/kg body-weight. This is repeated every 10 minutes of arrest time. For adults an 8.4% bicarbonate solution is used (this contains 1mEq/ml); however, this solution is generally too concentrated for small children, for whom a 4.2% solution should be used.
   (c) intravenous fluids as required, e.g. blood or plasma.
5. If intravenous access is not established, drugs may be given down the endotracheal tube directly into the patient's airway, where they work as quickly as when given intravenously. The exception to this is bicarbonate solutions, which must only be given intravenously.
6. As a last resort, drugs such as adrenaline may be given directly into the heart through the chest wall, though this may damage the heart muscle or cause a pneumothorax.

E. ECG (Electrocardiogram)
As soon as possible the ECG of the patient should be monitored:

Ventricular fibrillation should be treated by defibrillation.
Asystole should be treated with adrenaline and then defibrillation.
Ventricular tachycardias may be treated by defibrillation or verapamil.
Bradycardias may be treated with atropine.

F. Fibrillation Treatment (Fig. 7/5)
If coarse ventricular fibrillation or ventricular tachycardia are seen then clear the area and DC defibrillate the patient. Cardiac massage and ventilation should not be interrupted for more than a few seconds.

1. External defibrillation using 100–400J. Repeat shock as necessary.
2. Convert fine fibrillation to coarse fibrillation using adrenaline.
3. Lignocaine 1–2mg/kg intravenously as necessary. If a defibrillator is not available, then lignocaine intravenously or via the endotracheal tube may convert to a sinus rhythm.

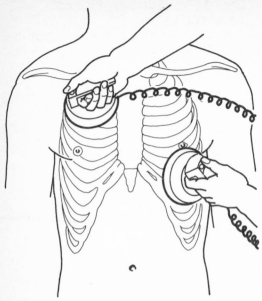

Fig. 7.5 External electrical defibrillation. After connecting the defibrillator to the power supply and switching on, it should be charged to give 200 joules (J), or roughly 3J/kg body weight. The electrodes should be well lubricated with conductive jelly and placed one just below the patient's clavicle and the other over the cardiac apex. Clear the immediate area, ensure that *no one* is touching the patient or the bed, apply firm pressure on to the patient's chest with the paddles and press the defibrillator button. Wait 5 seconds to confirm the resultant ECG and resume external cardiac massage and artificial ventilation as necessary. The latter should not be interrupted for more than 30 seconds after defibrillation

Prolonged Life Support (on intensive therapy unit)

G. Gauging
1. Gauge the likely outcome of resuscitation.
2. Gauge the cause of the cardio-respiratory arrest and treat it.

H. Human Mentation
1. Preserve cerebral function by maintaining normal cerebral blood flow and oxygenation.

   This may necessitate prolonged mechanical ventilation via a tracheal tube, or even the insertion of a tracheostomy tube in order to facilitate this.

   The patient may require oxygen to be added to the respiratory gas mixture in carefully controlled amounts, with repeated estimations of the oxygen content of the patient's blood.

2. Reduce and control intracranial pressure.

This may necessitate the insertion of devices through the patient's skull to measure intracranial pressure continuously so that therapy may be modified accordingly.

Mechanical ventilation is one of the most important ways to reduce and maintain stable the patient's intracranial pressure. If the intracranial pressure is allowed to rise due to swelling or bleeding, this will reduce the blood flow to the brain and, hence, also reduce the oxygen supply to it. The patient may also be given steroids and diuretics to reduce the swelling.

3. Monitor cerebral function.

The electrical activity of the brain may be monitored continuously with a variety of cerebral function monitors (CFMs). More specific information may be obtained with repeated electroencephalograms (EEGs).

Repeated neurological examinations by the doctors and careful observation of the patient by *all* members of staff will provide invaluable information on the degree of neurological damage or recovery exhibited by the patient.

I. Intensive Care

1. Provide intensive therapy.
2. Intensive nursing.
3. Intensive monitoring.

Patients who have undergone cardio-respiratory resuscitation need careful monitoring and care afterwards. They may have a further cardiac or respiratory arrest from the same cause as the original insult or as a result of its consequences. This will necessitate intensive monitoring of the patient's condition at all times and provision of immediate skilled resuscitation within seconds. He may require cardiac, as well as respiratory, support in order to maintain adequate tissue oxygenation. This cardiac support may be pharmacological, using drugs such as dopamine to increase cardiac output, or vasodilators such as sodium nitroprusside to reduce the work done by the heart. On the other hand, the support may be mechanical using the aortic balloon pump.

In a similar way, support for the patient who has had a respiratory arrest may be either pharmacological or mechanical. Pharmacological support may be provided with respiratory stimulants such as doxapram or, in the case of narcotic overdoses, by the narcotic antagonist naloxone. Mechanical support may be provided with ventilators.

One of the commonest problems encountered in these patients is acute renal failure, but with careful management function may be restored to normal. Patients with renal failure will require careful monitoring of their fluid input and urine output, serum and urinary electrolytes and osmolality. Fluid restriction, diuretics and, possibly, peritoneal or haemodialysis will be required.

Figure 7/6 summarizes action and management following cardiac arrest.

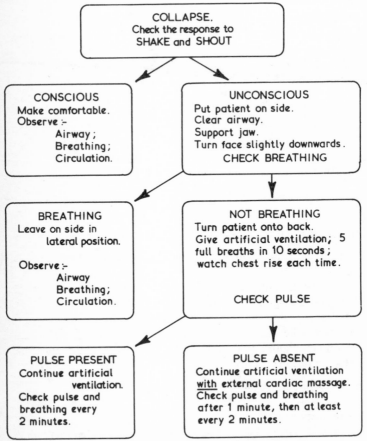

Fig. 7.6 Flow chart summarizing action and management following cardiac arrest

INFANTS AND CHILDREN

In this context, *infants* are aged less than 1 year and *children* aged 1 to 8 years. Over the age of 8, resuscitation may proceed as for a small adult. The most common causes of cardio-respiratory arrest in these groups are:

1. Asphyxia due to foreign bodies, near drowning or upper airway infection.
2. Trauma, burns or poisoning.
3. Sudden infant death syndrome.

In these groups, prevention of accidents will have the greatest effect on the overall morality.

There are certain key differences in the methods used to resuscitate infants and children compared with the scheme proposed so far. The overall 'ABC' plan, however, remains the same.

A. Airway

1. The neck should not be hyperextended, nor the head tilted, as far back as the adult as this will obstruct the upper airway.
2. Infants and small children are obligatory mouth breathers. During resuscitation the mouth should be kept open, using a pharyngeal airway if necessary.

B. Breathing

If the infant is not breathing begin artificial ventilation.

1. The infant's mouth and nose should be encircled with one's own mouth.
2. Small, gentle inflations should be given, puffing from the cheeks to avoid damaging the infant's lungs.
3. Watch the chest rise with each inflation and take the mouth off the face in between inflations to allow passive expiration.
4. An infant should be ventilated at a rate of 30/minute, and children at a rate of 20/minute.

Give 3–5 inflations of the lungs, then feel for a pulse.

C. Circulation

If no pulse can be felt, then give external cardiac compressions.

1. In infants, press the *mid-sternum* with 2 or 3 fingers. It should be depressed about 1.25cm(½in) at a rate of about 100/min.
2. In children, using the heel of one hand, press slightly *below the*

mid-sternum. It should be depressed about 2.5cm(1in) about 80 times per minute.
3. Ventilation should be continued at a rate of 1 inflation every 5 sternal compressions.

D. Drugs and E. ECG
Drugs and fluids used are essentially the same as those for adults except that the doses and volumes are scaled down to roughly 1/60th of the total adult dose per kilogram of the child's body-weight.

F. Fibrillation Treatment
1. Much smaller defibrillator paddles should be used than in adults.
2. In infants, 4.5cm diameter electrodes should be used and in children 8cm diameter ones should be used.
3. DC counter-shock should be applied using 2J/kg body-weight, repeating this, if necessary, with 4J/kg while taking steps to improve oxygenation, and giving adrenaline and bicarbonate as necessary.

Prolonged Life Support is similar to that of adults.

BIBLIOGRAPHY

Brophy, T. (1978). *Resuscitation in the Electrical Industry*. Handbook of the Brisbane Electrical Commission of Queensland, Australia.

Carden, N. I. and Steinhaus, J. E. (1956). Lidocaine resuscitation from ventricular fibrillation. *Circulation Research*, 4, 640.

Jennett, B. and Bond, M. (1975). Assessment of outcome after severe brain damage. A practical scale. *Lancet*, 1, 480.

Kirimli, B., Harris, L. C. and Safar, P. (1966). Drugs used in cardiopulmonary resuscitation. *Acta Anaesthesiologica Scandinavica*, 23, 255.

Redding, J. S., Asuncion, J. S. and Pearson, J. W. (1967). Effective routes of drug administration during cardiac arrest. *Anaesthesia and Analgesia*, 46, 253.

Safar, P. and Bircher, N. G. (1987). *Cardiopulmonary Cerebral Resuscitation*. W. B. Saunders, Philadelphia.

Tacker, W. A. (Jr) and Wey, G. A. (1979). Emergency defibrillation dose: Recommendations and rationale. *Circulation*, 60, 223.

Winchell, S. W. and Safar, P. (1966). Teaching and testing lay and paramedical personnel in cardiopulmonary resuscitation. *Anaesthesia and Analgesia*, 45, 441.

Chapter 8

General Surgery
by P. A. DOWNIE FCSP

Of necessity this chapter can only be superficial in content because the area of medicine concerned is a vast one. Successive chapters will concentrate on specific sub-divisions of surgery; this chapter outlines principles of care which may be offered by the physiotherapist to patients undergoing surgery.

The total care necessary for patients who undergo any form of surgery involves many people – the team. Not everyone will be required for each patient but all are available as and when necessary. The physiotherapist is included in this team and she, like all the team members, should be aware of the skills of the others and how they may be utilized to the best advantage of the patient and his family. She must realize that she herself may only have a minor part to play and in many instances no part at all. Some types of surgery will require that the physiotherapist is a very important team member, e.g. cardiothoracic and orthopaedic surgery, while other types of surgery, e.g. ear, nose and throat will only required limited physiotherapy. However much she is involved or not in the care of the patient the physiotherapist must always be prepared to co-operate with other members – for example she will need to discuss with the speech therapist what particular breathing exercises are most helpful for a patient who undergoes laryngectomy and subsequently requires to be taught oesophageal speech. Equally she will combine with the occupational therapist to ensure that patients can return home and that the necessary equipment and aids are provided.

In hospital the team will include the following:

1. The medical staff, e.g. the anaesthetist, the surgeon and his registrar and houseman, and in cases of malignant disease the radiotherapist and medical oncologist.
2. The nursing staff including nurse specialists such as stoma therapist, mastectomy liaison nurse, incontinence adviser.
3. The occupational therapist, speech therapist, remedial gymnast,

physiotherapist, and radiographer.
4. The social worker; the disablement resettlement officer (DRO).
5. The prosthetist will be a vital member of the team where mutilating surgery has been necessary, e.g. amputation of a limb or extensive head and face surgery.
6. The dietician.
7. Other ancillary staff including porters and cleaners.

There should also be links with the community team which will include:

1. The district nurse (community sister).
2. The health visitor.
3. The community physiotherapist.
3. The social services, who usually have an occupational therapist in their team.

At all times the patient, relatives and general practitioner are to be considered as the most important members of the team; the general practitioner (GP) can often act as the co-ordinator of services and the patient and relatives really determine the extent to which the team is required. The hospital chaplains and parish clergy and ministers should not be overlooked and they should be involved as and when required.

It is not proposed to discuss the individual roles of these team members but it is hoped that each physiotherapist will make it her responsibility to find out what everyone in the team is able to offer and how they can best be used. Participation in ward rounds, in clinics and in case conferences is to be encouraged. Whenever a patient is transferred either to a different hospital or back to the community full details of all treatment as well as an assessment of the patient should be sent to the relevant services.

There has been considerable discussion as to the value of physiotherapy for patients undergoing surgery. Nichols and Howell (1970) undertook controlled trials and the result showed that upper abdominal surgery in particular is likely to inhibit the function of the diaphragm. They concluded that physiotherapy had an accepted part to play in the treatment of established bronchitis by physically aiding the drainage and expulsion of bronchial secretions. They also felt that the problem of postoperative complications was more that of selecting those patients 'at risk', and treating them vigorously *before* surgery, rather than providing unnecessary postoperative treatment in a routine fashion to all surgical patients.

An Editorial (1982) in the *British Medical Journal* discussed postoperative pneumonias and came to the conclusion that prophylactic treatment of any kind was scarcely justifiable for all patients since more than 80 per cent suffer no complications.

Those patients who are referred for pre- and postoperative physiotherapy need to be adequately assessed so that unnecessary treatments are neither carried out nor continued indefinitely. Unless the surgical procedure is an emergency, it is to be hoped that when patients are referred for pre-operative training the physiotherapist will have sufficient time to prepare the patient adequately before the proposed surgery. Patients undergoing extensive abdominal surgery will certainly benefit subjectively and any patient who is known to be either a heavy smoker or who suffers from a chronic chest disorder should receive adequate pre-operative training. In many cases this preparation may be carried out as an outpatient, to save the patient occupying a hospital bed for a week prior to operation.

It is unlikely that patients undergoing minor surgery, endoscopic examination, haemorrhoidectomy, etc., will be ordered physiotherapy *unless* they are known to have a chronic chest condition.

PRINCIPLES OF PHYSIOTHERAPY FOR SURGICAL PATIENTS

The general principles involved are:

1. To prevent chest complications by maintaining lung function and aiding the clearance of secretions.
2. To prevent thrombosis of the legs by encouraging active leg movements, or, if necessary, by performing passive exercises.
3. To maintain muscle power and joint range by encouraging simple bed exercises.
4. To help maintain good posture by ensuring that pillows are arranged in a good supportive position.

The approach of the physiotherapist to the patient must be positive and firm, though sympathetic. Patients are very quick to sense when someone does not really know what she/he is doing.

Coughing

One of the invariable questions will be 'Will I burst my stitches when I cough?' All patients must be reassured about this and shown how they may themselves support their wound when coughing. A sensitive yet firm hand to support the patient's own hands as he holds his wound will give confidence as well as reassurance. The

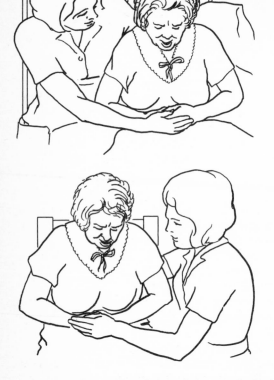

Fig. 8.1 Support from the physiotherapist following abdominal surgery while the patient coughs – in bed

Fig. 8.2 Support from the physiotherapist following abdominal surgery while the patient coughs – sitting in a chair

author has always found that sitting on the bed behind the patient, with the patient able to lean on her shoulder, enables her to use both hands to support the wound (Fig. 8/1). Sometimes patients are told to bend their knees up as they cough, but this is not always very easy. The head should be flexed as the patient coughs. Patients who undergo surgery are seldom in bed for very long and coughing is very much more easily performed when sitting (Fig. 8/2). Indeed, some patients will find sitting over the side of the bed with their feet supported on the locker a helpful position in which to cough. Sometimes it helps to give them a 'cough-belt' (Figs 8/3 and 8/4). These belts are very useful when the patient is a chronic bronchitic with a productive cough as well as being stout. They can be worn loosely and then pulled up tight when they want to cough (Barlow, 1964).

It is helpful to teach 'huffing' as a prelude to actually coughing. A 'huff' may be termed a type of forced expiration and is useful to

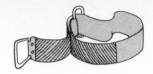

Fig. 8.3 A cough-belt

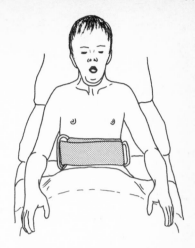

Fig. 8.4 A patient coughing with
the cough-belt in position

loosen secretions and initiate coughing. To 'huff' correctly the
patient should be taught to take a full inspiration using the diaphragm, and then to breathe out sharply contracting the abdominal
muscles as he does so. Following two or three good 'huffs' the
patient should then breathe in deeply and attempt two strong coughs
with the mouth slightly open.

In all teaching of coughing it is important for the patient to
appreciate the difference between an effective cough and a 'genteel'
clearing of the throat.

It is not the act of coughing which causes a wound to burst
occasionally, although it invariably seems to happen as the patient
coughs and he naturally assumes that the coughing was the cause. A
wound breaks down, i.e. the sutures give way, almost always
because there is an infection or an increased serous fluid collection.
Just occasionally the suture material may be faulty. If the patient is
stout or is known to have a chronic chest disorder, the surgeon may
insert some tension sutures as well. These are in addition to the
normal suturing of the wound, and are usually threaded through
thin rubber tubing so that they can remain in situ without cutting
through the skin.

General points to be noted by the physiotherapist

Pre-operative

1. Before the patient is seen by the physiotherapist, the notes should
   be carefully read and any relevant facts noted. For example he
   may be a heavy smoker, he may have a past history of a leg

thrombosis, he may have some disability which could influence his mobility, he may live alone and this could influence how independent he would need to be before being discharged.

2. Introduce yourself to the patient and explain in language which he can understand exactly what you are going to do and what he will have to do and why all this is necessary.

3. Assess the respiratory expansion of the patient and teach diaphragmatic and lateral costal breathing. It is wise to warn the patient that postoperatively it may be necessary to treat him in side lying and/or with the end of the bed tipped, and he should be shown how to reach this position. If this method has to be used, it is sensible to combine the physiotherapy at a time when the nurses are carrying out nursing procedures so that the patient is not moved unnecessarily.

4. As previously mentioned he should be shown how to hold himself when coughing.

5. Simple foot and leg exercises should be taught and the patient told why they are important. It is not necessary to talk about thrombosis; it is quite simple to explain that the legs will ache if they are kept still after the operation, and that if they are regularly moved this will not happen and they will feel less wobbly when he gets up. The patient should also be told not to sit in bed with his legs crossed at the ankles.

Postoperative

1. The notes must be read and the extent of the operation noted, together with the nursing record of the patient's condition since his return from the operating theatre.

2. The position of drainage tubes, intravenous lines, catheter and type of dressing should be noted.

3. If analgesic drugs have been prescribed, the physiotherapist should arrange that they are given *before* the physiotherapy. Occasionally Entonox (50% nitrous oxide and 50% oxygen) may be used – this has the advantage that the patient can control it, and its use can be very effective in pain relief where coughing is essential.

This chapter will now concentrate on some aspects of general surgical procedures and how the physiotherapist may find herself involved. Specialized care following gynaecological, plastic and cranial surgery in addition to amputations will be discussed in separate chapters.

SURGICAL PROCEDURES

The actual surgical procedures for different operations will not be described as these can be studied in surgical textbooks. There are, however, certain aspects about which it is useful for the physiotherapist to have some knowledge.

Incisions

Figure 8/5 shows some of the basic incisions which are used in surgical procedures. The decision to use which depends on the surgeon as well as the prime requirement of giving adequate access to the diseased area.

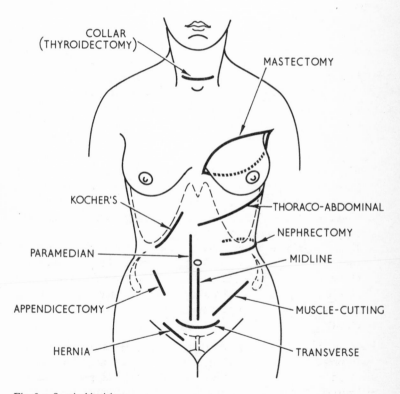

Fig. 8.5 Surgical incisions

Closure of the Incision

The incision may be closed in various ways:

1. Clips are used where an unsightly scar could be distressing to the patient, e.g. following thyroidectomy. They are removed 48–72 hours postoperatively.
2. Sutures can be absorbable, e.g. catgut; non-absorbable, e.g. silk or nylon; invisible intradermal absorbable sutures; or tension sutures (p. 97).
3. The sutures can be tied as single stitches, as a continuous suture or as mattress sutures. The advantage of single sutures is that alternate sutures can be removed and if there is any danger of the incision gaping, stitches in the area at risk can remain longer.
4. The size of the suture material will depend on the site at which it is used. Plastic surgery will require very fine material and more numerous stitches, whereas abdominal muscles will require a strong material. Steel wire is used to suture the sternum after the sternum is split in heart surgery, and in some jaw surgery when the mandible is divided and then resutured. If steel wire is used, it is necessary to drill a hole in the bone ends which are to be wired together, through which the wire is threaded.

Drains

Almost all operation sites will have some form of drainage left in situ, thus reducing the risk of haematoma formation and subsequent breakdown of wounds.

Drainage tubes can take several forms:

1. A Redivac drain, which is a closed system of drainage using a vacuum principle.
2. Corrugated drains which are either rubber or polythene drain into the dressing and can be shortened by pulling out gradually before final removal.
3. Intercostal drains which are inserted into the pleural cavity to drain blood and/or air following surgery involving the opening of the chest. They are attached to an underwater bottle(s) and this is a form of closed drainage. Where an empyema is being drained the wide-bore tubing is sometimes allowed to drain into a dressing. Occasionally, a suction pump may need to be used.
4. Internal drains such as a T-tube which is inserted into the common bile duct following an exploration of the common bile duct.

These are usually attached to a bottle or bag thus allowing the collection of bile or other fluid(s). They are usually in situ for 10–12 days.

A caecostomy is sometimes left following colon surgery – this is a drain inserted into the caecum which allows faecal fluid to escape instead of building up and possibly causing an obstruction. It is usually attached to a bag. It is withdrawn about 10–12 days post-operatively. It must *not* be confused with a colostomy. A caecostomy is essentially a safety valve.

Other tubes

Following surgery, the patient may also have an intravenous infusion – this is to maintain electrolyte balance as well as ensuring both nutrition and hydration. In surgery not affecting the alimentary tract such an infusion will be taken down the morning following surgery.

A nasogastric tube is almost always passed following surgery involving the alimentary tract. This has a dual purpose in that the stomach may be aspirated regularly and, at the appropriate time, feeding may be begun. The physiotherapist should acquaint herself with these essential nursing matters either by discussing them with her nurse colleagues or by reading about them in a nursing textbook.

A catheter may be passed while the patient is in the operating theatre, particularly where renal, bladder, rectal or very extensive abdominal surgery has been carried out. It will drain into a bag which hangs from the bed frame. Sometimes the catheter tube may be strapped lightly to the upper thigh and the physiotherapist must ensure that there is sufficient play on the tubing before she starts on too active leg exercises!

ABDOMINAL SURGERY

Unless the surgery is specifically for gall bladder disease, inguinal or femoral hernia, or nephrectomy, the incision will be a paramedian or mid-line with extension as necessary to allow for adequate exposure.

After gastrectomy, the patient may develop left pulmonary atelectasis and the physiotherapist needs to emphasize localized breathing to both lower lobes but particularly to the left. The diaphragm will have been handled in the operative procedure and the patient will be reluctant to breathe deeply.

Following cholecystectomy in which a Kocher incision is used, the danger of atelectasis is to the right lower lobe, and so the emphasis must be to the right lower lobe. In addition, if the common bile duct has been explored, there will be a T-tube in situ. This can cause pain and discomfort when the patient breathes deeply. Adequate analgesia must be given *before* the main treatment is given by the physiotherapist and the patient *must* be continually reminded by both nurses and the physiotherapist to breathe deeply.

ADRENALECTOMY

A bilateral adrenalectomy is most often performed for patients suffering from disseminated cancer and particularly for those with metastatic bone disease. It is also performed for primary tumours of the adrenal glands. The surgical approach is either through the abdomen when the physiotherapy will be as for any abdominal operation, or through bilateral loin incisions, i.e. through the bed of the 12th rib. If the latter approach is used there is always the danger of 'nicking' the pleura causing a pneumothorax which may require an intercostal drain to be inserted. Breathing exercises are most important when the loin incision is used.

In addition, if the patient has metastatic bone disease care must be exercised if the deposits affect the ribs. Clapping, shakings and vigorous vibrations must NOT be used; gentle vibrations and resisted bilateral costal breathing should be given. Bed exercises are important, but again these must be active and care must be observed if there are deposits in the weight-bearing bones, particularly the femora.

BREAST SURGERY

Perhaps no other surgery causes so many reactions. Mastectomy is performed most often for malignant conditions but it should always be remembered that it is also performed for benign lesions, e.g. multiple fibromata. The type of surgery varies nowadays from the removal of a lump – 'lumpectomy' – to the full radical mastectomy (Halsted's operation). Probably the most commonly performed operation is the simple or extended simple mastectomy (Patey operation). This latter allows for the removal of the axillary nodes with the breast tissue but without the excision of the pectoral muscles.

Whatever surgery is carried out, the physiotherapy allowed will be at the discretion of the surgeon and the physiotherapist MUST ascertain what each particular surgeon will allow by way of arm movement. If she is unfortunate enough to have little or no contact with the surgeon or if he tells her to 'do what you like', she will be well advised to steer a middle course with regard to arm movements. Basic guidelines may be summarized as follows:

1. Following lumpectomy, or wedge resection, no treatment should be required.
2. Following local or simple mastectomy without axillary clearance, no treatment should be necessary, but occasionally physiotherapy may be required to help the patient overcome her fear of movement and thus to encourage a full range of shoulder movements.
3. Following an extended simple mastectomy (Patey), the patient should be encouraged to use her arm for normal daily activities. If stiffness develops, pendular-type shoulder exercises are the most useful. In no circumstances must a shoulder be forced.
4. Following radical mastectomy (Halsted) physiotherapy will be aimed at restoration of shoulder movement, particularly elevation and rotation. The pectoralis major and minor muscles will have been excised and pure abduction of the shoulder should not be allowed until all the drains are out and the skin flaps firmly adhered to the chest wall. If abduction is allowed too soon, fluid will collect between the skin flaps and the chest wall and will require repeated aspirations. Apart from causing unnecessary discomfort for the patient, repeated aspirations carry the risk of infection. Pendular-type shoulder exercises are the most useful, and all exercises should be active and the shoulder must never be forced.

   Some surgeons will bandage the arm to the side for the first week, to prevent abduction and undue movement of the skin flaps. In this case finger, hand and wrist movements should be encouraged, also shoulder shrugging and isometric contractions of the deltoid.

Instruction should also be given in posture correction and how to lift without placing too great strain on the shoulder of the mastectomy side.

In all cases where the physiotherapist is involved in treating mastectomy patients, she must be prepared to enter into the total care of these patients. She should have a knowledge of breast prostheses, of how to adapt brassières and where to purchase suitable swimwear. She should be aware of the emotional problems which can arise following mastectomy (Downie, 1976; Maguire, 1975), and she should always be ready to listen and to help in any way possible. Co-operation with nurses, social workers, and patient volunteers as well as the doctors is very necessary in this field of care.

Lymphoedema

In some cases following mastectomy, and particularly following radical mastectomy or where the patient has undergone radiotherapy, lymphoedema may occur. Physiotherapy may well be ordered and various methods of treatment are available including massage in elevation, faradism under pressure and compression techniques. There is no firm evidence that any of these has a *lasting* effect though there is no doubt that all can help to relieve the condition. As well as such specific treatment, the patient should be taught exercises in elevation and how to posture the arm so that drainage may be helped; particularly useful to the patient is to be shown how to position the arm at night in bed, and while sitting watching the television. Precisely made pressure garments may be prescribed in severe cases.

COLONIC AND RECTAL SURGERY

As with all abdominal surgery physiotherapy will be directed towards the prevention of chest complications but with lower abdominal surgery special attention must also be paid to the prevention of thrombosis. Leg exercises must be taught and supervised thoroughly postoperatively.

Following surgical intervention on the bowel, a paralytic ileus can result leading to great discomfort for the patient with distension of the abdomen. It is important that breathing exercises are encouraged during this period as well as the patient being persuaded to move around in bed as much as possible.

Colostomy

A colostomy is the formation of an artificial anus on the surface of the abdominal wall which can be temporary or permanent. It is sited over the transverse colon or in the lower left quadrant of the abdomen. The lower the siting of the colostomy, the more formed will be the stool. The physiotherapist does not treat the colostomy itself but she should certainly have an understanding of the consequences of such an operation .

When the patient has undergone a combined synchronous abdomino-perineal excision for a carcinoma of the rectum, the colostomy will be permanent.

If a patient is admitted with an acute intestinal obstruction the first stage of relieving the obstruction is often the fashioning of a temporary colostomy. This is followed in about two weeks by an excision and end-to-end anastomosis of the affected colon and about two further weeks later the colostomy will be closed. Sometimes when a resection of the colon is carried out for a carcinoma of the colon, diverticular disease or Crohn's disease, a temporary colostomy may be fashioned so that the anastomosis of the colon can firmly unite before the continuity of the gut is re-established.

When the colostomy is permanent, the aim of rehabilitation must be to ensure that the patient can not only cope with the appliance but does return to a normal life and takes his place fully in society. The Colostomy Welfare Association has done great work in this area; their volunteers (all of whom have had a colostomy) are carefully selected and trained and are willing to visit any patient at the request of the surgeon or general practitioner. Unlike the Ileostomy Association they do *not* hold group meetings of colostomists. In recent years nurses, who have undergone a post graduate course in stoma care, have been appointed in many hospitals. These are clinical nurse specialists more commonly referred to as the stoma therapists. Their role is to advise patients and their families as well as ward and community nurses in the understanding of the colostomy and to ensure that the most suitable appliance is provided for each patient.

The physiotherapist should certainly teach these patients how to lift correctly and should help to ensure that they get dressed and are able to walk about not only in the hospital and its grounds, but out in the street as well, before being discharged home.

Ileostomy

Like the colostomy this is an artificial anus on the abdominal wall but is sited in the right lower quadrant of the abdomen. It is always permanent and is usually performed following a total colectomy or pan-procto total colectomy – the latter includes the excision of the rectum and anus as well as the colon. These very extensive excisions are performed for patients with ulcerative colitis or extensive Crohn's disease. These patients are often extremely ill before surgery and may require a great deal of physiotherapy to help them maintain a good respiratory function and leg mobility.

As they improve, and in many cases this improvement can be dramatic, the physiotherapist should teach lifting and generally help with total rehabilitation prior to discharge.

For these patients the Ileostomy Association organize volunteers to visit in hospital and after discharge and they have groups all over the country who meet regularly for social events, holidays, as well as to discuss new appliances, etc.

GENITO-URINARY SURGERY

Nephrectomy

The removal of a kidney may become necessary when it is diseased as the result of a malignant tumour; pyonephrosis (gross infection); tuberculosis; hydronephrosis (dilation of the renal pelvis due to obstruction, leading to atrophy of the kidney tissue and impaired renal function); and occasionally for calculi (renal stones).

The remaining kidney must be healthy before nephrectomy is undertaken. The incision is usually through the bed of the 12th rib but may be higher, through the bed of the 10th rib. Care of the chest is very important and it is not unknown for the pleura to be 'nicked' at operation and for a pneumothorax to occur. An intercostal drain will be inserted and physiotherapy will follow the pattern as for thoracic surgery (Anderson and Innocenti, 1987).

Whenever a loin incision is used, the physiotherapist should check carefully the posture of the patient, both when lying in bed and when he gets up and starts walking.

Prostatectomy

This operation is usually performed on elderly men, many of whom will have a chronic chest disorder. Chest physiotherapy is therefore very important, and this is an instance where the cough-belt could be used (p. 97). Prostatectomy is usually performed for benign enlargement of the gland and is carried out through a transverse suprapubic incision. Carcinoma of the prostate is usually treated by hormonal manipulation but if the condition is causing difficulty of micturition through pressure on the bladder neck, a transurethral resection (TUR) of the gland may be undertaken. This is performed endoscopically, and under direct vision the surgeon is able to resect the obtruding tissue.

Early ambulation of these patients is not only desirable but essential; drainage tubes and catheter will need to be secured safely and the elderly gentleman persuaded to walk. Nowadays catheters drain into bags which can be easily carried.

If there is subsequent incontinence, a course of interferential therapy or faradism may be necessary.

Cystectomy

Surgery for a carcinoma of the bladder will entail removal of the bladder (cystectomy) and the fashioning of an ileal conduit. Not all bladder cancers will need to be treated with radical surgery; radiotherapy is used quite extensively and it is often following such treatment that cystectomy and the formation of an ileal conduit is carried out. An ileal conduit is the formation of an artificial bladder on the abdominal wall, in a manner similar to that of forming a colostomy. In this case a small segment of the ileum is fashioned into a tube and brought out through the abdominal wall, thus forming a stoma. The two ureters are inserted into the ileal conduit and an appliance into which the urine will drain is attached to the stoma.

Physiotherapy for these patients will include care for the chest, and, more especially, teaching them to lift and generally helping them to become active, mobile and capable of being independent before discharge.

An ileal conduit may also be fashioned for patients suffering from chronic incontinence due to certain neurological conditions, e.g. children with spina bifida.

REPAIR OF HERNIAE

A hernia is a weakness in the musculature through which contents of a cavity may prolapse.

Herniae of the abdominal wall

1. A *femoral* hernia occurs at the femoral ring. It is more common in women.
2. An *inguinal* hernia occurs at the inguinal canal. It is more common in men. There are two types: *Direct*, which occurs in older people due to associated muscle weakness and increase in abdominal pressure; and *Indirect*, which is congenital and occurs in younger people.
3. An *umbilical* hernia or para-umbilical hernia occurs either in childhood or at the fifth decade. In adults they are more common in obese patients.
4. An *incisional* hernia occurs through a previous incision and can be found anywhere.

Repair for these herniae involves excision of the hernial sac where necessary and strengthening of the abdominal wall by means of sutures. Fascia lata may be used like a darn, to repair the groin herniae; this latter procedure is rarely performed now.

Apart from chest physiotherapy as required, hernia patients must be taught to lift correctly. They may also be given abdominal exercises – isometric or inner range exercises but not outer range exercises.

Two other types of hernia are:

1. A *hiatus* hernia which is the prolapsing of the stomach through the hiatus of the diaphragm. Repair is usually through a thoracotomy incision and physiotherapy will be as for patients undergoing thoracic surgery (Anderson and Innocenti, 1987).
2. A *strangulated* hernia which is always a serious surgical emergency. The contents of the hernia sac can become trapped if the neck of the sac is very narrow; if the blood supply is impaired, the trapped bowel can become gangrenous. Intestinal obstruction is a not infrequent complication of a strangulated hernia. Physiotherapy is as for abdominal surgery.

THYROIDECTOMY

Surgery of the thyroid gland can take the form of a partial, hemi- or total thyroidectomy. Total thyroidectomy is rare, except in the case of malignant disease when it may be combined with a bilateral block dissection of the cervical lymph nodes.

More often a partial or hemi-thyroidectomy is performed and is carried out through a collar incision (p. 99). Pre- and postoperative chest physiotherapy may or may not be given. If it is, particular attention should be paid to the upper lobes of the lung, for it is these that are most likely to develop atelectasis. Because of the close proximity of the recurrent laryngeal nerve to the thyroid gland, it may be bruised at operation thus making coughing more difficult, as well as giving the patient a degree of hoarseness of speech. Many patients are very frightened about coughing and one method of support is shown in Fig. 8/6. Clips are normally used to close the incision and will be removed very quickly – probably half on the first postoperative day and the remainder on the third day. Following thyroidectomy, patients are mobilized rapidly and can be discharged on the sixth postoperative day, unless after-treatment is required, e.g. radiotherapy or chemotherapy in the case of malignant disease.

Occasionally, a patient presents with a retrosternal thyroid and if this necessitates the splitting of the upper part of the sternum, then the physiotherapy care will be a modification of that given for a

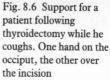

Fig. 8.6 Support for a patient following thyroidectomy while he coughs. One hand on the occiput, the other over the incision

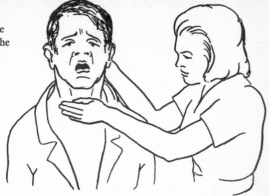

thoracotomy. Again, emphasis will be on the upper lobes of the lungs.

With any surgery in the neck region, patients are apprehensive about moving their heads. The physiotherapist should encourage head and neck movement and see that a correct posture is rapidly regained. The positioning of pillows is important and the physiotherapist can teach the nurse the best way to give maximum comfort and a good head position by the judicious placing of them.

Those readers who wish to read more deeply about techniques, etc., which may be used in the treatment of patients following surgery, are advised to refer to the companion volume *Cash's Textbook of Chest, Heart and Vascular Disorders for Physiotherapists*, 4th edition (ed. Downie, P. A.).

REFERENCES

Anderson, J. M. and Innocenti, D. (1987). Pulmonary surgery. Chapter in *Cash's Textbook of Chest, Heart and Vascular Disorders for Physiotherapists*, 4th edition, pp. 374–87 (ed. Downie, P. A.). Faber and Faber, London.

Barlow, D. (1964). A cough-belt to prevent and treat postoperative complications. *Lancet*, **2**, 736.

Downie, P. A. (1976). Post-mastectomy survey. *Nursing Mirror*, **142**, 13.

Editorial (1982). Postoperative pneumonias. *British Medical Journal*, **284**, 6312, 292–3.

Maguire, P. (1975). The psychological and social consequences of breast cancer. *Nursing Mirror*, **140**, 74.

Nichols, P. J. R. and Howell, B. (1970). Routine pre- and postoperative physiotherapy: A preliminary trial. *Physiotherapy*, **56**, 8, 356–9.

BIBLIOGRAPHY

Bailey and Love's Short Practice of Surgery, 20th edition (1988). H. K. Lewis, London.

Cotton, L. and Lafferty, K. (1986). *A New Short Textbook of Surgery*. Hodder and Stoughton, London.

Editorial (1989). Chest physiotherapy. *British Medical Journal*, **298**, 6673, 541–2.

Gray, R. C. (1987). The management of limb oedema in patients with advanced cancer. *Physiotherapy*, **73**, 10, 504–6.

Macfarlane, D. A. and Thomas, L. P. (eds.) (1984). *Textbook of Surgery*, 5th edition. Churchill Livingstone, Edinburgh.

Maguire, P. et al (1982). Cost of counselling women who undergo mastectomy. *British Medical Journal*, **284**, 1933.

Rennie, H. and Wilson, J. A. C. (1983). A coughing belt. *Lancet*, **2**, 138–9.

Chapter 9

Relaxation and Stress
by L. MITCHELL MCSP, DipTP

What is stress? Why teach relaxation? Does relaxation help stress? What type of person becomes stressed? When does stress occur? What is the role of the physiotherapist – if any? This chapter offers a discussion on these questions and indicates how relaxation may be adapted to other conditions as well as being applicable for stressed individuals.

STRESS

This is the body condition in which the physiology is geared for activity. Stress is usually considered useful if the amount of stimulation is suitable for the work to be done, and that work is then done, for example driving a car, giving a lecture, giving birth, and so on. The term *psychosomatic* dates from 1818 and is used to describe bodily diseases of mental origin (Taylor, 1979).

Stress has been described as 'the non-specific (that is, common) result of *any* demand upon the body, be it mental or somatic demand for survival and the accomplishment of our aims' (Selye, 1980). Over the years research into stress and stressors has abounded, and many papers and books have been published. Physiotherapists have been involved in several symposia notably the Fourth Congress of the World Confederation for Physical Therapy in Copenhagen in 1963 and the Annual Congress of the Chartered Society of Physiotherapy in 1977 (Mills, 1978). It is inevitable that such an airing of the subject should produce a descriptive title – stressology.

Stress may be considered as a state of being threatened, either by a life-shattering event or something absurdly small. It may be the death of a spouse with all the consequences of loneliness and poverty, or the dislike of the physiotherapist to whom the particular patient is referred. Indecision and the feeling of being trapped aggravate stress.

Holmes and Rahe (1967) drew up what has become a well-established scale of stress: it ranges from death of a spouse as 100 units to Christmas as 12 and minor violations of the law as 11. It demonstrates the point that stressors can arise through happy or unhappy circumstances (Benson, 1977). The menopausal woman may suffer stress not only through physical changes but also because of emotional changes such as children leaving home, death or disability of parents or spouse, or financial change.

Those who have become interested in stressology include doctors, sociologists, psychologists, physiologists, chemists, therapists (occupational, physical, music and art), as well as teachers of stress-relieving techniques.

There is some suggestion that there may be a virus causing a condition of appalling weakness associated with temperature following a period of overwork. The condition may be called myalgic encephalomyelitis (ME), and research is being carried out on this.

Burnout is the name now accepted for a condition in which someone gradually becomes less and less efficient and finally is incapable of carrying on their work. In the war years this condition was known as 'battle fatigue', sometimes 'a nervous breakdown' or 'overstressed' in peacetime. It is marked by periods of overwork, anxiety and lack of judgement alternating with periods of complete collapse (Squires and Livesley, 1984).

Physiology

Stressors may be classed as:

1. Physical, e.g. heat, cold, wind, bacteria.
2. Non-physical, e.g. mental, emotional, spiritual.
3. Social and psychological (Davison, 1978).

We depend upon our five senses, sight, hearing, smell, taste and touch to receive information from the environment, and relay it to the conscious brain. Information from within the body is conveyed to the mid- and hind-brain and spinal cord. Reflex actions determine the response to that information, e.g. an increase in the rate of breathing to remove the carbon dioxide due to increased muscle work. Joint position, skin pressure, pain and some temperature changes reach the conscious brain. As a result of all this information, plus the memory of past experiences (good and bad), mental and emotional states (grief, pain, happiness), so the state of stress, or lack of it, will be determined in a particular person at any particular moment.

Homeostasis

What then is the reaction of the body to stress? The most important function of the body is to remain in a state of homeostasis – the maintenance of constant conditions in the extracellular fluid derived from the blood that bathes all cells and upon which they depend for life (Guyton, 1974).

The Alarm Reaction When the body reacts to threat, the sympathetic nervous system goes into action for 'mass discharge', i.e. the 'fight or flight reflex', or stress reaction. This causes the anterior pituitary gland to secrete adrenocorticotrophic hormone (ACTH); the release of this into the bloodstream stimulates the thyroid gland to release thyroxine, and the medullae of the adrenal glands to release adrenalin and noradrenalin. These hormones will produce the following results:

1. Increase of heart action and blood pressure.
2. Increase in the metabolism of all cells particularly certain muscle groups to induce a definite position.
3. Increased carbon dioxide (CO_2) in the blood.
4. Increase in rate of breathing.
5. Increased dilation of the bronchioles and the eye pupils.
6. Increase in blood glucose from the liver, and, possibly, fatty acids from the fat reserves.
7. Increased sweating.
8. Increased blood supply to the voluntary muscles and the brain.
9. Decrease in the rate of peristalsis.
10. Decrease in gastro-intestinal glandular activity.
11. Decreased blood supply to the skin.
12. Decreased kidney and bladder function.

The sympathetic nervous system continues to act and enhances these results so that both hormone and nervous stimulation proceed simultaneously. Thus, in acute stress, homeostasis may be said to be endangered; in extreme cases actual pathology may result and death can occur.

General adaptation syndrome (GAS)

Selye (1975) showed that the body's resistance has a limit in its response to any stressor: he called it the General Adaptation Syndrome (GAS). This syndrome has three phases:

1. The alarm reaction (p.113).
2. The stage of adaptation or resistance.
3. If adaptation be chosen, then there can be a return to homeostasis. If resistance is offered and continued then exhaustion will follow, then pathology, and finally, possibly, death (Kelly, 1980).

Selye says 'There are two roads to survival: fight and adaptation. And more often adaptation is the more successful.'

It must be remembered that stress is a normal part of life, without it we are barely alive. What is a threat to one person is a challenge to another. It is the *response* to the stressor that determines its results. Carruthers (1974) found during his research into stress in motor racing that 'noradrenalin levels were doubled immediately before the race, and were often more than quadrupled by the end', and yet 'it seems unlikely that they damage their hearts by subjecting them [the drivers] to these brief episodes of stress, as the emotional relief appears to last for several days. It is the overall emotional climate that counts'.

The stage of resistance has been likened to a tightrope walker balancing a suitcase in either hand, one labelled *work* and the other *leisure*, each filled with the necessary constituents. If these activities and satisfactions keep balanced or suitably adapted, he can safely walk across the tightrope. If a change occurs in either which is greater than the individual is able to adapt to, then he may go into the *stage of exhaustion* and finally actual pathology will result. If, however, he can cope by restructuring his lifestyle, possibly including relaxation, then he will be able to continue a balanced life. Wright (1975) has said 'executive health involves what is coming to be called "the whole man". A full medical diagnosis depends on enquiry into, and assessment of, the individual in relation to his environment, his work, home, leisure and social pursuits.'

The physiotherapist having seen the medical diagnosis will need to carry out her own assessment dealing with the following.

Lifestyle

Lifestyle will include the amount and type of work, relationship with associates, conditions of work, degree of job satisfaction or undue competition, monotonous or dangerous work, amount of daily travelling or travel abroad, and so on. Having assessed all these, the individual can then decide whether it is possible to change any of it, or what he would like to change. Quite small and simple changes can alter the stress level dramatically, for example, wearing ear plugs in a noisy work area, taking a walk in the park instead of lunching at one's desk, and so on.

There may have been a sudden alteration in the pattern of life – promotion may entail a different method of working, including a change of work place and associates. Sometimes the gain in prestige and money is not worth the stress engendered, and it may be wiser to refuse promotion. Redundancy presents its own problems.

Women who look after a home, children, and also have a job may be quite unaware of their pattern. The author has been asked frequently by such women for help in relaxing: their comment may be 'Can you help me relax? I am always tired and yet never seem to get through all I have to do.' When the woman is asked to explain further it becomes patently clear that she has gradually taken on the work of several people without realizing it – home, children, husband, outside work, business entertaining and so on. To learn to relax at will is valuable, but it should be part of a pattern of healthy planning of work and leisure.

All this should be discussed with the patient who seeks your help; he will then come to understand what is meant by 'the whole man' approach to stress.

Home and social life

Personal relationships are the foundation of any life. If there is disharmony there will be stress. While physiotherapists must not probe into a patient's personal life, they can *listen*: everyone has to find his/her own solution, but it is often helpful to talk over difficulties. Advice should not be offered except to suggest that it might be wise to seek skilled help.

Creative, Artistic, Spiritual Pursuits   In the life of every human being some time must be given to these, for real balanced health of the 'whole man'. We are told that the right side of the brain controls imagination, and the left side reason. Both should be exercised daily.

A-Type People and B-Type People   These terms are now used to describe different types of people. The A-people appear to welcome stress, and are apt to cause it in other people by their forceful ways. They like to do several things at the same time, and are impatient of any delay. They are candidates for heart attacks.

The B-people are more balanced in their way of life but tend not to achieve so much.

There are now many stress consultants who give courses in

helping type A-people to change to a safer lifestyle, and to help type B-people to be more in charge of their own life. Sometimes the results are called type C-people.

Natural Surroundings   As we live in a world of earth, water, fish, plants, birds and animals, it follows that we should be in some contact with these natural surroundings and other creatures to maintain a balanced existence.

It is a personal choice as to how this is implemented; but there is no doubt as to the benefits derived by this intercommunication. Playing golf, gardening, or keeping a pet bird or animal, can all reduce stress and enhance the joy of living.

Disability

Disabled persons, whether long term or recently affected by accident or illness, are often stressed. For these considerable tact is required: heartiness from the able-bodied is not helpful. Always remember that the disabled person has a personality as well as a disability. Personal independence needs to be encouraged at all times. It is no use trying to relieve stress by relaxation if you (the helper) are part of the cause through unthinking, over-robust or domineering behaviour.

The physiotherapist can be a vital link in helping the disabled person and his family to resume a happy association after traumatic changes in circumstances; she can indicate to the family when to give help and when to withhold it. By patience, knowledge and a sensitive understanding of the individual's needs, the physiotherapist can help greatly in this process of re-orientation. A sense of humour can lighten many occasions, and when teaching the disabled relaxation, try teaching it to the whole family as well, or encourage the patient to do this. It encourages him to feel useful and increases his self-esteem.

Personal esteem

The sense of personal identity and being accepted by society are very important to the individual. The loss of either may well precipitate the onset of stress. Possible sources include pain, bereavement, disability, old age, lack of money or changed circumstances such as a mother having to cope with a handicapped child or an adult with elderly parents. The therapist has a great opportunity to help re-establish a sense of personal importance by encouraging a reassessment of the whole position and by teaching a method of relaxation to use when stressed. Other experts may be necessary to enable the patient to reach his own decision as to how best to improve conditions.

Diet: alcohol: smoking

There is much written about the value or otherwise of diet in stress, hypertension, and other metabolic disorders. There is conflicting evidence concerning cholesterol as a precipitating factor in coronary heart disease. Patients are best advised to be guided in all dietary matters by their general practitioner and/or dietician.

Alcoholic intake is difficult to assess, and is often a problem for those individuals who answer a stress situation with 'let's have a drink'. Although the physiotherapist does not deal with such matters she should know what treatment has been suggested for the individual alcoholic so that she may reinforce the advice. The same approach applies for those who smoke, and the physiotherapist can certainly reinforce the advice that any smoking is injurious to the breathing passages and lungs.

Exercise

Some form of physical activity is essential for a healthy body. A fit person tolerates stress better than an unfit person. Exercise leads to an increase in circulation and heart activity; increased carbon dioxide is given off by the working muscles, followed by increased breathing and general metabolic rate and a general sense of well-being. Exercise falls within the scope of the physiotherapist, though she must not be dogmatic. She should aim to help the patient understand why exercise, in some form, is necessary for everyone, and then help him choose whatever he prefers (Mitchell and Dale, 1980).

Probably the most important advice to give is to start any form of exercise gradually, and not rush from a lifetime of sedentary work to a marathon race overnight. Suggestions of walking one flight of stairs instead of taking the lift, of walking one fare stage instead of taking the bus from door to door, of standing up to dictate and so on; all these minor efforts may well prompt the businessman to take up more exercise and enjoy it. Swimming baths and gymnasia with well trained attendants are now very popular with both men and women.

Sleep and rest patterns (Hartman, 1973)

There is much discussion about sleep: some opinions say that it is necessary for 'biological restoration', others that it has no function. All agree that the length and depth of sleep is essentially individual. Certainly one of the rules of nature is a cycle of activity alternating with rest, for example the heart which *works* 0.5 second and *rests* 0.8 second in each beat.

Sleep may be classified as:

1. Orthodox or non-rapid eye movement for about one hour (NREM).
2. Paradoxical or rapid eye movement for about half an hour (REM).

It is thought that dreaming takes place during paradoxical sleep, because heart beat and breathing become faster and irregular, blood pressure rises and as more blood passes through the brain EEG waves show changes. It is not known whether the brain is sorting out past events or envisaging future ones. Dreaming is considered necessary for recuperation and emotional health. Some drugs interfere with sleep rhythms but the importance of this is not known. Other drugs are sometimes used to induce continual sleep for a limited period of enforced rest.

Regular sleep and rest periods interspersed with work and other activities appear to be normal, and a useful way of resisting stress. Both rest and sleep are essential to health. The substitution of physical effort for mental effort or vice versa, constitutes a rest; or rest may mean a period of calm from all kinds of activity during which relaxation techniques may be practised. For the busy person half an hour in the middle of the day or at the end of the day's work is the ideal routine. Stress is now almost a household word while relaxation is becoming more fashionable. No one will think less of anyone for practising relaxation during the day, indeed they may be envied.

Hobbies: holidays

Some form of recreation is essential for general well-being so beware of those who say they have no time for 'silly indulgences' such as hobbies or holidays. It is quite likely that such people have been sent to the physiotherapist because they are hypertensive or suffering from stress. The physiotherapist, in her assessment, may well enquire about such matters from the patient, and if this is found to be the attitude she will certainly have difficulty in teaching relaxation.

However, she can explain in simple language how the body is affected by tension and relaxation, for example she can explain and demonstrate how merely clenching the fist causes the blood pressure to rise. Thus the patient may appreciate the importance of reviewing his lifestyle and agree to learn relaxation.

Drugs

In the United Kingdom the taking of tranquillizers and sedatives has reached appalling heights: in 1979 prescriptions for sedatives and tranquillizers numbered 24 million at a cost of over 24 million pounds; similarly prescriptions for hypnotics numbered 17 million at a cost of over 19 million pounds. Many patients are unhappy about taking drugs and prefer to stop them as soon as they begin to feel better; however, there are others who become addicted.

There is considerable interest in the discovery that the body itself is capable of manufacturing its own pain relievers and tranquillizers; endorphins are produced in the brain and considerable research is now being undertaken to ascertain how they function and how they can be stimulated to provide effective pain relief in patients.

The prescribing of any drug is the responsibility of the doctor but it is reasonable to assume that if tense and stressed patients could be encouraged to try 'relaxation' then the need to prescribe drugs could be reduced considerably.

Doctors are now much more aware of the dangers of abuse of drugs, and are prescribing less than was the custom some years ago. I have assisted at a group trying to come off drugs ordered by their doctor and continued for years without supervision. Some had been taking sedatives for 20 years. Of course the reduction of dosage must be carefully controlled by a doctor.

Let us consider the work of the American psychologist Abraham Maslow (1908–70). He taught that human beings have a hierarchy of needs, and that until the lower level was satisfied a person could not easily achieve the next development, although there may be some overlap (Fig. 9/1). I have found these ideas to be useful in dealing with stressed people, especially encouraging them to reach the stage of self-esteem.

One has to be aware of the danger of stressed patients seeking safety by becoming dependent on the physiotherapist. They must be helped to discover their own strengths, and thus advance towards self-fulfilment. Maslow tells us that only 2–10 per cent of people

Fig. 9.1 A hierarchy of needs (*after* Maslow, 1954)

Self-
fufilment

Esteem of others

Self-esteem

Interchange of affection

Safety

Physical needs: heat, cold, food, drink

achieve this (Maslow, 1954).

Considering this, I have been given suicide figures from the General Register Office for Scotland, General Register Office, Belfast, and the Office of Population Surveys (England and Wales).

TABLE I   SUICIDES IN THE UNITED KINGDOM

1976		*1986*	
Total	4314	Total	4839
Men	2621	Men	3391
Women	1693	Women	1448

One wonders how much stress and of what kinds contributed to these dreadful figures.

RELAXATION

As this chapter is essentially for physiotherapists who may wish to apply the principles of relaxation to pathological as well as physiological circumstances, it is proposed to discuss fully the author's physiological method. This is suitable for all postoperative conditions involving stress, obstetrics, chest and heart conditions, arthritis where there is pain and tension, the terminally ill and patients with psychiatric conditions. It is a perfectly safe technique for anyone to use. Many physiotherapists, occupational therapists, nurses, and social workers use it daily to rid themselves from undue stress while working.

THE MITCHELL METHOD OF RELAXATION
(Mitchell, 1987a)

This method was devised by the author during the period 1957 to 1963 when the author was invited to demonstrate her method at the WCPT Conference in Copenhagen. It is now widely used throughout the world. It is based on three premises:

1. That stress causes anyone to adopt a certain posture that is recognizable. Therefore not all muscles are tense – only those controlling the posture.
2. That by the application of physiological laws this posture can be changed at will to a position of ease. The muscles holding the tense positions relax by reciprocal innervation.
3. That the changes of stress physiology gradually subside.

Posture of Stress Sitting　The typical features of tension include:

Face is frowning; the jaw is clamped shut; the tongue is on the roof of the mouth, and there is possibly grinding of teeth.
The shoulder girdle is raised.
The upper and lower arms are adducted and flexed.
The hands are clenched.
The legs are adducted and flexed so that one crosses the other.
The upper foot is held rigidly in the dorsiflexed position or is moved up and down continuously.
The head and body are held flexed.
Breathing is of a rapid sighing nature, or intermittent gasping associated with diaphragmatic spasm.
The person sits on the edge of the chair, often twisted on one buttock.
He may, when not sitting, walk up and down continuously.

Teaching　When teaching the Mitchell method of physiological relaxation either individually or in a class, it is helpful to ask people to build up a picture of the tension position by asking them to remember what happened in their own bodies or what they have seen in others who were suffering from stress. In this way they are enabled to recognize the stress posture and to be encouraged to observe others for signs of stress. They are always able to remember the positions of shoulders, arms and hands, often head, body and breathing changes, usually facial changes but seldom leg and feet changes although when demonstrated they are usually recognized.

Physiological Laws Applied

1. The brain does not order muscle work; it only understands movement (Basmajian, 1982). Therefore orders which are given to the body must be for positive activity in joints. They must not be for muscle action or relaxation, for example the command might be 'stretch your fingers', but not 'relax your fingers'.
2. The body is accustomed to receive precise orders from the brain for specific performance, e.g. hop, skip, jump. These actions are brought about by different muscle work which has been learned by the body receiving exact orders carried out repetitively and enjoyably. The patterns are stored in the sensory areas of the brain as engrams (Guyton, 1972). After much repetition it is thought they may be transferred to the motor cortex or basal ganglia.
3. Sherrington's law of reciprocal innervation which states that if one group of muscles is voluntarily contracted, the opposite group relaxes.
4. Sensation from muscle contraction does not reach the conscious brain, only joint position and skin pressure are recognized by the cortex (Buchwald, 1967). The sensations become more appreciated as they are repeated, and produce an engram of the ease position.
5. What the body has enjoyed it will remember and ask for repetition. What has been unpleasant it will forget, avoid or reject.

Treatment

The patient may be in bed, on the floor or sitting in a chair with a tall back and arms; he may be lying, side lying or sitting leaning back or forward on to supporting pillows on a table.

The head should be supported by pillows, one only if lying on the floor. The arms rest on pillows if leaning forward, while if sitting leaning backwards or lying the hands rest on the thighs or abdomen and do not touch each other.

The principle of this treatment is to teach the patient body awareness following the physiological rules of the body. Therefore no added pillows for so-called comfort are used as this confuses the patient. The lighting should be normal and even bright. There should be no attempt at silence and the physiotherapist should use a normal voice, rather firm and exact, as no attempt is being made to soothe the patient. Music is never used.

The patient is learning to feel joint positions exactly and skin pressures. Probably he has never felt these before, so it is a completely new experience and always pleasurable as the tense muscles relax due to the in-built reciprocal relaxation. He must concentrate and realize he is in charge of his own body. The teacher is not giving him orders but simply saying them so that he may give the orders to his own body as he does every day when changing any position to another.

If a group of people is being taught, they should not lie in rows, but should be scattered on the carpeted floor so that each person concentrates on his own body reactions. It is usual in any group for people to be in various positions to suit themselves, and to change position during the class if they wish. The orders will always fit.

Orders   These self-orders are as follows:

1. Make an exact small movement in every joint in turn. I have worked out these orders by reciprocal innervation so that they will induce relaxation in the tensed muscles. They will fit any position of the body and the words must *never* be changed. They are in lay language.
2. Stop the movement: the part remaining where it has arrived. The muscles used are now relaxed.
3. Feel the exact position of the joints in the new position and the skin pressures. All muscles in the area are now relaxed. Do not attempt to feel them.

Sequence

Shoulders:	*Pull* your shoulders towards your feet. *Stop*. *Feel* your shoulders are farther away from your ears.
Elbows:	Elbows *out* and *open*. *Stop*. *Feel* your upper arms touching the support and away from your sides. Feel the open angle at the elbows.
Fingers and thumbs:	*Long and supported*. The fingers and thumbs are stretched out 'long' with wrists extended. *Stop*. The fingers fall back on to the support. *Feel* the fingertips touching the support and the thumbs heavy.
Legs:	*Roll* your thighs outwards. *Stop*. *Feel* your turned out legs.

Knees: *Move* your knees very gently if not comfortable. *Stop*.
            Feel your comfortable knees.

Feet: *Push* your feet away from your face, bending at the
            ankle. *Stop*. *Feel* your dangling feet.

Body: *Push* your body into the support. *Stop*. *Feel* your body
            lying in the support.

Head: *Push* your head into the support. *Stop*. *Feel* your head
            lying on the support (pillow).

Breathing: Breathe in gently, lifting your lower ribs upwards and
            outwards towards your armpits, and a slight bulging
            above your waist in front. Breathe out easily and feel
            the ribs fall back. Repeat *once* only.

Face: Keep your mouth closed and drag your jaw down. *Stop*.
            Feel your separated teeth. Place your tongue low in
            your mouth. *Close* the eyes by lowering the top eyelids
            only. *Stop*. *Enjoy* the darkness. *Smooth* the forehead up
            into the hair, continue over the top of the head and
            down backwards. *Stop*. *Feel* the hair move.

(A full description of these sequences may be found in *Simple
Relaxation* (see Bibliography).)

The Mitchell method of relaxation can be adapted for any stressed
patient – two groups of patients, obstetric and psychiatric, are
discussed briefly.

Obstetric patients (See also Chapter 11)

Antenatal Expectant mothers may be treated singly or in a group.
It is wise to emphasize to them that fear of delivery is quite usual,
and that this method will help the mother to cope with it. Relaxation
is therefore given with the following objectives:

1. To obtain rest during pregnancy.
2. To help the mother during all stages of delivery by inducing rest
   when possible.
3. To help the mother regain normal health afterwards by preventing unnecessary fatigue.

Pregnancy: The mother should practise the whole technique
thoroughly in many positions. It is often helpful to rest kneeling
forward on to one's arms on a cushion placed on the seat of a chair;
the knee and hip joints are at a right angle. The weight of the fetus
lies on the anterior abdominal wall.

Another useful position for a rest after activity, is kneeling forward on to one's arms on a cushion on the floor, with the buttocks high. The weight of the fetus lies on the diaphragm.

In both positions the pelvic floor is given a rest from the weight of the fetus. The self-orders work as usual.

Delivery: The mother begins relaxation as soon as the first contraction starts. She remains wherever she happens to be. As she has already learned many positions in which to perform the technique, she should adopt whichever is convenient. The mother maintains a slow sustained relaxation throughout the contraction. Immediately the contraction is over she moves and does whatever she wishes. At every contraction, no matter where she may be, she repeats the performance.

The final dilation of the cervix may be prolonged; she should try to obtain, and continue, total relaxation, checking each joint for '*move*', '*stop*', '*feel*' continuously, while breathing high in the chest 'pant, pant, sigh'.

During the second stage of labour, the mother may be in a variety of positions, and may or may not be pushing during the contractions. Immediately the contraction *begins* to pass off she seeks rest for her whole body and flashes the massages of relaxation in a wave down arms, legs, body and head all at once. She rests totally until the next contraction begins and is ready to resume relaxation for the birth of the baby's head. All this should be practised in the antenatal class.

Psychiatric patients

The physiotherapist in a psychiatric hospital or unit works as part of a team so that her part in treatments will dovetail with others.

She usually treats patients in a group for relaxation, and this consists of the usual techniques allied with varying suggestions, for example 'Think of the happiest moment of your life', 'Think of any unhappy experience you had last week', etc. Discussion is intermingled with bouts of relaxation, and each patient is encouraged to talk. Music is never used in these sessions as the patients are concentrating and thinking of body reactions, feelings and controls. If music therapy is used it would be at a different session (Mitchell, 1987b).

Results of teaching relaxation

1. Tension and ease cannot exist at the same time in one section of the body. As the relaxation proceeds the physiological processes of stress subside. Noticeable changes are the alteration in the rate of breathing, often preceded by a long sigh, and the eyes closing before the order for this is given. The blood pressure and heart beat are lower.
2. Patients enjoy the treatment, find it easy to learn, and practise willingly by themselves. They often willingly change their lifestyle for the better.
3. The technique can be used to ward off stress during work by using selected orders to relax some parts of the body, while continuing activity on others, or the full treatment can lead to sleep.
4. Often after practice, the patient can discontinue sedatives or tranquillizers under medical supervision.

Other treatments which physiotherapists may encounter are briefly discussed.

PROGRESSIVE RELAXATION (Jacobson Method)
(Jacobson, 1977)

The idea is to teach the patient to be aware of voluntary muscle contraction and relaxation of the same muscle group. 'Doing away with residual tension is the essential feature of the method' (Jacobson, 1977). The physician trained in this method teaches the patient for about an hour, and the patient is then asked to practise by himself for one or two hours a day between sessions. The sessions are continued for several months.

Practice consists in contracting a selected group of muscles, for example the wrist extensors by bending the hand back at the wrist and noting the sensation. Jacobson describes this as 'diffuse, indistinct and characterless'. He asks the patient to ignore the feeling of movement at the appropriate joint, in this case the wrist (Jacobson calls this 'strain') and says these and skin sensations are more noticeable than are the sensations from muscle. This is true because joint and skin sensations, but not muscle tension, are relayed directly to the cortex.

The patient then lets the hand fall back to its resting position on the couch and registers the lack of tenseness, i.e. relaxation in the same muscles. This is called 'going negative'. After repeating this several times, the patient rests for the remainder of the hour. This sequence is taught in subsequent sessions to all parts of the body.

An amended form of this system was taught in the United Kingdom in the 1930s and 1940s and often called 'tense and let-go'.

BIOFEEDBACK

This technique has been developed over the past 20 years and is now coming into the repertoire of the physiotherapist (see *Cash's Textbook of Neurology for Physiotherapists*). By the use of electrodes attached to the body and led into a machine (often portable) the patient is made aware of physiological effects. For stressed patients the electrodes register the amount of dampness on the fingers; a light or a buzzer indicates that sweat is present, and as the individual seeks to control his stress by thought, the light or buzzer becomes dimmer or more quiet indicating the measure of success.

MASSAGE AND HANDLING

In time past this was a frequent order in the treatment of patients suffering from stress – then called neurasthenia. It consisted of making the patient comfortable, using pillows and possibly some form of infra-red irradiation, then giving effleurage and stroking to each part of the body but concentrating upon the back. Such a treatment lasted about one hour; there appeared to be good immediate results, but long-term effects did not justify its continuance.

Today, massage is seldom prescribed, although it is still taught in the syllabus of training. There is little doubt that massage teaches the physiotherapist the skilful use of her hands, the awareness of touch and the ability to handle patients comfortably. Massage applied judiciously to a frightened and tense patient can work wonders. As physiotherapists we must remember that our methods of handling patients can cause distress or considerable relief. No machine can really be a substitute for a sensitive pair of hands (Pratt and Mason, 1981).

Comfort of the patient extends to ensuring that he is properly supported when sitting up in bed and adequately covered. The head should be supported in the mid-position and not pushed forward or allowed to fall into extension. The physiotherapist should be able to spot the uncomfortable patient and help him, without asking the somewhat fatuous question 'Are you comfortable?' when it is clearly apparent that he is not. Skilled handling establishes the necessary trust and confidence between carer and patient which enables treatments, especially those to reduce stress, to be more effective.

HYDROTHERAPY

Hydrotherapy is exercise involving partial or complete submersion of the body in water, with active or passive movements of body parts, usually carried out by a physiotherapist. It is regarded as a useful method of developing movement and body awareness while supported. All physiotherapists are taught the principles and methods of hydrotherapy as part of their training.

While most patients enjoy relaxing in warm water and carrying out exercise, some do not: therefore be sure the patient will welcome the treatment before attempting it. For those patients who really enjoy water, hydrotherapy can provide an excellent form of exercise and stress relief.

Other techniques which are said to aid relaxation include hypnosis, breathing methods, autogenics, distraction and visualization, meditation, yoga and so on, but all these fall outside the scope of this chapter.

I would like to give a warning about some cassettes advertised for sale, in which the voice seeks to dominate the listener, and make him dependent on the tape. I consider this dangerous. There are others full of vague advice, which hardly helps the patient to deal with his stress.

Since stress has been widely accepted, many untrained people are selling tapes. Please select with care.

REFERENCES

Basmajian, J.V. (1982). *Primary Anatomy*, 8th edition. Williams and Wilkins, Baltimore.

Benson, H. (1977). *The Relaxation Response*, pp. 39–41. Fount Paperbacks, London.

Buchwald, J.S. (1967). Proprioceptive reflexes and posture. *American Journal of Physical Medicine*, 46, 104–13.

Carruthers, M. (1974). *The Western Way of Death*, pp. 44, 45. Davis-Poynter Ltd, London.

Davison, W. (1978). Stress in the elderly. *Physiotherapy*, 64, 4, 113.

Guyton, A.C. (1972). *Structure and Function of the Nervous System*, pp. 211–12. W.B. Saunders Co, Philadelphia.

Guyton, A.C. (1974) *Function of the Human Body*, 4th edition, p. 4. W.B. Saunders Co, London.

Hartman, E.L. (1973). *The Function of Sleep*, pp. 23–5. Yale University Press, London.

Holmes, T.H. and Rahe, R.H. (1967). Social readjustment scale. *Journal of Psychosomatic Research*, 2, 213.

Jacobson, E. (1977). *You Must Relax*. Souvenir Press, London.

Kelly, D. (1980). *Anxiety and Emotions*, pp. 88–91. Thomas, USA.

Maslow, A.H. (1954). *Motivation and Personality*, pp. 91–2. Harper and Row, New York.

Mills, I.H. (1978). Coping with the stress of modern society. *Physiotherapy*, **64**, 4, 109.

Mitchell, L. and Dale, B. (1980). *Simple Movement*, chapter 7 and appendix. John Murray, London.

Mitchell, L. (1987a). *Simple Relaxation*, 2nd edition. John Murray, London.

Mitchell, L. (1987b). *Simple Relaxation*, p. 110. John Murray, London.

Pratt, J.W. and Mason, A. (1981). *The Caring Touch*. HM&M Publishers, London.

Selye, H. (1975). *Stress Without Distress*, p. 38. Hodder and Stoughton, London.

Selye, H. (ed.) (1980). *Selye's Guide to Stress Research*. Von Nostrand Reinhold Co, New York.

Squires, A. and Livesley, B. (1984). Beware of burnout. *Physiotherapy*, **70**, 6, 235–8.

Taylor, G.R. (1979). *The Natural History of the Mind*, p. 135. Secker and Warburg, London.

Wright, H.B. (1975). *Executive Ease and Dis-ease*, p. 11. Gower Press, Epping, Essex.

BIBLIOGRAPHY

Bolton, E. and Goodwin, D. (1983). *Introduction to Pool Exercises*, 5th edition. Churchill Livingstone, Edinburgh.

Brooks, V.B. (1986). *The Neural Bases of Motor Control*. Oxford University Press, Oxford.

Clare, A. (1980). *Psychiatry in Dissent*, 2nd edition. Tavistock Publications Limited, London.

Fenwick, P.B.C. et al (1977). Metabolic and EEG changes during transcendental meditation: An explanation. *Biological Psychology*, **5**, 101–18.

Gowler, D. and Legge, K. (eds) (1975). *Managerial Stress*. Gower Press, Epping, Essex.

Illman, J. (1978). *Masks and Mirrors of Mental Illness*. National Westminster Bank on behalf of MIND, London.

Kearns, J.L. (1975). *Stress in Industry*. Priory Press, Hove, Sussex.

Kelly, D. (1980). *Anxiety and Emotions*. Thomas, USA.

McLean, A. (1977). *Occupational Stress*. C.C. Thomas, Springfield, Ill.

Maslow, A.H. (1973). In *Self-esteem, Self-actualization* (ed. Lowry, J.R.). Monterey, California.

Mitchell, L. (1984). *Healthy Living Over 55*. John Murray, London.

Mitchell, L. (1987). *Simple Relaxation*, 2nd edition. John Murray, London.

Norfolk, D. (1979). *The Stress Factor*. Hamlyn Books, London.

Skinner, A.T. and Thomson, A.M. (eds) (1983). *Duffield's Exercise in Water*, 3rd edition. Baillière Tindall, London.

Cassettes, a booklet and video on the Mitchell method of relaxation are available for purchase. All enquiries should be addressed to the author at 8 Gainsborough Gardens, Well Walk, Hampstead, London NW3 1BJ United Kingdom (a stamped addressed envelope will be appreciated).

ORGANIZATIONS

International Stress and Tension Control Society, United Kingdom Branch,
The Priory Hospital, Priory Lane, London SW15 5JJ

Heartcare, 72 Park Lane, Congleton, Cheshire CW12 3DD, United Kingdom

Remedial Swimming   Association of Swimming Therapy, 10 West Way, Wheelock,
Sandbach, Cheshire

Hypnosis   The British Society of Medical and Dental Hypnosis, PO Box 6,
Ashstead, Surrey KT21 2HT

Margaret Morris Movement   International Association of MMM Ltd, Suite 3/4,
39 Hope Street, Glasgow G2 6AH, United Kingdom

Chapter 10

Aspects of Obstetrics and Gynaecology

by MARY ANDERSON MB, ChB, FRCOG

Obstetrics concerns itself with pregnancy, labour, delivery and the care of the mother after childbirth. *Gynaecology* is the study of diseases associated with women – which in effect means conditions involving the female genital tract. It is usual for a specialist to practise both these specialties although nowadays the emphasis is often on one particular aspect of the combined specialty so that a doctor may spend the greater part of his or her time dealing with, for example, urodynamics (study of disorders of the urinary tract) or colposcopy (a study of the unhealthy cervix) or ultrasound, particularly in relation to obstetrics – and so on.

Clearly it is an impossible task to cover the whole of obstetrics and gynaecology in one chapter. What will be described are the commoner conditions and surgical procedures particularly where the physiotherapist is concerned. Mention will also be made of some of the moral and ethical problems which face the gynaecologist nowadays – not because the physiotherapist will have to become directly involved but because it may help her to have a wider understanding of her gynaecological and obstetrical patients.

ANATOMY AND PHYSIOLOGY

The anatomy of the pelvic floor musculature will be familiar to the student of physiotherapy (Figs 10/1, 10/2, 10/3). The relationship of the uterus and cervix to the pelvic floor and to the bladder in front (Fig. 10/4) is of great importance both in certain gynaecological conditions and in childbirth and some of its effects. The physiotherapist should have a clear picture of these structures and their relationship to each other when she comes to the treatment of various problems.

So far as physiology is concerned we shall consider only those aspects which are relevant to certain areas of obstetrics and gynaecology – again particularly with relevance to the physiotherapist.

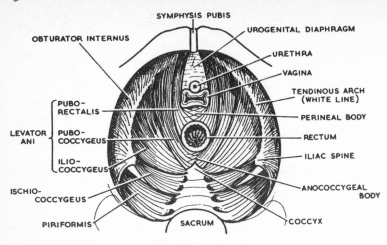

Fig. 10.1 The levator ani muscles and urogenital diaphragm

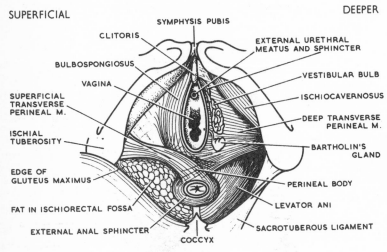

Fig. 10.2 The superficial muscles of the pelvic floor

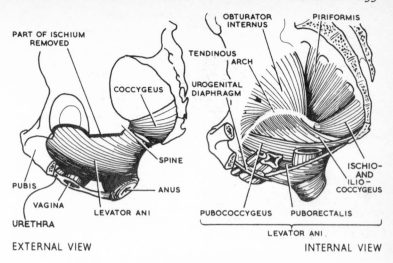

Fig. 10.3 Lateral view of the pelvic diaphragm, showing the urogenital diaphragm

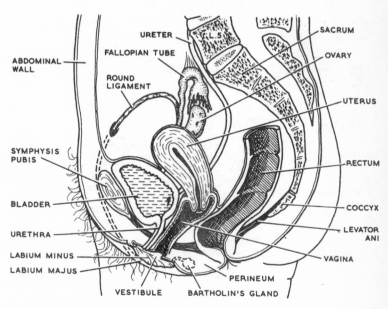

Fig. 10.4 The relationship of the various pelvic organs

OBSTETRICS

Anatomy

The Pelvic Floor This consists essentially of the levator ani muscles which lie like a sling over the floor of the pelvis (Fig. 10/1). It is an incomplete floor since various structures pass through it – the urethra in front, the rectum behind and the vagina between these two structures.

During pregnancy the pelvic floor stretches and this is particularly the case in labour. This is partly explained by mechanical stretching as the uterus grows but also partly by the hormonal changes which take place in pregnancy. The main hormone concerned is progesterone which has a relaxing effect on muscle. It also has a relaxing effect on the ligaments of joints and this explains why many women experience a lot of joint discomfort particularly so far as the pelvic joints are concerned. Low back pain and sacro-iliac discomfort are common and pain and tenderness over the symphysis pubis may be particularly disturbing.

Treatment: There is not a great deal that can be done for these joint discomforts of pregnancy which, after all, exist so long as the pregnancy continues and will recede after delivery. Physiotherapy may have some part to play in the form of gentle passive and active exercises and possibly some heat (see also Chapter 11).

Labour

Clearly the maximum stretching effect on the pelvic floor and pelvic joint ligaments will take place during labour. The passage of the fetus through the pelvis during what may be a long first stage produces continuing pressure and stretching. This is where the relaxation effect of progesterone on the pelvic joints is beneficial in that it will gain some extra 'space' for the fetus during its progress through the pelvis.

Nowadays the duration of labour is monitored closely and lengthy labours (of 18–24 hours) are no longer acceptable. The average duration of labour in a primigravida (a woman pregnant for the first time) is now probably 8–12 hours while for a multigravida it is 6–8 hours.

Labour is divided into stages. The *first stage* is from the onset of labour until the full dilatation of the cervix which then allows the passage of the fetus out of the pelvis. The *second stage* is from the full dilatation of the cervix until the delivery of the baby. This is the 'active' stage in that maternal effort is required to help the uterine contractions deliver the baby. The duration of this stage should be under an hour in a primigravida and about half an hour in a multigravida. If these times are exceeded then the obstetrician will aid the delivery by the application of forceps. These instruments are devised to create a protective metal cage for the fetal head and traction is made to coincide with each contraction and continuing maternal effort.

Big babies and prolonged maternal effort may result in a degree of prolapse, where either the anterior or the posterior wall of the vagina 'drops'. Occasionally the uterus itself may prolapse to some extent presumably due to over-stretching of the main uterine supports – the cardinal and utero-sacral ligaments (Fig. 10/5).

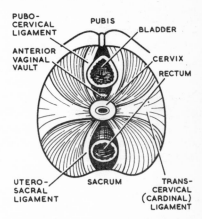

Fig. 10.5 The ligaments of the cervix

Physiotherapy has much to offer both in antenatal preparation and in the postnatal period.

The *third stage* is the delivery of the placenta.

Antenatal preparation

The value of the physiotherapist here is in teaching relaxation techniques and in teaching the 'control' of the body at each stage of labour. Women who have been prepared in this way have shorter labours requiring less analgesia than those who are unprepared and often tense and unrelaxed. Of course, the use of epidural anaesthesia helps in this respect but preparation classes also have a major beneficial psychotherapeutic effect and should be encouraged for all women – certainly for primigravida. Physiotherapists taking part in such classes should have a special interest and training.

Postnatal exercises

These are of benefit to all women and most maternity units arrange for a physiotherapist to visit the postnatal wards on a daily basis.

Perineal muscle (pelvic floor) exercises will clearly help to restore the strength and function of these muscles stretched as they have been by both pregnancy and the process of labour.

Bladder 'weakness' with leakage of urine on coughing or sneezing or even on walking may also be part of the weakening of the pelvic floor musculature after childbirth and pelvic floor exercises with perhaps faradism or interferential treatment at a later date may be all that is necessary to restore continence (see p.167). Surgery is rarely if ever indicated in the young woman of childbearing years and total reliance is placed on physiotherapy.

Incontinence of this kind and, indeed, prolapse may be wrongly related to childbirth particularly where there is a history of large babies or forceps deliveries. It is not true to say that these events will automatically lead to prolapse and incontinence later. Intrinsic weakness in ligamentous supports and musculature must be the basic background and certainly in these cases (which cannot be identified in advance) good physiotherapy with encouragement to maintain exercises after discharge from hospital will do much to avoid later problems.

Special problems

Infection Infection of the genital tract after childbirth is not uncommon. Nowadays, however, it is routine in most maternity units to take a high vaginal swab for culture towards the end of pregnancy. The significant organism is the Group B haemolytic streptococcus and if discovered a course of antibiotics (usually amoxycillin) is given to the mother, often to the partner and always to the newborn infant. This has avoided a lot of the problems of puerperal sepsis seen previously.

Infection arises because if contaminants such as Group B haemolytic streptococcus are in the vagina then the uterus following childbirth with its raw placental site offers an ideal focus for infection, and organisms which have only been contaminants before become pathogenic.

This is more likely if many vaginal examinations have been carried out during labour and if instrumental delivery has been required.

The treatment of such infection which is usually ascending, involving the uterine cavity and out into the tubes, is firstly with antibiotics.

Pelvic short wave diathermy may have some part to play but usually at a later date if the infection has produced the condition known as chronic pelvic inflammatory disease (see p.144).

Episiotomy An episiotomy is a deliberate surgical incision made to ease the birth of the fetal head (or breech). It is made through the perineum either centrally or, more usually, medio-laterally on the right side.

Obstetricians and midwives are often accused of carrying out episiotomies too frequently not allowing enough time for the perineal muscles to stretch adequately. This is not true in most cases. But equally it is true to say that a clean surgical incision can be repaired more easily and heals better than a jagged tear, so that if a tear seems inevitable it is advisable to carry out an episiotomy before tearing occurs. By the time the fetal head is stretching the perineum there is undoubtedly relative anoxia for the baby and to wait too long for the perineal muscles to stretch adequately is therefore inadvisable.

Although an episiotomy wound is not in a site that is ideal for quick and uncomplicated healing, nevertheless healing is usually very satisfactory. If suturing is done by someone experienced, without delay, so as to avoid too much anatomical distortion, and the correct tension used for the sutures, then healing should be uncomplicated. Infection, with breakdown, may occasionally occur and although antibiotics and local swabbing are the mainstay of treatment the physiotherapist may be asked to help by using heat or ultrasound therapy.

Caesarean Section This operation is done for many reasons. For example, for the sake of the mother in conditions such as hypertension or diabetes, or for the sake of the fetus where it becomes distressed during labour or where it is growing inadequately and early delivery before term is deemed advisable. There are other conditions and abnormalities for which delivery by caesarean section may be indicated.

The operation used is the lower segment procedure – the lower segment of the uterus being the area which becomes markedly thinned and stretched out during the growth of the uterus throughout pregnancy. A transverse incision is made in the lower segment and this usually heals well because the lower segment provides an inactive area for healing to take place as distinct from the upper segment which remains active even after delivery and this muscle activity is not conducive to sound healing. The abdominal incision used is usually the transverse lower abdominal one – or Pfannenstiel incision as it is called. Like any other surgical scar this may become infected, develop a haematoma or break down and then physiotherapy in the form of heat or ultrasound may be helpful.

As in any other surgical procedure, postoperative care in general is of the utmost importance. Early mobilization, leg exercises and breathing exercises are important and the physiotherapist plays a major role in the management of the puerperal mother following caesarean section.

GYNAECOLOGY

There are several gynaecological conditions which are of relevance to the physiotherapist. The most frequently occurring will be considered.

Prolapse

This has already been mentioned. There are several types of prolapse:

(a) *Vault prolapse*: Or uterine prolapse (Fig. 10/6).
(b) *Rectocele*: A prolapse of the posterior wall of the vagina including the rectum.
(c) *Cystocele* (Fig. 10/7): A prolapse of the anterior wall of the vagina including the bladder and frequently associated with stress incontinence or other urinary difficulties.
(d) *Enterocele*: A true herniation of peritoneum through the uterosacral ligaments appearing as a high rectocele and often containing small bowel.

As has already been indicated, if prolapse appears in a young woman still of childbearing years, it is better to avoid surgery and use physiotherapy instead – and frequently that is successful. Once childbearing is completed and if the problem remains, causing symptoms, surgery can be undertaken. Symptomless prolapse does not require treatment.

The surgical procedures used are:

1. *Anterior repair*: This means excising the redundant skin over the 'bulge' of the cystocele, plicating the bladder ('tucking it up') and bringing together the anterior fibres of levator ani under the bladder neck area in particular so as to form a buttress for the bladder.

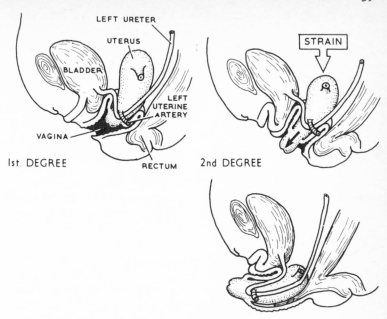

LEFT URETER

UTERUS

BLADDER

LEFT
UTERINE
ARTERY

VAGINA

RECTUM

1st. DEGREE

STRAIN

2nd DEGREE

3rd DEGREE
COMPLETE PROCIDENTIA

Fig. 10.6 Degrees of uterine prolapse

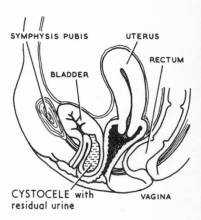

SYMPHYSIS PUBIS

UTERUS

RECTUM

BLADDER

CYSTOCELE with
residual urine

VAGINA

Fig. 10.7 A cystocele

2. *Posterior repair*: This means removing the 'bulge' of redundant skin over the rectocele and repairing in two layers so as to support the rectum. The final stitches of this procedure are in the levator ani fibres to draw them more closely together and rebuild what is almost always a deficient perineum.

3. A *'Manchester' or Fothergill repair*: This operation is not so popular as it once was. Here the cervix is usually enlongated and the mainstay of the procedure is to amputate the cervix thereby shortening the cardinal ligaments on either side, and, in recovering the cervix with the vaginal skin, the shortened cardinal ligaments are picked up and brought together on the front of the cervical stump which has the effect of pushing it upwards.

4. The preferred operation nowadays is the *vaginal hysterectomy and repair*. Here, as the name suggests, the uterus is removed by the vaginal route, the pedicles formed thereby on either side (cardinal ligaments, and broad ligament pedicles) are sutured together in the mid-line to close over the vault, the utero-sacral ligaments are sewn together also in the mid-line to prevent later enterocele formation, and the anterior vaginal wall closed in the usual way. If a rectocele co-exists this is then repaired as described before, taking great care not to tighten the vagina too much if the woman is still sexually active – a fact that should be ascertained before the operation.

5. Other operations are carried out for specific variations in the condition of prolapse. Repair of an enterocele basically consists of dissecting out the peritoneal 'hernial' sac, excising it, having ligated it at its 'neck' – just as in a routine hernial repair.

Various operations are done now for urinary stress incontinence, the anterior repair not having proved very successful. Basically the 'wet' woman must first be investigated to elucidate which type of incontinence she suffers from – urge incontinence, for example, where the woman must pass urine whenever she feels the urge otherwise dribbling incontinence will occur, is due to instability of the bladder muscle, the detrusor, and will not be helped by surgery.

Colposuspension is an operation which pulls up the vault of the vagina and therefore the urethra and fixes it to the back of the pubic symphysis. Sling operations are done using material such as nylon to pull up the bladder neck and again fix it to the back of the pubic symphysis.

Physiotherapy After Repair Operations   Like any surgery early mobilization and leg exercises are most important after any of the above procedures. Gentle abdominal and pelvic floor exercises are also helpful but clearly vigorous exercising should not be encouraged until healing has taken place. See Chapter 12 for full details.

Abdominal hysterectomy

This is one of the commonest operations in gynaecology, carried out for many reasons – fibroids, heavy periods and carcinoma of the endometrium being commonly the indications for the operation.

The operation is nowadays a total one, that is the body of the uterus and the cervix are removed. If the tubes and ovaries are also removed – because they are unhealthy, or in an older, especially postmenopausal, woman – the operation is described as a total abdominal hysterectomy and bilateral salpingo-oophorectomy.

After the operation active physiotherapy in the form of leg, breathing and abdominal muscle exercises is desirable. Early mobilization is imperative. Very often these women are overweight and anaemic – both precursors of deep vein thrombosis. Various steps are taken to avoid this complication nowadays – pressure stockings, 'mini' doses of subcutaneous heparin – but physiotherapy plays a major part in prophylaxis.

Pre-operative preparation for gynaecological procedures is important but gone are the days when a hospital can spare beds to admit women several days before surgery for preparation, including physiotherapy. But pre-operative counselling is important since many women still believe that the operation of hysterectomy will produce a major change in their appearance and their psychology. They must be reassured that this is not so. If in a premenopausal woman the ovaries have to be removed then it is customary to place an implant of 50 or 100mg oestradiol in the fat of the abdominal wall during closure of the wound. This acts as a reservoir of oestrogen which is slowly absorbed over the following six months or so when it can be replaced, or tablets of oestrogen taken or skin patches used. In this way acute menopausal symptoms, especially hot flushes, can be avoided. Women do *not* put on weight after hysterectomy which so many believe. As a woman gets older her metabolism changes and most women begin to put on weight rather easily at this time of life. Attention to diet and to exercise will help and in the latter respect the physiotherapist can be of great value in giving advice in the post-operative period.

The menopause

In addition to the foregoing remarks it is of some interest perhaps to add some further comments on the 'natural' menopause (as distinct from the iatrogenic surgical menopause mentioned above). It is a topic on which there is a lot of myth rather than fact but fortunately with increasing publicity in recent years, understanding is getting greater. The physiotherapist is frequently involved in discussion about the features of the menopause as she treats women for example with pelvic floor exercises. She should therefore be aware of the facts rather than join the mythologists.

Salient points are as follows but short useful pamphlets and books are available for further reference.

1. Not every woman automatically experiences adverse symptoms so that they should not be anticipated as inevitable.
2. Other changes take place in a woman's life at this stage (family leave home, husband away a lot on business, for example) so it is not surprising that minor degrees of depression result leading to lassitude, sleeplessness and so on.

   Hormone replacement therapy (HRT) can do a lot to help the general well-being of these women especially where a genuine background of the effects of diminished oestrogen production exists (such as hot flushes and atrophic vaginitis).
3. Small joint pains are common and may be helped by hormone replacement.
4. Osteoporosis has now been shown to be a most important feature of menopausal changes. It is not possible to identify which women are likely to suffer from it (although a family history is important) nor is there as yet a simple clinical test to detect it at an early stage. It is however an important cause of morbidity among elderly women who are liable to fractures with the resultant possible complications. Hormone replacement can effect improvement and should certainly be given to the following categories:
   - the woman with a family history of osteoporosis
   - women reaching menopause at a comparatively young age. The average age for the cessation of menstruation is 50 with a range 45–55. If a woman stops menstruating at a much younger age than this or has to have the ovaries removed then hormone replacement therapy should be given. It is believed, and research is increasingly supporting the belief, that the use of HRT will significantly diminish the risk of osteoporosis.

It has always been thought that a good diet and adequate exercise will help in avoiding osteoporosis but studies have shown that this is not so important as appropriate hormone replacement. This is not to say that diet and exercise should not be encouraged in the postmenopausal women as they are obviously of the greatest importance in controlling weight which as we have seen is so often a problem in this age-group.

Menstruation and its problems

This aspect of gynaecology occupies a lot of the gynaecologist's time. Menstruation commonly occurs in a cycle of 28 days, that is from the first day of one period to the first day of the following one. It lasts for three to five days and is not unduly heavy although 'heaviness' varies from woman to woman and is a very subjective assessment. Menstruation should not, however, produce anaemia, the body making adequate adjustment for the cyclical blood loss (average 40 ± 20ml). Variations in cycle length are common and may be normal for the individual woman.

Common problems of menstruation are:

(a) *Menorrhagia*, or heavy menstruation. Here anaemia is likely to result. Causes vary from fibroids or endometrial polyps to hormonal causes such as is described as 'dysfunctional uterine bleeding'. The cause of menorrhagia must be sought – dilatation and curettage to obtain endometrium for study in the laboratory, ultrasound scan of the pelvis to exclude fibroids and so on. Then the appropriate treatment is given – surgery for a physical cause such as fibroids, conservative treatment, usually hormonal (such as the pill in younger women or the progesterone-like hormones in the older woman) for dysfunctional bleeding.

(b) *Dysmenorrhoea*, painful periods. Commonly the aetiology of *primary* dysmenorrhoea which means periods that are painful almost from the menarche (the onset of menstruation) is unknown but it is rarely due to a physical cause. Treatment, of necessity, is somewhat arbitrary varying from simple analgesics to the contraceptive pill. Local heat may be helpful but the wider use of physiotherapy has not proved to be of value.

Secondary dysmenorrhoea means painful periods developing years after normal pain-free menstruation. This implies pathology, and the two commonest conditions resulting in secondary dysmenorrhoea are *endometriosis* and *pelvic inflammatory disease*.

Endometriosis is a condition in which pockets of endometrial tissue grow outside the uterine cavity – the ovaries and the utero-sacral ligaments being common sites. Its aetiology is unknown and its treatment is either hormonal in the younger woman with limited disease, or surgical, especially in older women where the loss of uterus and ovaries is not a disaster.

Pelvic inflammatory disease (PID) is a title given to what is chronic post-infective inflammation involving the tubes and ovaries almost always bilaterally. It can be an acute illness with fever and systemic upset or chronic, presenting with painful periods, dyspareunia and sometimes a mass in the pelvis representing a tube and ovary 'stuck down' together by adhesions or actual abscess formation. The condition is synonymous with salpingitis.

At the present time (1989) PID is a major problem, the aetiological background being sexual activity, virus infections, the use of intra-uterine contraceptive devices and termination of pregnancy. It can, however, follow an intercurrent illness such as appendicitis or even normal childbirth.

Diagnosis is made both clinically and at laparoscopy.

Treatment is difficult and frequently unsuccessful necessitating ultimate removal of the tubes and ovaries – a personal tragedy for a young woman. The mainstay of treatment is (apart from education) antibiotic therapy, analgesia and, in the chronic case, physiotherapy in the form of short wave diathermy. Prolonged treatment with the latter can often effect very good clinical improvement.

These then are the most common gynaecological and obstetrical conditions with which the physiotherapist will become involved. She will play an important part in the team treating and caring for such women.

MORAL AND ETHICAL PROBLEMS

The physiotherapist will be aware of these issues as they affect the gynaecologist at the present time. She will not get directly involved unless in the after-care of some of the patients about whom these issues are raised. She may well become more closely involved, however, in discussion with the patients themselves and it is as well to look at these questions briefly so that she can begin to evolve her own thoughts and opinions.

ABORTION

The deliberate termination of a pregnancy is permitted by law under the provisions of the Abortion Act 1967 under four headings:

- that a continuing pregnancy would involve risk to the life of the pregnant woman
- that a continuing pregnancy would injure the physical or mental health of the woman
- that a continuing pregnancy would injure the physical or mental health of any existing children in the woman's family
- that there is a substantial risk that if the child is born it would be seriously handicapped.

The law is quite clear and although the second clause is open to wide interpretation this is not in the strict legal sense correct and there is no such thing as a 'social' abortion or abortion on demand.

Many doctors feel unable to take part in implementing the Abortion Act either for religious reasons or other reasons of conscience, and many nurses feel likewise. This is understandable. Where all efforts must be directed is towards the education of young people particularly with regard to sexual promiscuity and its risks, and to contraception, understanding it and using it.

The operation of abortion has many potential risks and perhaps one of the most common long-term complications is pelvic inflammatory disease with its possible outcome of blocked tubes and infertility.

INFERTILITY

This problem, particularly so far as the female is concerned, has been very much in the forefront of medical progress in recent years. Because of the successful advances in treating infertility no couple need despair when all the signs are that they will not achieve a pregnancy by natural means.

The subject is a vast one but the important aspects can be summarized as follows:

Aetiology of infertility

1. *Male causes*: A separate entity which will not be discussed further.
2. *Blockage of Fallopian tubes*: This can follow chronic infection as we have seen. Surgery is possible but not often successful. The

newer option which is proving successful is *in vitro* fertilization (IVF). Here the ovum is taken from the ovary via the laparoscope, fertilized with the husband's sperm in the laboratory (hence the popular description 'test-tube baby') and when successfully fertilized implanted back into the mother's uterus hormonally primed for its reception. This procedure has given otherwise infertile women much success and happiness but it has raised some ethical and moral objections. Is man justified in intervention with natural processes to this extent? Does such a procedure lend itself to 'research' on the developing embryo? But the regulations guiding the conduct of such infertility units are quite specific and any 'research' has only been into improving techniques to make them more successful.

3. *Anovulation* (lack of ovulation): Great advances have been made here in drugs used to stimulate the non-functioning ovary. But in some women the ovaries remain refractory and now the technique of 'donor eggs' is being explored. This again raises many issues – genetic and ethical – and is not widely acceptable as yet.

4. *Other causes of female infertility*: There are many, and not the least common is the unknown.

Hostility of cervical mucus to the partner's sperm with an immunological background may necessitate offering *artificial insemination* either with the partner's sperm (injected directly into the uterine cavity at the time of ovulation) or with donor sperm if the partner is infertile. This latter again raises moral issues but it has been an accepted practice for many years.

GIFT – gamete intra-fallopian transfer – is a new technique particularly suitable for patients with male causes of infertility, immune factors or infertility of unknown origin. In this technique both the ova and the sperm are placed together (via the laparoscope) in the lateral end of the tube where fertilization can take place. Here again the question of unnatural intervention could be raised. Although it is up to each individual to consider their response to these developments and be guided by religious rulings or conscience or whatever, it is difficult to see how the benefit such techniques have brought can be outweighed by hypothetical considerations of 'embryo research' and 'genetic engineering' particularly when one considers the strict ethical and moral protocols observed by the workers in this field.

Surrogate motherhood is another question. Tantamount to 'womb leasing' this involves a healthy woman being inseminated by another woman's husband's sperm so as to 'carry' the pregnancy for that infertile woman. This raises enormous ethical problems particularly where payment may be involved.

All these issues were examined by a Government committee chaired by Lady Warnock which reported in 1984. For those interested, this report or its summary is well worth reading and pondering over.

RAPE

Rape is a difficult and ugly problem which the gynaecologist may have to face. It may involve older or younger women and sometimes even children. It plays a conspicuous part in the topical issue of child abuse.

Defined as 'unlawful sexual intercourse with a woman by force without her consent' it is a legal not a medical diagnosis. Detailed assessment of these patients is imperative particularly with the medico-legal implications in mind.

So far as the management of the victim of rape is concerned repair of injuries, draining haematomata, taking swabs for bacteriological culture, antibiotic therapy, sedation and pain relief are all important aspects. The physiotherapist may be involved in the postoperative care of such patients.

Psychotherapy may be necessary and certainly social workers need to be involved and long-term follow-up of such cases by doctors and social worker teams is desirable medically, psychologically and socially.

Permanent damage to such women is not likely in a physical sense apart from the risk of ascending infection with involvement of the tubes. With adequate management this should be avoided. It is the psychological trauma which is the greatest problem and must be handled expertly and sensitively. In this way the woman's sexual and childbearing future potential may be rescued.

AIDS

AIDS – acquired immune deficiency syndrome – is a new and potentially devastating disease of which all health care workers must be aware. It is mainly described in homosexual men but also found in heterosexuals, drug addicts, haemophiliacs and the female partners of affected males. It can be transferred via blood and body secretions and presents in a variety of ways – pneumonia, fever, parasitic or fungal infections for example. The death rate from the active disease is high. Much has still to be learned about aetiology, causation, prevention and treatment but clear guidelines are now available for those working with patients among whom may be 'at risk' groups. The physiotherapist in her handling of patients and their wounds must be aware of this and take all necessary precautions. To date we are not allowed to screen for the disease without the patient's permission but the observance of strictest hygiene at all times with other 'no touch' techniques for handling of wounds, sputum and so on should give protection.

BIBLIOGRAPHY

Adler, M.W. (ed.) (1988). *ABC of AIDS*. BMA, London.

Anderson, M. (1987). *Infertility: A guide for the anxious couple*. Faber and Faber, London.

Anderson, M. (1986). *An A–Z of Gynaecology: With comments on aspects of management and nursing*. Faber and Faber, London.

Anderson, M. (1983). *The Menopause*. Faber and Faber, London.

Anderson, M. (rev.) (1978). *The Anatomy and Physiology of Obstetrics: A short textbook for students and midwives*. Faber and Faber, London.

Committee of Enquiry into Human Fertilization and Embryology (*Warnock Report*) (1984). HMSO, London.

Kenyon, E. (1986). *The Dilemma of Abortion*. Faber and Faber, London.

Pepperell, R.J., Hudson, B. and Wood, C. (eds) (1987). *The Infertile Couple*, 2nd edition. Churchill Livingstone, Edinburgh.

Warnock, M. (1988). A national ethics committee - Editorial. *British Medical Journal*, 297, 1626–7.

ACKNOWLEDGEMENT

Figures 10/1, 10/2, 10/4, 10/5, and 10/6 have appeared previously in *An A–Z of Gynaecology* by Mary Anderson, and are reproduced by permission of the publisher, Faber and Faber, London.

Chapter 11

Obstetrics

by J. McKENNA MCSP

In the United Kingdom physiotherapists have been involved in parenthood (mothercraft) education from the early 1900s. Since that time midwives and physiotherapists have worked with other members of the obstetric team in providing a pre- and postnatal service. Most parents derive maximum benefit from this team approach with each member giving of their expertise and all working in harmony. It is particularly important that those responsible for the delivery should be closely involved so that all advice is directly related to labour ward policy.

In this chapter reference will be made to the midwife who, in the United Kingdom, has the responsibility for normal deliveries. She works under the direction of the obstetrician who heads the team and is available as required.

The role of the physiotherapist in obstetrics may be considered under three headings: pregnancy, labour and puerperium, although this demarcation should not be emphasized. The pregnant woman should be encouraged to look forward to her postnatal recovery and the pleasures of her new family relationships, and this attitude will help her to face labour. In hospital the physiotherapist is often the one person who sees her through the whole period and is therefore in a position to encourage this positive approach. As well as being a physical experience, childbirth is a deeply emotional one. Brice Pitt (1978) in his book *Enjoying Motherhood* cites *anxiety* as the prevailing emotion. Since a major aspect of parenthood education is encouragement and reassurance the physiotherapist, as well as the whole team, must be sensitive to the very special needs of the parents.

PREGNANCY

Antenatal education is best given in the form of classes of, ideally, not more than a dozen people so that they can be conducted informally with time and opportunity for discussion. Small groups also ensure that those with special needs, such as single parents or those with language problems, can be given particular attention. If convenient, classes may be held in the evening so that both expectant parents can attend, otherwise there should be at least one evening session for partners. Since discussion forms an integral part of the programme, each member of the team must have a basic knowledge of the others' specialties. It is particularly important that the physiotherapist and the midwife work closely together; ideally the physiotherapist should have access to the delivery suite to keep in touch with procedures and see the results of her work.

The aim of the course of classes is to give a full account of the physical and emotional aspects of pregnancy, labour and the puerperium (including diet, clothing – both for the mother and the baby, preparing the home for baby, types of carrying sling, prams, cots, coverings, etc.). Relaxation techniques and postnatal exercises will be an integral part of the classes.

The specific role of the physiotherapist in pregnancy is to promote good health and a sense of well-being, to prevent or alleviate the physical stresses and instigate a training for labour. The physical stresses are caused by the increase in weight with an altered centre of gravity, increased blood volume and hormone changes.

Back problems

The weight increase and the ligamentous laxity caused by hormone change can lead to postural problems if a woman is not helped to compensate. The commonest problem is backache, which is often considered an inevitable consequence of pregnancy. However, the physiotherapist can bring knowledge and skill to refute this view. Good posture must be encouraged throughout, and recent studies point to the benefits of prophylactic care early in pregnancy (Mantle et al, 1981). An introductory class around the 12th–14th week of pregnancy gives an opportunity for advice and instruction to be offered as well as a chance for the parents-to-be to meet members of the obstetric team involved in the preparation programme.

The physiotherapist starts by giving a brief description of normal posture and the changes which will occur as the pregnancy proceeds. This is followed by advice on activities of daily living applied to the pregnant state. Mantle (1988) suggests taking the class through a hypothetical day discussing the various areas of potential problems. The following points might arise from this:

1. *Getting out of bed*: This should be done with the knees bent and gripped together to protect the vulnerable sacro-iliac joint and

avoid straining the abdominal muscles and the lumbar spine.

2. *Posture in standing and walking*: The instruction to 'walk and stand tall' is a useful guide. An early look in a long mirror during this posture correction will reveal the resultant improvement in appearance.

3. *Sitting positions at home and the place of work*: For the office worker, desk chairs may need to be adjusted and the lumbar supportive roll (as recommended by McKenzie, 1980) is particularly appropriate in pregnancy where there is a tendency for an increased lumbar lordosis. The roll should be approximately 31cm long and 10cm in diameter, and may be made from foam rubber or similar material. At home, hard supportive chairs are often found to be more comfortable than armchairs.

4. *Working surfaces and equipment in regular use*: These should be of the right height at home and at work so that bending is avoided.

5. *Heavy lifting*: This should be avoided as far as possible and where necessary performed correctly with knees bent and a straight back.

6. *Shopping*: If heavy, should be divided between both hands to balance the weight.

7. *Back to bed at night*: The mattress should be firm and supportive. Additional pillows may be necessary to help achieve a suitable position for sleeping, e.g. in side lying, a pillow under the upper knee can be comfortable.

It will be helpful to ask those who have backache whether this is worse in the morning or at the end of the day. If the former it may be related to the type of mattress or sleeping position; if the latter to some daily activity or to fatigue. Adequate rest is essential in pregnancy.

If this prophylactic advice is not effective in preventing/curing backache, a full back assessment will be necessary. Once serious pathology has been excluded the usual modalities of treatment (rest, infra-red, massage, etc.) may be employed. Deep heating (SWD, etc.) is contra-indicated in pregnancy but manipulations and mobilizations are safe in skilled hands up until the last month of pregnancy. Sacro-iliac torsion is claimed by some to be a common cause of obstetric backache. Fraser (1976), a Canadian practitioner, describes the following exercise which has been found to be effective where this diagnosis has been reached (the description is for the *right* side): 'In the supine position, the right ankle is grasped by the left hand and pulled into the groin. The right hand is placed below the right knee and the knee is pulled firmly towards a point just outside the right shoulder, while maintaining the heel's position in the groin'. This has the advantage that it can be performed unaided and, if it brings relief, may be repeated two or three times daily. Intransigent back pain, especially if associated with diastasis of the pubic symphysis, may be relieved by some form of support belt.

Circulation

Increased blood volume and the effect of hormones on the elasticity of the vessel walls can cause circulatory problems. The woman should be advised to avoid standing for long periods and, where possible, to rest with the legs elevated. She should be shown how to do vigorous foot and ankle exercises and be given advice regarding the wearing of support tights. It is important that she reports any sudden excessive swelling of her ankles because of its possible relevance to pre-eclampsia. Carpal tunnel syndrome may occur and, if severe, may be relieved by the use of night splints allowing the wrists to rest in a mid-position.

The pelvic floor

Frequency and/or stress incontinence may occur in pregnancy due to hormone change, increased renal activity and pressure of the gravid uterus on the bladder. At an early class the physiotherapist can give welcome reassurance that these symptoms are normal and usually temporary. She should give a simple explanation of the anatomy and function of the pelvic floor muscles related to childbearing and teach how to perform a contraction of these muscles as follows: 'With the knees slightly apart (this prevents any action of the adductors) tighten the muscles around the back passage as if stopping a bowel action and then bring the action forward as if stopping passing water. Draw these tightened muscles up and hold if possible for a count of *four* – then slowly let them down.' This is an opportunity to start a regime of regular practice of the exercise. (A good routine is four to five contractions after each use of the toilet.) This will help to build up an awareness of these important muscles as well as forming an exercise habit to be continued in the postnatal period.

Relaxation

The ability to relax has far-reaching benefits towards an improved lifestyle apart from its particular application to the childbearing period. Relaxation ensures that maximum advantage results from the periods of rest so necessary both in pregnancy and the busy postnatal period. The method most generally taught is that of Laura Mitchell (see Chapter 9). In antenatal classes it is practised in various positions and the women are encouraged to have a daily session at home. Its application as an important component of labour training is discussed later.

General activity

The physiotherapist is the ideal person to give advice on general physical activities which may be continued through pregnancy. Swimming and walking are especially recommended. The advice regarding other sports should take into account the very differing habits of individual women. Fatigue and indulging in highly competitive sports should be avoided. The importance of interspersing activity with rest cannot be over-emphasized.

Specific exercise for pregnancy

An obstetrician, Professor Norman Morris, has commented: 'I am very aware that knowledge of the proper function of muscles and joints helps them to apply the skills of breathing, relaxation and muscular co-ordination during labour in a very practical and effective way' (Morris, 1982).

In many units today the woman is encouraged to participate actively in her labour and, within the bounds of safety, to make choices as to its management. This might include positions for delivery. In order to make these choices and also to use to greatest advantage the skills as described by Professor Morris during labour, the woman needs to have a knowledge of the workings of her body and how to respond to the changing demands of labour. Various schemes of antenatal exercise are designed to achieve this 'body awareness' as well as enhancing general health and laying the foundations of postnatal recovery. The vulnerability of the body in pregnancy makes it advisable that this teaching should be in the hands of skilled professionals.

Exercise in water for pregnancy is becoming increasingly popular. Vleminckx (1988) gives an account of the 'Association Nationale Natation et Maternité' – an association with an international membership for those involved in this type of preparation. She also describes a full programme of exercise and relaxation in water as well as practical information for those wishing to set up such a service.

Schemes overseen by the physiotherapist might include the following items:

Breathing Awareness   A brief description of the organs of respiration is followed by practice of diaphragmatic and costal breathing. Shortness of breath (common as the gravid uterus enlarges) is explained and slow natural breathing associated with relaxation.

Body Awareness   Exercise for the abdominal muscles is adapted to the pregnant state. The following are suitable:

1. Pelvic rocking with abdominal contraction.
2. Alternate hip hitching.
3. Crook lying – rolling the knees slowly to alternate sides.
4. On all-fours – back rounding.

Starting positions may have to be adapted – supine lying in pregnancy can result in pressure on the venae cavae. Exercises which strain the increasingly stretched abdominal muscles must be avoided (e.g. sit-ups and straight leg raising).

Stretching Exercises and Postures (to prepare for delivery positions).

1. Cross-leg sitting – changing the front leg periodically.
2. Tailor sitting with soles of the feet together.
3. Long sitting – stretching the legs apart.
4. Squatting (this position should be held for an increasing length of time each day – support may be had from a chair or against a wall).

In addition to the above, every exercise session should include practice of pelvic floor contractions, relaxation and posture correction.

LABOUR

A programme of labour training forms an important element of the antenatal classes. Today's methods have evolved from various past trends and no doubt will continue to be changed and modified. Instruction must always be directly related to the labour ward routines of the unit concerned and ideally given in co-operation with the midwife. The overall aim is to give a woman confidence in herself and a trust in those caring for her. Rehearsals for labour embody the skills learned of relaxation, breathing and body awareness and they should, where possible, involve the partner.

Throughout the training the unpredictability of labour must be emphasized. The woman should be taught about the methods of pain relief available in her unit and be ready to take advantage of them where necessary. The concern of all should be for her to have the best possible labour experience. For some this will be achieved with the learned physical skills alone; others may need varying amounts of analgesia. If TENS is available the physiotherapist may instruct the parents-to-be and the midwife in its use. It has the advantage of being non-pharmacological and allowing the woman to remain mobile.

In the class programme a session in the use of inhalant analgesia may be included. The most usual agent used is Entonox (50% oxygen and 50% nitrous oxide). Using a disconnected machine the woman is taught the technique of inhaling and advised that this should be started at the very beginning of a contraction.

Relaxation for labour

Some form of neuromuscular control has been part of the programme since the earliest days of antenatal education. During all stages of labour an ability to relax will help to conserve energy and is an aid to emotional stability. It can also have the effect of raising the pain threshold as it overcomes the body's natural 'fight or flee' reaction to pain. Thus it may be described as the first defence against the pain of contractions. However, physical relaxation can never be completely achieved in a state of anxiety; the ease of mind acquired with knowledge and understanding, reinforced during labour by caring staff, is essential.

In the early part of the first stage of labour the woman may be encouraged to keep active and mobile, which has been shown to be advantageous regarding the length of labour and the need for analgesia (Flynn et al, 1978). During contractions she may feel the need to take up a comfortable resting position and relax. As the strength of the contractions increases she will help herself further by concentrating on the slow natural breathing which complements the relaxation. If she has learned the Mitchell method she will recognize at the end of each contraction if she has picked up any tension and will quickly check through her body re-adjusting all her joints to the position of ease. This is important so that a gradual build-up of tension is avoided.

During the second stage she will welcome periods of relaxation to recover from each pushing effort and conserve energy for the next.

Breathing for labour

Formal breathing patterns to be practised during first stage contractions have featured in many of the teaching programmes of the past. There seems to have been scant physiological basis for them and they have gradually been abandoned. A research project by St John Buxton in collaboration with the Obstetric Association of Chartered Physiotherapists to investigate the effects of different types of breathing being taught at that time found that the rigid pattern of differing levels, such as featured in the psychoprophylaxis method, caused hyperventilation and increased the stress and anxiety they purported to relieve (Buxton, 1965). This view is further supported by Stradling (1983) who commented that 'it is likely that the mother's physiology knows best during labour, and that a better pattern of breathing that she could be taught, does not exist'. Rather than impose a regime of breathing patterns it is preferable to encourage the woman to be sensitive to the demands of her body and to concentrate on the *natural* breathing rate during her contractions. During the antenatal relaxation sessions she will have experienced the slow easy breathing associated with complete relaxation and realized the importance of avoiding the fast shallow breathing or breath-holding common in tension situations. She is taught to 'listen in' as she relaxes through her first stage contractions to the rhythm of slow natural breathing. She may be shown a special 'pattern' to use when the build-up of the strength of contractions in late first stage makes the deep breathing impossible and threatens to result in breath-holding. A popular pattern is gentle 'sighing-out' breaths through parted lips – S.O.S. (sigh out slowly). If she needs to control a premature urge to push due to an anterior lip (at the end of the first stage) this same breathing may help her.

In the second stage of labour studies have indicated that breath-holding and forced pushing with a closed glottis is unproductive and may cause compression of the uterine blood vessels (Stradling, 1983). This can result in problems to an already compromised fetus. A deep breath at the start of the contraction should be followed by pushing with slight expiration interspersed with new breath intakes.

Body awareness and labour

In the first stage of labour sensitivity to her body will help the woman to take up positions of comfort during her contractions. While she is mobile the following may be tried:

(a) sitting with head and shoulders resting on a table.
(b) standing leaning against a wall – either facing or with back supported.
(c) stride sitting across a chair resting the head and arms on the back.
(d) on all-fours on the floor.
(e) supported by partner, standing resting head on his shoulder.

When in bed, assisted by a sympathetic midwife (with a supply of pillows) she also has a range of possible positions for relaxation. 'Listening' to her body helps her to find the most comfortable one and also to be ready to change position to suit her needs. If she has the problem of premature urge to push this can often be controlled by adopting a forward kneeling position with her hips higher than her head.

For the second stage the work of Russell (1982) has brought about a revolution in delivery positions. He found that the increased mobility of the pelvic joints gave the possibility of a 28 per cent increase in the pelvic outlet in upright (primitive) positions such as squatting, kneeling, all-fours. Antenatal instruction should discourage a woman from planning beforehand precise details for delivery; rather she should be ready to 'listen' to her body and move into appropriately comfortable positions. The stretching exercises practised antenatally will help her to sustain these positions.

Rehearsals for labour

Where possible these should include the partner or other supporter in labour. *Emotional* support is the most important aspect of partner participation but there are also many practical aids.

1st Stage The partner can support the various resting positions already described as well as providing distraction and company for what can be a lengthy period. Later, when the contractions become stronger and painful he can encourage relaxation, help her to move around the bed into positions of comfort, watch her breathing and remind her to keep it calm and slow, and massage her back. If she is needing the S.O.S. breathing (p. 156) in any crisis he can do this with her while having eye-to-eye contact.

2nd Stage The woman will need support in the various upright positions for delivery (see above) and again will need to be reminded of the techniques of breathing and pushing she has learned in the classes.

The advantages, both emotional and practical, of the presence of a sympathetic partner or other chosen companion cannot be over-estimated. In addition parents today appreciate the sharing of the birth experience.

THE PUERPERIUM

The best use of the physiotherapist in the postnatal period is in taking group sessions. This enables her to give more time and attention to the mothers who will also benefit from each other's company. Formal exercise should be kept to a minimum bearing in mind that the early weeks after delivery can be the busiest time in a woman's life. During the first 24 hours post-delivery the physiotherapist should see each woman individually. The following may be practised:

1. Deep breathing and circulation exercises for feet and ankles.
2. Pelvic rocking with abdominal contraction.
3. Pelvic floor contractions – these may be started within hours of delivery; those who have had stitches need to be reassured that no harm will come to them.

In the following days during group sessions a few carefully chosen exercises are better than a long list. Each woman should be tested for diastasis (divarication) of the recti in crook lying. The physiotherapist or the woman herself measures, with the fingers, the gap between the recti as the head is raised. If the gap is greater than two fingers' breadth, twisting and bending exercises should be avoided. Carefully controlled inner range exercise only for the recti should be practised until the gap closes sufficiently.

The following are suggested exercises for the abdominal muscles:

1. Crook lying, abdominal contraction – stretching hands towards knees (this can be progressed by lifting the head and shoulders up during the action).
2. Lying with one leg bent and one straight – shortening the straight leg with abdominal tightening.
3. Crook lying – rolling both knees to alternate sides. This should be done slowly, contracting the abdominal muscles before each action.
4. For cases of diastasis recti (divarication of the recti): crook lying – abdominal contraction using crossed hands to pull the recti together.

The foundations of postnatal recovery are best laid in the antenatal period when the woman is receptive and not yet involved in the many occupations of motherhood. Ideally she will form habits of good posture ('walk tall') as well as regular practice of the important pelvic floor muscles ('four contractions after each use of the toilet') which will benefit her postnatally. The main part of the postnatal group sessions should be devoted to daily living advice with special reference to the new mother's commitments. Much of this is similar to the antenatal instruction related to correct lifting, correct heights of working surfaces, protection of the sacro-iliac joint (remembering that the hormone imbalance causing ligamentous laxity can remain for many weeks after delivery). New mothers should be reminded how periods of relaxation can relieve tiredness and a practice session should be included. Breast feeding can cause muscle tension and the physiotherapist can give invaluable help by teaching good positioning with shoulder joints in the ease position and support for the back. Backache can cause fatigue and add to the considerable pressures on the new mother. Individual advice and treatment is similar to that given antenatally (p. 150). Special cases will also need the individual care of the physiotherapist. A woman who has had a caesarean delivery will need postoperative chest and circulation care although the increasing use of epidural anaesthesia has reduced chest problems. A sore perineum following a tear or episiotomy is usually relieved by salt baths or ice application. Pulsed electromagnetic energy (PEME) and ultrasound may be effective, but it is not possible to give precise details of dosage. There are numerous models of machines available and the therapist is advised to read the treatment instructions carefully and to consult with colleagues who have experience of the particular machine. Careful records of the treatment given, including dosage, should be kept so that results may be evaluated. With both PEME and ultrasound, treatment should not be started before 12 hours postpartum; in both cases the current used should be sub-thermal.

The success of postnatal rehabilitation depends largely on the enthusiasm of the physiotherapist who must supply the motivation to women who are often overwhelmed by the experience of motherhood. Sometimes it can be many weeks before a woman is sufficiently settled into her new life to think about herself. Later postnatal support groups (in the United Kingdom often held in the community) are invaluable, particularly if a physiotherapist can be involved. This gives an opportunity to check for any outstanding problems such as backache, incontinence, dyspareunia, and give appropriate advice and treatment.

The recovery of the pelvic floor muscles may be checked in the following way – with a half-full bladder the woman 'bounces' up and down and gives a strong cough. Any leakage indicates a further need for exercise. If after three months the problem persists, the woman should be referred to the gynaecologist to be assessed and treated (see Chapters 10 and 12). An enjoyable scheme of later exercise with the baby is described in *Postnatal Exercise* (Whiteford and Polden, 1984) and these are ideal for use in community clinics. Relaxation and posture correction should be part of each session.

Today every woman looks forward to the birth of a normal healthy baby. In the event of an unhappy outcome of infant death or congenital disability the physiotherapist can give much-needed emotional support. In cases of certain curable conditions such as talipes, congenital dislocation of hip, it can be reassuring to show the mother a series of photos of cures resulting from treatment. She may also be put in touch with an appropriate support group, meeting those with similar problems. Obstetric physiotherapists are becoming increasingly aware of this important aspect of their work and are taking courses in counselling skills.

In the United Kingdom the obstetric physiotherapist often works in the gynaecology ward/clinic as well which enables her to view a wide span of a woman's life. Stress incontinence is an example of a condition met with both obstetrically as well as in the gynaecology unit. The physiotherapist knows that good training following childbirth results in far-reaching benefits; it is her responsibility to apply her skills in the ante- and postnatal periods thus making an important contribution to the realm of preventive medicine and general health care.

REFERENCES

Brice Pitt, D. (1978). *Enjoying Motherhood*. Sheldon Press, London.

Buxton, R. St J. (1965). Breathing in labour: the influence of psychoprophylaxis. *Nursing Mirror*, **120**, 3128, 8–9.

Flynn, A. M., Kelly, J., Hollins, G. and Lynch, P. F. (1978). Ambulation in labour. *British Medical Journal*, **2**, 591–3.

Fraser, D. (1976). Postpartum backache: a preventable condition? *Canadian Family Physician*, **22**, 1434–6.

Mantle, M. J., Holmes, J. and Currey, H. L. F. (1981). Backache in pregnancy: prophylactic influence of back care classes. *Rheumatology and Rehabilitation*, **20**, 227–32.

Mantle, M. J. (1988). Backache in pregnancy. Chapter in *Obstetrics and Gynaecology*. *International Perspectives in Physical Therapy*. Churchill Livingstone, Edinburgh.

McKenzie, R. (1980). *Treat Your Own Back*. Spinal Publications, Waikanae, New
Zealand. (UK distributor – Spinal Publications (UK), PO Box 275, West Byfleet,
Surrey KT14 6ET)

Morris, N. (1982). Introduction to *Exercises for Childbirth* (Dale, B. and Roeber, J.).
Century Publications, London.

Russell, J. G. B. (1982). The rationale of primitive delivery positions. *British Journal
of Obstetrics and Gynaecology*, **89**, 712–15.

Stradling, J. (1983). Respiratory physiology in labour. *Journal of the Association of
Chartered Physiotherapists in Obstetrics and Gynaecology*, **53**, 5–7.

Vleminckx, M. (1988). Pregnancy and recovery: the aquatic approach. Chapter in
Obstetrics and Gynaecology. International Perspectives in Physical Therapy. Churchill
Livingstone, Edinburgh.

BIBLIOGRAPHY

The titles marked * are particularly recommended.

Bourne, G. (1984). *Pregnancy*, revised edition. Pan Books, London.

England, M. A. (1983). *A Colour Atlas of Life before Birth*. Wolfe Medical
Publications, London.

Grieve, G. P. (1988). *Common Vertebral Joint Problems*, 2nd edition. Churchill
Livingstone, Edinburgh.

Kitzinger, S. (1984). *The Experience of Childbirth*, 5th edition. Penguin Books,
Harmondsworth.

Llewellyn-Jones, D. (1986). *Fundamentals of Obstetrics and Gynaecology*, vol. 1.
Obstetrics, 4th edition. Faber and Faber, London.

Llewellyn-Jones, D. (1989). *Everywoman: A Gynaecological Guide for Life*, 5th
edition. Faber and Faber, London.

McKenna, J. (ed.) (1988). *Obstetrics and Gynaecology. International Perspectives in
Physical Therapy*. Churchill Livingstone, Edinburgh.

Mitchell, L. (1987). *Simple Relaxation*, 2nd edition. John Murray, London.

Noble, E. (1988). *Essential Exercises for the Childbearing Year*, 3rd edition. Houghton
Mifflin Company, Boston, USA.

*Whiteford, B. and Polden, M. (1984). *Postnatal Exercises*. Century Publications,
London.

*Williams, M. and Booth, D. (1985). *Antenatal Education: Guidelines for Teachers*, 3rd
edition. Churchill Livingstone, Edinburgh.

Chapter 12

Gynaecology
by S. M. HARRISON MCSP

Physiotherapy cover on gynaecological wards varies throughout the country. In some hospitals the physiotherapist will only treat patients who develop a chest infection with an accumulation of secretions after a general anaesthetic; other hospitals will have a therapist in attendance for a short period every day.

Statistics indicate that 90 per cent of the major operations in a gynaecology unit are hysterectomies and vaginal repairs. Most of these women will have borne children; thus there are a large number of women, of all ages, whose pelvic floor and abdominal muscles and backs have been subjected to the strains of childbearing. It can be argued that these women will achieve a more complete recovery if they are shown how to strengthen their pelvic floor, abdominal and back muscles, and be given advice on self-care at home. The following points indicate differences in treatment regimes which may be used for other surgical patients.

Deep vein thrombosis

Patients who have had a pelvic operation appear to be more susceptible to deep vein thrombosis, therefore special precautions should be taken:

1. If Tubigrip or anti-embolic stockings have not been applied prior to operation or in the theatre, the physiotherapist may be asked to do this when the patient returns to the ward.
2. The foot of the bed can be elevated and a bed cradle used to facilitate frequent foot and leg movements. These are most effective if practised slowly and strongly.
3. Extra emphasis should be placed on full chest breathing, practised frequently, to improve venous return and move secretions in readiness for coughing.

Coughing

Secretions are most effectively dealt with if a patient is in a curled-up position sitting up, or in side lying, with forearms 'cuddled' over the incision to prevent movement. They should be shown (preferably pre-operatively) how to move the secretions towards the bronchi with long, easy, slow breathing. Repeated 'huffs' (see p. 96) will project the mucus into the mouth with the minimum of discomfort. For vaginal operations, one hand should be placed on the sanitary towel with firm pressure upwards when coughing.

Pelvic rocking

This activity encourages the viscera to move away from the incision, prevents protective muscle spasm in the abdomen and back and decreases the pain from flatulence by speeding the dispersal of gases. Pelvic rocking should be commenced as soon as possible on recovery of consciousness. It is most easily taught as follows:

The patient is in crook lying with hands resting on hip bones; she is then told to 'Tilt your hip bones towards your face – hold for four seconds and put it down slowly.'

Repeat in a rocking rhythm several times an hour. The patient will also feel the tilting of her pelvis under her hands and notice her lumbar spine flattening and hollowing. This is a simple, non-threatening and comfortable activity which can give patients confidence to make other movements even after extensive surgery, e.g. Wertheim's hysterectomy.

Correction of posture

As soon as drainage tubes allow ambulation the patient should be encouraged to adopt an upright posture using the phrase 'stand tall'. As the top of the head is pressed upwards, the vertebral column is stretched and opened, the pelvis tilts back and alignment of hips, knees and ankles is corrected automatically. This becomes the 'new posture' after a few days if it is practised whenever upright.

Further activity

The provision of an illustrated leaflet can be useful to promote further activity. If such a leaflet is available it should be given to patients in the pre-operative period so that they are able to understand that a programme of continuous care and activity in hospital and at home will reduce the effects of an anaesthetic and surgery and speed their restoration to normality.

Suggested Contents of Leaflet

1. Pre- and postoperative breathing and coughing.
2. Foot and leg movements.
3. Pelvic rocking.
4. Posture correction: 'stand tall'.
5. Pelvic floor information and exercises. Starting dates to be discussed with surgeon after vaginal repairs.
6. Graduated exercises to strengthen abdominal and back muscles.
7. Advice for home care, see below.

Advice for Home Care   In addition to your exercises:

1. When you go home you will tire easily – lie on your bed for an extra rest during the day – for several weeks.
2. Do not return to full-time work until after your post-operation clinic visit (about six weeks after the operation).
3. It is common to have twinges of pain around the site of your wound for a few weeks.
4. Forceful pulling or pushing (vacuuming or opening swing doors) will seem difficult – start when you feel able.
5. Avoid straining to open your bowels – seek advice if necessary.
6. Your bladder will take a week or two to settle down – pelvic floor exercises will help.
7. No heavy lifting. Moderate lifting and carrying must be avoided for six to eight weeks. After this, if the pelvic floor is braced when lifting – especially after vaginal repairs – the effect of the downward thrust in the pelvis is reduced. Get help to lift whenever possible.
   Always remember:
   Bend your knees, hold heavy objects close to you, and twist from your feet and not your spine.
   Teach your family the 'safe' way as well!
8. All operations are different, so it is better not to compare your progress with friends.

Infra-red irradiation and short wave diathermy

Heat can be very effective in speeding the healing of infected and slow-healing wounds. Care should be taken to ensure that an adequate area of skin around the incision is exposed to the heat, as thermal sensation in the proximity of a wound is frequently impaired. The presence of metal within the tissues or in the form of metal clips or buttons anchoring a continuous suture is a contra-indication to any form of heat treatment.

Infra-red irradiation has been found to be particularly useful in promoting granulation of the open areas after a radical vulvectomy. Twice-daily treatment, seven days a week, is recommended.

Short wave diathermy for an infected abdominal wound is most easily carried out using a co-planar method with medium sized disc electrodes placed over normal skin either side of the incision. After an initial thermal treatment of 10 minutes, a 20-minute period repeated twice daily seems most satisfactory. Further details and contra-indications are on page 181.

PHYSIOTHERAPY FOR GYNAECOLOGY OUT-PATIENTS

The following additional comments relating to the pelvic floor anatomy should be read in conjunction with the diagrams and description on pages 132–3.

The pelvic floor comprises three layers:

1. *Superficial* (perineal): Bands of striated muscles radiating outwards to the pelvic bones from the central tendinous point of the perineum (perineal body).
2. *Middle* (urogenital diaphragm): A sheet of fascia filling the triangular space below the symphysis pubis and the pubic rami. It is pierced by the urethra and vagina and contains some muscle fibres in the urethral portion (compressor urethrae) and below the vagina (deep transverse perineal). The latter are inserted into the perineal body.
3. *Deep* (levator ani): A composite group of striated muscles which form the sling-like base of the pelvic floor. They are made up of types I and II fibres (Gosling et al, 1981). There is a predominance of type I fibres throughout; the proportion of I:II varies in different parts of the muscle group.

   The muscles originate from bone and fascia on each side of the pelvic brim and pass backwards towards the coccyx and insert centrally into the anococcygeal raphe (levator plate). The central portions (the pubococcygeii) have free inner borders as they do not meet around the urethra and vagina anteriorly, the gap being greatest when the muscles are stretched and weak. They are innervated by the pudendal nerve (S 2,3,4). The puborectalis is different. It is a single continuous U-shaped loop of muscle originating from the posterior aspect of the pubis passing behind the rectum to form the acute anorectal angle and returning to the pubis for insertion.

The anorectal angle is an efficient flap-valve mechanism due to the pull of puborectalis and the sealing effect of raised intra-abdominal pressure.

The puborectalis lies in a vertical plane below the rest of levator ani so its upper fibres are apposed to the latter muscle (Shafik, 1975; Swash, 1985). Innervation of the puborectalis is from a branch of the sacral nerve (S 3,4) which lies above the pelvic floor (Percy et al, 1981).

Urethral Musculature The middle third of the female urethra contains a striated muscle collar, thicker anteriorly, which forms the external urethral sphincter (not to be confused with levator ani). The sphincter is made up of type I fibres and assists in maintaining urethral closure over long periods. Innervation is via the pelvic splanchnic nerves from S 2,3,4.

Figure 12/1 shows how additional pressure to maintain urethral closure is obtained from rises in intra-abdominal pressure – providing the bladder neck lies above the pelvic floor. When the bladder descends this cannot occur.

Fascia plays an important role in the pelvic floor as it ensheaths the muscles and forms most of their origins and insertions. Surgeons report that the proportion of muscle tissue to fascia is very variable. It is also known that the thinning and loss of muscle fibres laterally is

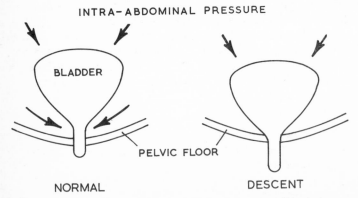

Fig. 12.1 The effect on the urethra of the transmission of intra-abdominal pressure

accentuated in obese women and women of advancing age. After the menopause this can be due to substitution of muscle fibres by collagen tissue. There is also a correlation of levator muscle mass to general body musculature (Zacharin, 1980).

Comparative studies of the quality of the levator muscles in Occidental and Oriental women have highlighted the greater muscle bulk and less deterioration of the muscles with age in the latter group. Explanations to account for these changes include adoption of squatting positions for many daily activities, physically hard lifestyle, a diet which discourages obesity, and genetic differences (Zacharin, 1977).

One cause of dysfunction of the pelvic floor muscles is difficult childbearing; similarly, straining due to chronic constipation. Both can cause damage to the innervation of the pelvic floor muscles. It seems likely that this damage is cumulative and more likely to be irreversible as childbearing continues (Parkes et al, 1977; Snooks et al, 1984).

Function of the Pelvic Floor Muscles

1. Support of the viscera.
2. Compressive action as part of the closure mechanism of the urethra, vagina and bowel.
3. Reflex action in maintenance of intra-abdominal pressure.

INCONTINENCE

Incontinence is a symptom – not a diagnosis. By definition it is the inability to control the passing of urine and faeces so that either or both excretions are passed at inappropriate times or places.

During the past 15 years this topic, previously hidden by sufferers and largely ignored by health professionals, has become a subject for research, education and discussion. International and national organizations have members with enthusiasm and dedication whose aim is to ensure incontinence is identified, then cured, reduced or managed well; but above all they want to 'promote continence' and this commences with prevention.

To be continent a person has to:

– register the need to pass urine or faeces
– know where the toilet or receptacle is located – or be able to summon assistance
– be able to reach the toilet
– undress adequately

– sit or stand safely
– and perform all these activities in time!

A sudden or gradual change in a person's health status or her/his environment can precipitate her into a cycle of events in which incontinence becomes a dominant and distressing factor.

Incontinence is a complex subject and the following discussion is designed to assist physiotherapists distinguish between the various types of incontinence when assessing patients. This will enable an effective physiotherapy treatment programme to be given or onward referral to a more appropriate adviser.

(In this text information about urinary incontinence predominates. Faecal incontinence will be mentioned when appropriate.)

Types of incontinence

Stress Incontinence   This may be a symptom, sign or a condition.

The *symptom* is an involuntary loss of urine on exertion, e.g. coughing or running. The *sign* is the observation of loss of urine from the urethra when coughing or straining, sometimes only when upright. As a *condition* 'genuine stress incontinence' (as defined by the International Continence Society) is 'the involuntary loss of urine when pressure in the bladder exceeds maximal urethral pressure in the absence of a detrusor contraction'. When genuine stress incontinence is accompanied by a minor degree of vaginal wall prolapse, re-education of the pelvic floor muscles can alleviate the incontinence. The exercises can also assist when surgical correction of the condition is only partially effective.

Idiopathic stress incontinence of faeces (particularly in the post-partum period) responds well to re-education of the puborectalis.

Urge Incontinence   This is the involuntary loss of urine associated with a strong desire to void. It is most easily understood if it is divided into motor and sensory types.

Motor urge is characterized by uninhibited detrusor contractions (detrusor instability). It is responsible for at least 30 per cent of gynaecological referrals (Frewen, 1978). It is more common in the elderly as it can be secondary to atherosclerosis. In many women the cause is never found. Bladder training can be used to good effect (p. 176).

Sensory urge is generally related to an acute or chronic infection, urinary calculi or bladder tumour. Treatment is with antibiotics or by surgery.

Overflow Incontinence This is the involuntary loss of residual urine in dribbles or jets (on movement) when the bladder is unable to empty completely. The condition is often caused by an obstruction to the outflow of urine, e.g. enlarged prostate gland or impacted faeces (especially in the elderly), a retroverted gravid uterus, pelvic tumour or urethral stenosis. But it can also occur in people who have overstretched atonic bladders that are unable to contract, e.g. after repeated overdistension or linked to diabetic neuropathy.

Reflex Incontinence (neurogenic) This is the voluntary loss of urine due to abnormal reflex activity in the spinal cord in the absence of sensation usually associated with the desire to micturate. It is associated with a wide range of disorders which affect the brain and spinal cord, including trauma, e.g. paraplegia.

Each type requires its own special management.

Continuous Incontinence This may result from pathological or structural abnormality or be related to major trauma or surgery, e.g. a fistula.

Frequency This is usually defined as the passage of urine seven or more times during the day and waking twice or more at night to void. It often presents with other types of incontinence. 'Self-induced' frequency is found in patients who make a habit of voiding regardless of a desire to do so because they are frightened of leaking urine. They can develop small 'just in case' bladders which become very inconvenient with ageing as frequency will increase. The condition often responds well to bladder training (p. 176).

In some patients urodynamic, radiological and electromyographic studies are necessary to complete a diagnosis.

PATIENTS REQUIRING RE-EDUCATION OF THE PELVIC FLOOR

These fall into two groups – postpartum and menopausal. This means that the age of patients being treated may vary from the early twenties to the late seventies. Referrals may come from many sources, e.g. gynaecologists, urologists, general practitioners, postnatal clinics, family planning clinics, health visitors and self-referral by women. The latter is particularly relevant for women who have their babies in hospitals where physiotherapists give them postnatal advice and exercises to combat the effects of childbearing. In such instances, if problems then arise at home in respect of these activities self-referral allows the woman to contact the physiotherapist quickly and receive further advice. Liaison with the general practitioner by the physiotherapist will follow when necessary.

Presenting symptoms

1. Pelvic floor laxity.
2. Stress incontinence.

One or both of these symptoms may be present in the menopausal group as a result of progressive oestrogen deficiency. Changes in the vaginal mucosa lead to the hot, dry irritation of senile vaginitis, while in the urethra the mucosa shrinks and allows urine to escape more easily. Oestrogen therapy in the form of implant, oral tablets or topical cream is frequently beneficial.

Pelvic Floor Laxity When the pelvic floor muscles are stretched and weak the support for the pelvic organs is poor and patients complain of 'heaviness' in the perineal area. Varying degrees of overstretch of the walls of the vagina and urethra (cystocele, rectocele and urethrocele) and uterine supports (1st, 2nd and 3rd degree uterine prolapse) may be found (Chapter 10).

Re-education of the levator muscles will relieve these symptoms if they are mild. If there is severe fascial stretching (e.g. gross cystocele or 2nd or 3rd degree uterine prolapse) surgery is required. Pre-operative pelvic floor exercises are worthwhile in most cases.

Sexual problems can arise as a result of pelvic floor laxity. The vagina will feel slack and lacking in 'squeeze' as the weak muscles are unable to compress the vagina during intercourse. There is also likely to be difficulty in retaining a contraceptive diaphragm or tampon.

Some women find air becomes trapped inside the slack vagina and become very distressed and embarrassed when this 'vaginal flatus' escapes noisily as they move about.

Stress Incontinence (p. 168)

ASSESSMENT AND TREATMENT OF THE PELVIC FLOOR

Quiet, comfort, privacy and time are essential for the patient's first visit; wherever possible the patient (client) should be seen in a consulting room as curtained cubicles are not acceptable. At least 45 minutes is required for the initial interview.

History An assessment chart is a useful way of recording the relevant facts about all aspects of the client's history, lifestyle and the results of the digital assessments (Fig. 12/2). In some cases an accurate record of the woman's bladder function in the form of a urinary diary is necessary to determine if bladder training or other advice is required. This can be completed for five days and brought to the first appointment or between first and second visits.

Explanation This should include simple details about the anatomy of the pelvis with a diagram. Two cupped hands, palms uppermost, hypothenar eminences touching, and a 2.5cm (1in) gap between the little fingers is the best way of illustrating the levator muscles. The compression of the rectum, vagina and urethra by the pubococcygeus and puborectalis is shown by bringing the little fingers together and raising the central portion of the hands to simulate the 'squeeze and lift' the woman is expected to feel. The function of the muscles is explained mentioning the different sensations when the muscles are weak and strong and relating this to the person's symptoms and the need for a re-education programme.

Assessment of the pelvic floor muscles and initial instruction

This is an essential part of the treatment. The muscles are not visible so the therapist must use a digital check and/or a vaginal pressure gauge (perineometer) to monitor the strength of the pelvic floor muscles and whether the exercise is being performed accurately.

During this period the therapist must be particularly mindful of the woman's sensibilities and use her words and actions with care.

Method The woman is positioned on a couch in crook lying with her knees and feet apart and suitably covered. Additional lighting may be required to illuminate the perineum. Wearing disposable gloves and using the thumb and finger of her left hand the therapist separates the labia and notes any sign of inflammation, discharge or uterovaginal prolapse. She asks the woman to cough twice and 'strain' downwards, noticing any bulging at the introitus or leakage of urine. She then applies some vaginal lubricant to her fingers. With the phrase 'I am going to slide two fingers into your birth canal, so make room for my fingers', she introduces the index and middle fingers of her right hand into the vagina – *slowly*. This is not a

PHYSIOTHERAPY WOMEN'S HEALTH ASSESSMENT FORM - Gynaecology and Promotion of Continence

NAME: _Mary Brown_   AGE: _38_   WEIGHT: _75 kg target 65 kg_

ADDRESS: _2, Main St. Benton_   TELEPHONE: H _123 9876_ W

OCCUPATION: _Shop Asst. (heavy lifting)_   DOCTOR: _Johnson_   DATE: _10·8·88_

---

1. PRESENTING PROBLEM (As described by patient)
   Leaks Urine on exertion
   Duration: _13 yrs - worse since doing_
   present job.
   Referral Comments:
   GP- Cystocele & S.I

2. OBS - GYN. HISTORY

   Parity: _2 + 1 miscarriage_

Date	Weight	Delivery	Epidural	Epis	2nd Stage
1975	8-1	Forceps	✓	✓	2 hrs
1977	Misc				
1978	8-6	SVD	—	✓	10 mins

   Menarche: Age _13_   Cycle: _4-5 / 30_
              Perimenopausal (o)
              Postmenopausal (o)
   Effect of menses on condition _Worse 7 days_
   before.
   Breastfeeding ....

3. SURGERY
   Type _D + C_
   Date _March '77 after misc_
   Outcome _—_

4. MEDICAL HISTORY

   Diabetes   ( )   Hypertension   ( )
   Cystitis   ( )   Hay Fever   (✓)
   Chronic Respiratory Disease ( )
   Back Pain   ( )   Effect ....
   Trauma _MVA_ (✓)   Other ....
   Whiplash

5. MICTURITION PATTERN:
   Frequency: (hours) _1½ - 2_
   Nocturia: .... _× 2_
   Nocturnal Enuresis (o)
   Dysuria: _o_   Haematuria: _o_
   Urgency (o) Hold Time ....
   Urge Incontinence (o)

True Stress Incontinence

Mild	( )	Mod	(✓)	Severe	( )
Cough	(✓)	Sneeze	(✓)	Laugh	( )
Run	( )	Jump	(✓)	Orgasm	( )

Sport ... _aerobics_ ....

S.I. + Detrusor Instability (o)

Protective Underwear - Pads/day _1 aerobics_
                         Pants/day _2_

Bladder function chart _passes small amounts_
'just in case'. leakage shown

Urinalysis: (Yes) No Result _clear_

Urodynamics: Yes (No) Result ....

---

6. FLUID INTAKE

Liquid/day: _5_ Cups   _No water_

Caffeine/day:

coffee (4) Cups   Cola ( ) Cups

Chocolate ( ) Cups   Tea (1) Cups

Alcohol:

Amount: _minimal_

---

7. BOWEL PATTERN

Loose ( )   Normal ( )   Constipated (✓)
Strain (✓)   Haemorrhoids ( ) Soiling ( )

Diet _low fibre & fluid ↓_

---

8. Coitus _Sensation ↓ - 'slack'_
   Contraception _Condom_

---

9. DRUGS _occ. for Hay fever_

Fig. 12.2 Assessment chart for re-education of pelvic floor muscles (PFM)

10. PERINEAL/VAGINAL EXAMINATION

VISUAL	DIGITAL
Nil relevent	*Slack*
Cough *Perineal descent*	Cough ⎫ *cervix descends to 1cm*
Effort *anterior vaginal wall bulge*	Effort ⎭ *of introitus .*

STATUS P.V.:   Cystocele   (✓)   Min/(Mod)/Severe/Nil

Rectocele   ( )   Min/Mod/Severe/(Nil)

Uterine descent   (✓)   1°/(2a)/ 2b/ 3 / Nil

Other   ( )   ....

PELVIC FLOOR MUSCLES:

Muscle	Good	Mod	Weak	None	Comment
Perineal			✓		
Pubococcygeus			✓		
Puborectalis P.V (✓) P.R ( )		✓			

Date	*10·8·88*	*31·8·88*	*28·9·88*	*26·10·88*	*30·11·88*
Perineometer	*3*	*3*	*6*	*7*	*8*
Hold Time	*2 secs*	*5 secs*	*4 secs*	*6 secs*	*6 secs*

Wt - 68 kgs .

COMMENTS: *Well motivated lady . referred by G.P*
Needs to change lifestyle & work practice

INITIAL ACTION:

1. *PFX with leaflet - fill in record chart*
2. *Diet change - fibre ↑ water ↑ (3-4 glasses/day) constipation leaflet*
3. *Brace PFM when lifting - share loads*
4. *Retrain bladder by timed micturition delay — aim for 4 hrs*
5. *Low impact aerobics - reduce weight. See monthly*

difficult procedure if the direction of the vagina is visualized and the muscles relaxed by the use of the afore-mentioned phrase.

Keeping her fingers in place, the therapist asks the woman to 'strain' and cough again – any descent of the base of the bladder, the cervix or anterior and posterior vaginal walls will be noted. If there is a large degree of uterovaginal prolapse the therapist's fingers may be pushed out of the vagina.

To assess the strength of the pelvic floor muscles the following phrases are useful:

(a) With fingers *open* palpating the pubococcygeii: 'Close my fingers'.
(b) With fingers closed: 'Don't let me pull my fingers out'.
(c) With fingers closed: 'Squeeze my fingers'.
(d) With fingers palpating posterior vaginal wall: 'Imagine you have diarrhoea so close your back passage'.

Phrase (d) will elicit a contraction of puborectalis.

If the woman's problem relates more to poor bowel control it is advisable to add another component to the assessment. In the side-lying position using new gloves check the strength of the pubo-rectalis by inserting the index finger through the anus to the anorec-tal angle. Using (d) the muscle strength can be assessed and re-educated in this way.

Using the woman's best visualization and contraction from (a) to (d) she must now learn to formulate this into an exercise which can be repeated many times a day.

Most people find this phrase useful: 'Close your back and front passages, draw them up inside so you feel a squeeze and lift – hold for four seconds and let go slowly'. Some women will only start with a two- or three-second hold – all should aim to progress to 10 seconds.

When the therapist is satisfied the woman can do this, she concludes the assessment. A vaginal pressure gauge or perineometer is valuable as a teaching aid and over a period of time will demonstrate an improvement in the strength of the muscles as the readings on the gauge increase. Initially it should be used early in the assessment before the muscles become fatigued. A few service units have their own perineometers; the Bourne Duo unit is made in the United Kingdom and has large and small diameter sensors (see p. 185). Women are encouraged to check their own pelvic floor muscles digitally at home.

Finally, explain to the woman that a definite daily routine must be followed if the treatment is to be effective.

Routine for exercises

It has been found that a position of sitting or standing with thighs slightly apart is most effective, as the weight of the pelvic contents acts as a resistance to the muscles. An effective command is, 'Close the back and front passages, draw them up inside, hold this squeeze and lift for up to six seconds – let go slowly'.

Some women find it necessary to concentrate on closing the 'back' and 'front' components separately at first, combining them at a later date.

The therapist should check that the woman understands that she should not contract her glutei or abdominal muscles or hold her breath while practising pelvic floor contractions. This is not easy at first, especially if the muscles are very weak, but if she concentrates her attention on the central area from her coccyx to symphysis pubis she will find she can gradually feel the 'squeeze and lift' in this area alone. As the muscles tire after five or six contractions, the exercise needs to be repeated frequently each day. Discussion with the therapist will ensure that a routine is worked out to suit the person's everyday activities.

It has been found useful to relate contractions to the clock, e.g. practice on the hour every hour (using an alarm clock or cake timer as an aural stimulus); or linking contractions to activities, e.g. at the sink, having coffee, on the lavatory. Reminders should be given to the woman to brace her pelvic floor (to reduce the downward thrust) whenever she coughs, sneezes or lifts heavy objects. Stopping and starting a flow of urine while micturating is a good 'awareness' test and provides an indication of progress if the stream of urine is stopped more completely, but it should not replace the exercises. The use of a daily record chart is advisable for at least the first week of the pelvic floor exercise programme as it serves as a reminder to do the exercises until they become part of the daily routine.

Obesity: If the patient is overweight she needs encouragement to reduce weight or be referred to a dietician.

Persistent cough and sneezing: Chest or allergy clinics may be of assistance. Smoking must be reduced if that is the cause of the coughing.

Follow-up appointments: Patients return for assessment three weeks after the first appointment. Subsequent appointments are at four- to six-week intervals. Those with less severe symptoms will be ready for discharge after about three months.

Progression of the exercise programme is important so that the muscles re-learn how to contract reflexly in response to a threat, as detailed in group therapy.

Group therapy

When several women living near the hospital require treatment weekly exercise sessions as a group can be very beneficial. Much can be gained from contact with others who have similar problems and an element of competition enters for the overweight patients during the weekly 'weigh-in'. The 'pelvic floor group' meets once a week for about 20 minutes. Very little equipment is required; any moderate-sized room is suitable.

Exercises

Pelvic floor contractions are practised in all the variations of lying, sitting and standing, making the positions relate to the woman's daily life. To prevent fatigue of the pelvic floor muscles, strengthening and mobilizing for the abdominal and back muscles are interspersed. Posture correction is also taught.

As the pelvic floor muscles increase in strength the contractions can be made more difficult to sustain by practising them while skipping, running or jumping. Coughing, sneezing and lifting with the pelvic floor contracted must also be taught. Duplicated reminder lists of exercises will aid the woman's memory as great emphasis is laid on home practice. The overweight women are weighed each week and their weight is recorded.

In very recent times, a few centres have begun assessing the use of 'vaginal cones' in cases of stress incontinence. Readers who wish to know more are referred to the papers listed in the Bibliography, p. 184, i.e. Bridges et al, 1988; Peattie and Plevnik, 1988; Plevnik, 1985.

Bladder retraining

Physiotherapists who are able to teach re-education of the pelvic floor can be involved in bladder retraining. This may be done in the ward or in the outpatient department. Each time the desire to pass urine is felt the pelvic floor is contracted in an effort to delay micturition. If the delay time is slowly lengthened an appreciable improvement in urgency and frequency can be obtained in a few weeks.

Pre- and post-treatment bladder function charts can motivate women to continue the retraining.

Geriatrics

If elderly people become inactive the pelvic floor muscles may atrophy through lack of stimulus of changing intra-abdominal pressure, which leads to difficulty in stopping the act of voiding. Practice to 'stop and start' a stream of urine can lead to greater awareness and increased confidence in controlling bladder and bowel. Inactivity is a contributory factor to stasis in the gut, constipation and impaction of faeces. General exercise programmes can be designed (even for the chairbound) for individuals or groups. Brisk walking and swimming for the 'well-aged' benefits all the body systems (Pardini, 1984).

ELECTRICAL TREATMENTS

Short wave diathermy

The resolution of some gynaecological conditions can be accelerated by the application of heat. The short wave diathermic current is of high frequency and alternating and does not stimulate motor or sensory nerves. It is therefore ideal for heating tissues as deeply placed in the pelvis as the female reproductive organs.

Treatment of infected wounds (p. 23)

Pelvic Inflammatory Disease (p. 144)   This responds well to short wave diathermy. It is best treated by the cross-fire method with the patient in lying and side-lying positions on a couch or in a canvas and wood deck-chair. In most cases a thermic initial treatment of five minutes each way followed by treatments of 10 minutes each way daily for two weeks, then three-times weekly for two or three weeks is required. There has been a tendency to stop treatment too early with long-standing pelvic inflammatory disease.

Precautions especially relevant in the treatment of gynaecological patients by short wave diathermy

Clothing   The patient should remove all her garments from her waist down to her feet. The skin of the abdomen, buttocks and thighs can then be adequately inspected for scars or other blemishes.

Skin Sensation Every area that is to be treated should be tested for sensation to heat and cold, paying particular attention to any scarred area which may show altered reactions.

Moisture Great care should be taken to see that the perineum and inner aspects of the thighs are dry, as moisture will cause a concentration of the electric field. If the patient is obese a dry Turkish towel could be placed between her thighs.

Intra-uterine Devices These contraceptive devices have been found to lose their shape when subjected to short wave diathermy. Metal devices like the 'Copper 7' concentrate the field.

It is the author's opinion that short wave diathermy is *contra-indicated* for a patient fitted with an intra-uterine device.

Menstruation It has been the practice not to treat a patient who is menstruating. The author has found it unnecessary to suspend treatment at this time unless the patient has very heavy periods or secondary dysmenorrhoea. The sanitary protection should be removed before treatment, whether it is a pad or tampon, and the perineum thoroughly dried. The patient can sit on a paper towel if she feels she may soil the towelling. A clean pad or tampon can be replaced after treatment.

Pregnancy The effects of short wave diathermy on a fetus are unknown, therefore pregnant women should not be treated. Patients anticipating or suspecting pregnancy should inform the therapist.

Laparoscopic Sterilization If the Fallopian tubes have been occluded by plastic or metal ring clips, short wave diathermy is contra-indicated.

The presence of pacemakers, hearing aids or items of replacement or fixation surgery should be checked by the physiotherapist.

Faradism and interrupted direct current (IDC)

If the pelvic floor muscles are very weak patients can experience difficulty in practising exercises; the resultant contractions are so small that the effect on the surrounding tissues and, therefore, the patient's sensation is minimal. Faradism and IDC are still used by therapists to enhance weak contractions of the pelvic floor muscles, and thus encourage patients to greater awareness and voluntary effort. It is not clear whether the modalities are used by choice or because an interferential unit is not available.

The placement of electrodes is variable. A vaginal or rectal electrode with a large indifferent over the sacrum or lower abdomen is one option. It is the author's experience when using faradism that two metal electrodes each in a sponge sleeve placed either side of the perineum, parallel to it, stimulate the pelvic floor muscles effectively. A routine of 10 contractions and one minute rest repeated 10 times for 12–14 treatments (3 times weekly) is proving useful.

Electronic stimulators for the pelvic floor muscles, either as implants or vaginal/rectal electrodes connected to batteries worn around the waist are still the subject of experiment with indefinite results at present.

Interferential therapy

This modality is used in many parts of the world to treat a variety of conditions including genuine stress incontinence of urine and detrusor instability.

Interferential therapy appears to facilitate healing by utilizing the bio-electric effect. Bio-electric currents occur throughout the body, but when tissues are damaged the bio-electric profile is altered. Tissues in the body, categorized as excitable and non-excitable, respond to stimulation by electrical energy within a given frequency range. At present for practical purposes this range is from 0.1Hz to 200Hz (De Domenico, 1987).

In the treatment of micturition disorders interferential (IF) is generally used in conjunction with pelvic floor exercises to increase the efficiency of the treatment. Confirmation of this theory is proving difficult: one study has already found that the addition of interferential or faradism to pelvic floor exercises in the treatment of genuine stress incontinence did not improve the results (Wilson, 1984). Research continues and Laycock (1988) has described a study where interferential therapy was being used alone in the treatment of stress incontinence with some success.

Application As treatment profiles for micturition disorders vary and the efficiency of each is unproven, the target tissues will be identified and interferential stimulation options given.

Genuine stress incontinence
(a) *Urethra*: external urethral sphincter; smooth muscle walls. Low frequency range required.

(i) 0.5–15Hz or (ii) 0–100Hz – using slow rhythmic sweep.
(b) *Pelvic floor muscles*: Medium frequency range required. Surge facility required to prevent tetanic contraction.
(i) 40–80Hz – fast sweep or (ii) 50Hz. Two seconds on and six seconds off.

Electrodes: Four plates or suction cups – place medial to ischial tuberosities and obturator foramina.
Two plates (pre-modulated approach is more convenient) – place either side of the perineum (medial to the ischial tuberosities).

Intensity: Maximum that is comfortable – work up to it slowly.

Duration: (a) 15–20 minutes for plate electrodes; 10–15 minutes for suction cups.
(b) 40–50 contractions in groups of 10 with a rest between each group.

Detrusor instability: Interferential stimulation is reported to be useful in inhibiting the contractions of an unstable bladder. Two methods are described:

1. This method originates from the treatment of clients with detrusor instability who have multiple sclerosis where stimulation over the thoracic outflow may have an effect on motor neurones from spinal segments beginning below this level; also a direct action on the autonomic system is possible (van Poppel, 1985).
   Position: Client in lying or half lying.
   Electrodes: Two large plates (13×8cm). One is placed horizontally over the vertebrae T12–L1 and the other anteriorly at the same level and held in place with Velcro bands.
   Current: 10–110Hz fast sweep with intensity up to 40mA within 2–4 minutes.
   Duration: 30 minutes, three times weekly for 12 treatments.

2. Originates from the treatment protocol of Laycock (1988).
   Electrodes: Two or four are placed as for genuine stress incontinence.
   Intensity: 5–10Hz fast sweep, intensity maximum to tolerance.
   Duration: 30 minutes, three times weekly for 12 treatments.

In all treatments using interferential therapy minor adjustments may be required to pad placement and current intensity to ensure a safe, comfortable treatment which gives optimum results.

Precautions and Contra-indications

Short wave diathermy interference: Interferential machines should *never* be operated close to active short wave diathermy units as the radio energy transmitted by the short wave diathermy can cause the interferential machine to malfunction or cause 'surges' of current in the patient's circuit. A minimum of 3 metres distance is suggested with a reservation that this may not be enough for some machines and separate operating times or rooms would be safer (De Domenico, 1987).

Interferential is a relatively safe treatment as thermal and electrochemical build-up does not occur. Normal safety checks for operating equipment are necessary and observation for adverse skin reactions due to sensitivity to electrical currents or high current density in the pad area.

Consideration should be given to the following:

1. Check condition of the skin (avoid or insulate open areas).
2. Skin test for sharp/blunt sensitivity to pain.
3. Avoid febrile conditions, malignancy, pulmonary tuberculosis or purulent conditions.
4. Interferential is contra-indicated to the back, abdomen or pelvis in pregnancy or during menstruation.
5. Interferential is contra-indicated in severe cardiac conditions, severe hypotension.
6. Interferential is contra-indicated if cardiac pacemakers are in use.
7. Avoid using interferential on anyone who has comprehension difficulties.
8. Avoid using interferential in areas of excessive bleeding.

Ultrasound

Ultrasonic energy is a form of mechanical energy with frequencies beyond the range of audible sound, i.e. greater than 20 000Hz. Varying frequencies of ultrasound are used in medicine (Sanders and James, 1980):

Medical usage	Intensity (watts/cm²)
Surgical	>10
Therapeutic	0.5–3.0
Diagnostic	0.001–0.1

Therapeutic ultrasound is widely used in the treatment of recent injuries for its beneficial effect on pain, traumatic and inflammatory conditions and on scar tissue. The immediate effects of childbearing on the perineal area are frequently pain, trauma and inflammation and these respond readily to isonation. Unfortunately that is not the end of the problem; the resulting scar tissue often gives rise to varying degrees of dyspareunia and distress and thus becomes a gynaecological problem.

New scar tissue will always shorten unless it is repeatedly stretched. This is due to the property of collagen to gradually shorten when it is fully formed. This occurs from the third week to the sixth month after the injury (Evans, 1980). This scar tissue may be superficial as a result of an episiotomy, or perineal tear, or in deeper tissues, perhaps the posterior vaginal wall.

Treatment   The combination of pulsed ultrasound and stretching message on perineal scars make this a successful treatment despite the absence of clinical trials.

Alternate daily pulsed ultrasound of 1MHz between 0.5 watts/cm^2 and 0.8 watts/cm^2 for five minutes with a pulse ratio of 2:1 works well. The transducer is applied in contact with a suitable coupling agent. The woman is generally most comfortable in open-knee crook lying. Firm stretching massage by the therapist over the scarred area completes the treatment. The client is instructed to repeat the massage herself twice daily at home. On average about four treatments are required before the client can resume coitus using a suitably adapted position.

The softening and stretching of the scar tissue which follows isonation appears to be permanent. Lehmann (1965) and Patrick (1978) report this 'softening' effect, but opinions vary about the efficacy of isonation on scar tissue over six months old.

Precautions
Burns: Pain or pins and needles are warning signs – care should be taken over de-sensitized areas.
Cavitation: A non-thermal effect where bubbles are generated in sound field – it can be stable or transient. Movement of the transducer lessens the chance of this occurring (Coakley, 1978).
Overdose: Opinions differ as to a safe dose, but it is generally advisable to increase duration of treatment rather than intensity.
Damage to crystal: Tests should be carried out in the normal way prior to treatment. The transducer must remain in contact with coupling medium while emitting.

Contra-indications
Deep venous thrombosis
Acute infections
Pregnant uterus (in area to be treated)
Tumours
Radiotherapy to the areas requiring treatment (for six months)
Cardiac patients should be treated with care
There are differing opinions as to excluding all patients with pacemakers from treatment

The role of the physiotherapist does not only lie in the assessment and treatment of the patient's symptoms as mentioned in this chapter.

Prophylaxis must be her aim. Her knowledge of the musculo-skeletal changes in pregnancy, labour and the puerperium should be used to minimize the effects of these processes on women.

Patient care starts during antenatal classes and should include instruction to the student midwives, district midwives and health visitors who have no obstetric physiotherapist working with them. Constant attention should be given to postnatal advice, particularly exercise schemes and booklets to ensure they are accurate and realistic in teaching self-care to the patients.

Patients in the postnatal ward who have a history of stress incontinence or pelvic laxity should be checked in the physiotherapy outpatient department until they are symptom free. Antenatal, postnatal and gynaecology clinics should have access to a physiotherapist for consultation and referral of patients.

It is by this combination of prophylaxis and active treatment that the physiotherapist can contribute so much to the alleviation of many of the physical problems of modern women of all age-groups.

REFERENCES

Coakley, W. T. (1978). Biophysical effects of ultrasound at therapeutic intensities. *Physiotherapy*, **64**, 6, 168.

De Domenico, G. (1987). *New Dimensions in Interferential Therapy: A theoretical and clinical guide*. Chapters 1, 5. Reid Medical Books, Australia.

Evans, P. (1980). The healing process at cellular level: a review. *Physiotherapy*, **66**, 8, 256.

Frewen, W. K. (1978). An objective assessment of the unstable bladder of psychosomatic origin. *British Journal of Urology*, **50**, 246–9.

Gosling, J. A., Dixon, J. S., Critchley, H. O. D. and Thompson, S. A. (1981). A comparative study of the human external sphincter and periurethral levator ani muscles. *British Journal of Urology*, **53**, 35.

Laycock, J. (1988). Interferential therapy in the treatment of genuine stress incontinence. Paper in *Proceedings of the 18th International Continence Society Conference*, Oslo.

Lehmann, J. F. (1965). Ultrasound therapy. Chapter in *Therapeutic Heat and Cold*, 2nd edition, pp. 321–86 (ed. Licht, S.). Williams and Wilkins, Baltimore.

Pardini, A. (1984). Exercise, vitality and aging. *Aging*, April–May, 19–28.

Parkes, A. G., Swash, M. and Urich, H. (1977). Sphincter denervation in anorectal incontinence and rectal prolapse. *Gut*, 18, 656–65.

Patrick, M. K. (1978). Applications of therapeutic pulsed ultrasound. *Physiotherapy*, 64, 4, 104.

Percy, J. P. et al (1981). Electrophysiological study of motor nerve supply of pelvic floor. *Lancet*, 1, 16–17.

Sanders, R. C. and James, A. E. (1980). *Principles and Practice of Ultrasonography in Obstetrics and Gynaecology*, 2nd edition. Appleton-Century-Crofts, New York.

Shafik, A. (1975). A new concept of the anatomy of the anal sphincter mechanism and the physiology of defaecation. *Investigations in Urology*, 12, 412–19.

Snooks, S. J. et al (1984). Damage to the voluntary anal and urinary sphincter musculature in incontinence. *Journal of Neurology, Neurosurgery and Psychiatry*, 47, 1269–73.

Swash, M. (1985). *Coloproctology and the Pelvic Floor*, chapter 8, p. 131. Butterworths, London.

Van Poppel, H. et al (1985). Interferential therapy for detrusor hyperreflexia in multiple sclerosis. *Urology*, 25, 6, 607–12.

Wilson, P. D. et al (1984). The value of physiotherapy in female genuine stress incontinence. Paper in *Proceedings of the 14th International Continence Society Conference*, Innsbruck.

Zacharin, R. F. (1977). A Chinese anatomy: the pelvic supporting tissues of the Chinese and Occidental female compared and contrasted. *Australian and New Zealand Journal of Obstetrics and Gynaecology*, 17, 1–10.

Zacharin, R. F. (1980). Pulsion enterocele: review of the functional anatomy of the pelvic floor. *Obstetrics and Gynaecology*, 55, 2, 35.

BIBLIOGRAPHY

Books

Collins, M. (ed.) (1978). *Women's Health Through Life Stages: the physiotherapist's contribution*. Australian Physiotherapy Association, New South Wales, Australia.

Govan, A. D. T., Hodge, C. and Callander, R. (1985). *Gynaecology Illustrated*, 3rd edition. Churchill Livingstone, Edinburgh.

Henry, M. M. and Swash, M. (1985). *Coloproctology and the Pelvic Floor: Pathophysiology and Management*. Butterworths, London.

Llewellyn-Jones, D. (1986). *Fundamentals of Obstetrics and Gynaecology*, 4th edition, Vol 2, *Gynaecology*. Faber and Faber, London.

Mandelstam, D. (ed.) (1986). *Incontinence and Its Management*, 2nd edition. Croom Helm, London.

Savage, B. (1984). *Interferential Therapy*. Faber and Faber, London.

Zacharin, R. F. (1972). *Stress Incontinence of Urine*. Harper and Row, New York.

Papers

Bridges, N., Denning, J. et al (1988). A prospective trial comparing interferential therapy and treatment using cones in patients with symptoms of stress incontinence. Paper in *Proceedings of the 18th International Continence Society Conference*, Oslo.

Harrison, S. M. (1988). Promotion of continence in mobility groups for elderly people. *Australian Journal on Ageing*, 7, 1, 3–6.

Harrison, S. M. and Mandelstam, D. (1982). The use of exercises in pelvic floor re-education in women: an analysis of technique. Paper in the *Proceedings of the World Confederation of Physiotherapy* (Stockholm Conference).

Jordan, J. A. and Stanton, S. L. (1982). The incontinent woman. Paper in *Proceedings of a Scientific Meeting of the Royal College of Obstetricians and Gynaecologists*, London.

Laycock, J. and Green, R. J. (1988). Interferential therapy in the treatment of incontinence. *Physiotherapy*, 74, 4, 161–8.

Peattie, A. B. and Plevnik, S. (1988). Cones versus physiotherapy as conservative management of genuine stress incontinence. Paper in *Proceedings of the 18th International Continence Society Conference*, Oslo.

Plevnik, S. (1985). The use of cones in the re-education of the pelvic floor muscles. Paper in *Proceedings of the 15th International Continence Society Conference*.

Apparatus   The Bourne Duo Perineometer may be obtained from: Dr D. Withey, 56 Chaldon Common Road, Chaldon, Caterham, Surrey CR3 5DD.

ACKNOWLEDGEMENT

The author thanks Mr J. Carron Brown, consultant obstetrician and gynaecologist, Norfolk and Norwich Hospital, who gave her so much assistance and encouragement with the original chapter. In this revision she has appreciated the advice and co-operation of colleagues in both the United Kingdom and Western Australia.

Chapter 13

Skin Conditions

revised by J. BURGESS MCSP

Today, few patients are referred to physiotherapy departments for the treatment of skin disease. The range and efficacy of other methods of treatment (drugs and dressings) have reduced the need for physiotherapists to spend their time in treating these conditions. However, a small number of patients are still referred. This usually occurs where drug treatment alone has proved inadequate to alleviate the condition, or where drug treatment is more effective if combined with ultraviolet irradiation.

In order to treat these patients effectively, the physiotherapist needs to have an appreciation of the methods of treatment available to her and a knowledge of the skin conditions concerned. She should also appreciate that the skin is frequently a mirror of the mental state of the patient: she should therefore treat the patient as a whole rather than confining her attention exclusively to a localized area.

METHODS OF TREATMENT

Relaxation

If the patient is being treated by tranquillizer drugs, instruction in relaxation techniques may be of great benefit as an adjunct to treatment. Many physicians now believe that the ability of the patient to relax without recourse to sedative drugs (which may become addictive) is of prime importance. Because of this more patients who find it difficult to relax may be referred for instruction in the future. Physiotherapists should ensure that they are skilled in communicating the art of relaxation and should use this in the treatment of skin conditions particularly if the condition is related to mental stress (see Chapter 9). Training in relaxation is also important where the skin condition causes itching, e.g. eczema. The patient's natural desire to scratch will cause further skin irritation and the ability to relax will be of great benefit in controlling this.

ULTRAVIOLET IRRADIATION

Ultraviolet light (UVL) consists of electromagnetic waves in a band between visible light and x-rays. The wavelengths are measured in nanometres (nm). The division of ultraviolet light into three parts (A, B, C) is important when considering biological effects.

UVC (short wave UV) 100 to 290nm. UVC is present in solar radiation, but is absorbed by the ozone layer.

UVB 290 to 320nm. UVB produces sunburn.

UVA (long wave UV) 320 to 400nm. UVA is not biologically active under normal circumstances. Because of its longer wavelength UVA can penetrate through window glass, thin clothing, and atmospheric conditions which would absorb UVB.

The beneficial effect of natural sunlight and the improvement seen in many skin diseases during the summer months are sufficient indications of the value of ultraviolet light. Physiotherapists have traditionally used artificial sources of ultraviolet rays in the treatment of skin diseases. Dosage can be varied from the sub-erythemal dose, that is, 75 per cent of a first degree (E1) erythema dose, through all the degrees of erythema according to the desired effect. In clinical practice the effect aimed for is most likely to be increased cell production leading to thickening of the skin, increased desquamation, increased blood supply to the skin or increased pigmentation. Irradiation of the whole body is said to have a tonic effect. The usefulness of ultraviolet irradiation on areas denuded of skin, e.g. infected wounds, is doubted by many. It seems to be more logical and effective to culture the bacteria and apply the appropriate antibiotic. However, in a few cases, use of the abiotic rays of the spectrum may be appropriate.

When applying treatment the most appropriate ultraviolet source must be used. Treatment given with an air-cooled source of ultraviolet may be either from a mercury vapour lamp or fluorescent tubes. The spectra of these differ. The mercury vapour lamp gives rays from 184.9nm to 390nm (1849 Å–3900 Å) while the fluorescent tube gives rays from 280nm to 390nm (2800 Å–3900 Å). Where an erythema reaction is desired, irradiation from a fluorescent source will probably be the best choice as there is a higher percentage of the longer wavelengths. The initial choice of source is important as the same lamp must be used at subsequent treatments.

Definition The nanometre (nm) is now the official Standard

International Unit of wavelength and has replaced the Ångström (Å).

1 Ångström = one ten-millionth of a millimetre
1 nanometre = 10 Ångström
1 nm   = 10Å

Prefix: nano
Symbol: n

Heat

The physiotherapist may also find that the application of mild heat has beneficial effects in the treatment of localized skin infections, such as boils, carbuncles or infected wounds. Heat may be applied superficially using infra-red rays or more deeply by short wave diathermy or microwave diathermy. The rationale underlying the use of heat is that increased metabolic activity and increased blood supply will aid the local tissues to combat the infection. The heat should be directed to the area of blood supply rather than towards the infection, so that the rate of bacterial growth is not stimulated (for example, heat could be applied to the forearm in the case of an infection of the hand). This type of treatment should be given in association with localized and systemic antibiotics.

Cold

An effective erythema can be obtained by massaging the local area with an ice cube. This may be preferable to the use of dry heat and is useful in the treatment of an area of skin which threatens to break down into a pressure sore.

Tissue mobilizing techniques

Where the skin condition has led to fibrosis and thickening of the tissues, with the possibility of contracture and deformity, the mobility of the tissues must be maintained, and deep localized massage, with active movements, ultrasound and possibly passive stretchings, may be appropriate.

ASSESSMENT AND RECORDING

In this field no less than in other areas of physiotherapy, the pre-liminary assessment of the patient's condition is essential. Careful observation of the affected skin area should be made and the extent, type and severity of the eruption should be noted. Standard diagrams of the anterior and posterior aspect of the body are useful, so that the affected areas can be outlined and the pre-treatment record kept with the patient's treatment card.

A careful scrutiny of the patient's notes will be made in order to determine relevant points in the history of the condition, especially so that the type of medicaments being given can be known. Some of these may be sensitizers, e.g. coal tar, which will alter the patient's reaction to ultraviolet radiation. The patient's skin reaction to sunlight should be tested if the treatment prescribed includes ultraviolet irradiation. The result of this test and the other findings should be carefully recorded on the patient's treatment card. A special note should be made concerning the extent of the area treated so that at subsequent treatments the possibility of overdose because of altered screening is avoided.

In the treatment of most skin conditions re-assessment of the affected area should be made at each attendance, and the treatment should be based on the findings. A careful recording of the day-to-day condition and the consequent modifications to treatment is therefore of prime importance. Objective evidence such as a tracing of a wound, or the extent of an active area of acne, should be recorded rather than subjective assessments such as 'patient improved'. The physiotherapist should be in a position to base her reports to the dermatologist on factual evidence rather than optimism.

SKIN CONDITIONS REFERRED FOR PHYSIOTHERAPY

Acne vulgaris

This is a chronic inflammatory disease of the sebaceous glands. The condition most commonly affects those parts where the glands are large, i.e. the face, chest and upper back, and is seen in adolescents and young adults primarily, though very occasionally the condition may persist into later life. The essential lesion of the condition is the blackhead, or comedo, a firm mass of keratin which blocks the follicular pore. This may cause inflammation of the surrounding tissues or it may become secondarily infected with eventual fibrous tissue formation and unsightly scarring.

In mild cases no treatment other than careful skin toilet is required. Severe cases respond well to a prolonged course of a tetracycline antibiotic. The few patients who are referred for physiotherapists to treat are those who have severe acne which is not responding well to other forms of therapy. The rationale underlying this referral is that cases of acne improve in the summer months and therefore ultraviolet irradiation from an artificial source can be used to supplement the effects of natural sunlight. Exceptions to this are patients who have fair or sensitive skins, as they are often made worse by local ultraviolet radiation.

The affected skin should be washed with soap and water prior to treatment and gently dried with a clean towel and then irradiated by an air-cooled mercury vapour lamp. A first degree erythema is given to improve the condition of the skin and this is repeated when the reaction has died down. A first degree erythema is preferred to a second degree as the aim of the treatment is to stimulate skin metabolism rather than produce desquamation. The technique of ultraviolet irradiation will vary with the area being treated. The physiotherapist must ensure that her screening techniques are such that there is no possibility of 'overlap' dosage. In the interests of the patient it is as well to screen to the natural bony features of the body, such as the jaw line or the clavicular line. A more acceptable cosmetic effect can be obtained by allowing a natural fade-off of irradiation, but this can only be done where screening is not essential.

Psoriasis

This condition affects approximately 1–2 per cent of people with white skin. The cause is unknown but the abnormality results in unduly rapid cell division within the epidermis. Normally the cells reproduce at such a rate that the epidermal turnover takes approximately 28 days. In psoriasis the turnover rate is seven times as fast, i.e. every four days. The amount of skin area affected varies from trivial to extensive. Characteristically, initial lesions are on the extensor aspects of elbows and knees and in the scalp, or over the sacral area. Severe cases may have total skin involvement, although the face is usually spared. The condition appears to be adversely affected by mental stress, although the course of the condition is typically unpredictable and exacerbations cannot always be attributed to this factor.

The affected area shows a slightly raised red plaque, with a sharp margin between it and healthy skin. The plaque is surmounted by dry silvery grey scales. If the scales are removed the underlying skin bleeds easily.

Medical treatment for psoriasis is usually by the administration of local or, very occasionally, systemic agents which contain a toxic substance to slow down the rate of cell division. Where these fail, or in the case of a patient whose condition is becoming rapidly worse, admission to hospital may be advised. It is in the intensive treatment of patients with psoriasis that the physiotherapist is most likely to become involved. The usual treatment is a modification of the Ingram regime. The patient bathes first thing in the morning in a tar bath and scrubs off his psoriatic scales. He then attends the physiotherapy department for general ultraviolet irradiation from the fluorescent source. As the irradiation is given daily, no more than a first degree erythema should be achieved and some authorities believe that a sub-erythemal dose only should be given. The lesions are then covered with dithranol paste and a suitable dressing until removal the next day prior to bathing. Removal of the paste can be facilitated by the use of liquid paraffin. This treatment is effective in nearly all cases, though many relapse again.

PUVA

Photochemotherapy describes the combination of a photo-active chemical and light. Phototherapy of UVA is combined with the chemotherapy of psoralen. An abbreviation of psoralen (P) + UVA produced the acronym PUVA. Psoralen is a drug which makes the skin and the lens of the eye temporarily sensitive to UVA. The drug alone is inactive in the skin; it becomes activated in the presence of UVA and binds to the DNA thiamine bases. Psoralens can also intercalate with two base pairs and give interstrand cross-linkages (Pathak and Kramer, 1969; Cole, 1970; Dall'Acqua et al, 1971); this inhibits DNA synthesis and cell division.

The psoralen drug is taken by mouth (or applied to the skin as a lotion). Two hours later (or 30 minutes after applying the lotion) the maximum concentration of the drug is present in the skin. At this time exposure to UVA is given. Over 90 per cent of orally administered psoralen is excreted in the urine within 12 hours. Oral psoralen is made up in tablets of 10mg, and the prescribed dose is calculated on the patient's body-weight.

Source of irradiation

Most UVA sources used in photochemotherapy use the fluorescent tube. The tubes in UVA sources are coated with a phosphor with an emission spectrum between 310–380nm. The tubes are usually housed in a hexagonal-shaped cubicle. For treatment the patient stands undressed in the machine and receives a general irradiation.

Smaller machines are available which allow treatment to localized areas, e.g. hands and feet, without irradiating the whole body.

PUVA treatment

PUVA should only be prescribed by a dermatologist. The treatment and long-term side-effects should be explained by a doctor and the patient should sign a consent form before treatment commences.

During experiments on animals using excessive doses of PUVA the development of cataracts was observed. Although there is no evidence to suggest that therapeutic doses of PUVA will cause cataracts, it is advisable that the medical examination of the patient includes an ophthalmological test.

Dosage and Duration of Treatment   The dosimetry used for PUVA is the joule (J).

The *initial* dose is determined by the patient's skin type. At each subsequent treatment the UVA dose may be increased by one half to a maximum of $2J/cm^2$.

There are no hard and fast rules regulating the increase in dosage and the frequency with which this should be done. If the initial UVA dose is determined on the basis of skin type it should not be increased before 72 hours have elapsed to allow the erythema to reach a peak. Patients who tan well tolerate greater increments at more frequent intervals than those who do not.

A treatment regime of two or three times a week is recommended. The duration of the treatment is variable depending on the skin condition and the time it takes for the lesions to clear.

After clearance has been achieved some patients are placed on maintenance therapy. The last effective dose of PUVA in the clearing phase is used as the maintenance dose. Maintenance doses are initially given once a week for a month. If the remission is maintained the frequency of treatments is reduced.

Instructions to Patients Having PUVA

1. Take the prescribed dosage of tablets with food two hours before treatment.
2. Wear protective sunglasses as soon as the tablets are taken and keep them on for 12 hours. (The glasses should be tested by the physiotherapist using a UVA meter and a UVA source.)
3. Avoid exposure to sunlight for 12 hours after treatment. Shield yourself from sunlight with clothing or sun-screening creams.

4. Inform the physiotherapist about any pills or creams or ointments that have been prescribed elsewhere.
5. Avoid any other form of ultraviolet treatment or relaxation, e.g. solarium, sun-bed or sun-bathing.
6. Use moisturizing creams and ointments on your skin since the treatment tends to make your skin dry.
7. Do not use topical treatments such as tars and cortisone creams during PUVA treatments unless prescribed by your consultant.
8. Females of reproductive age should use contraceptive measures during the course of treatment.

Conditions treated with PUVA

PUVA has been shown to be a useful and acceptable treatment for a growing number of skin conditions. The most common treated with PUVA are as follows:

Psoriasis: A clearance and maintenance course is used as previously described.

Atopic eczema: Eczema is a condition which results in red, itchy and often weeping rashes on the skin. In recent years PUVA has been used with good results. The regime used is similar to that of psoriasis, except that the maintenance period is much more prolonged (six months to one year).

Vitiligo: This is a disorder of skin pigmentation which is more pronounced in darker skin. The lesions present as white patches of irregular shape, and are symptomless apart from being sensitive to sunlight.

A prolonged course of PUVA is sometimes beneficial. The duration may be two treatments a week for over a year. Initial dosage must be based on the vitiliginous areas and not on the patient's general skin type. The vitiliginous area is treated as a skin type I. An E1 dosage is recommended. Re-pigmentation is usually patchy appearing first as small dark freckles in the white areas.

Polymorphic light eruption (PLE): This is the most common photosensitive eruption. It is becoming more widely recognized with the increased exposure to the sun. The condition can begin at any age but the teens and twenties are most common. The rash erupts within 2–48 hours of exposure to the sun. The intensity and the duration of the rash is variable.

A six-week course of PUVA in the Spring (or before a holiday in a hot climate) using initial low doses of UVA may give protection for the summer.

Mycosis fungoides: This is a rare skin condition. It is a reticulosis or lymphoma which starts in the skin. The most common lesions are red, scaly patches which can appear on any part of the body. Diagnosis is confirmed by skin biopsy. In the majority of cases the disease progresses slowly over a number of years. The skin lesions can develop into plaques or nodular tumours. Eventually the disease may spread to involve the lymph nodes and internal organs, and cause death.

PUVA in the early stages of the disease can be effective in clearing the lesions. The lesions tend to be more sensitive to UVA than the normal skin and so the initial dose is less than the patient's skin type would indicate. Maintenance PUVA is usually very prolonged to try and keep the condition under control. Some patients may need maintenance over a period of years.

SKIN INFECTIONS

Furuncle

A furuncle or boil is an acute staphylococcal infection of the hair follicle. The infection discharges through the hair follicle after a series of inflammatory changes in which necrotic tissue is broken down into liquid pus. Any area of the body can be the site for a boil but areas of friction such as the back of the neck are the most likely. A series of boils affecting different parts of the body is known as a furunculosis.

The patient is first aware of pain and an area of redness is visible over the site of the infection. This becomes a raised area which quickly shows a yellow centre. After a short while the skin over this central core breaks down and pus is discharged onto the surface. Frequently a solid core of unliquefied pus is also discharged. The affected area is quickly repaired by fibrous tissue and a scar is left to mark the place where the boil existed.

A single boil is very often left to run its own course. Patients who are obviously prone to this kind of skin infection may be treated with appropriate antibiotics, such as penicillin. Only a few patients will ever find their way to a physiotherapy department. The treatment for those who do will depend upon the stage in which the boil presents itself. In the early stage before the boil has started to discharge mild co-planar short wave diathermy should be given. This aims at providing heat to the base of the boil, and the electrodes should be positioned so that the field passes deep to the boil. The treatment by heat accelerates the metabolic processes and encourages discharge of pus. Once discharge has occurred, the localized area may be treated by a more superficial type of heat such as infra-red radiation in order to aid the healing process. Boils which do not drain freely or do not discharge their contents completely may be treated by local ultraviolet irradiation using the sinus applicator.

Carbuncle

If the infection spreads subcutaneously to affect a group of hair follicles a large area of skin may break down to reveal a deep slough which may take a long time to heal. This kind of skin infection requires the administration of antibiotics. The patient may be referred to the physiotherapy department when the objects of physical treatment will be to aid the rapid breakdown of slough and assist in the healing of the affected area.

Treatment will be along the lines already indicated for a boil except that initially there is a wider breakdown of the skin and the area of infected tissue thus revealed should be treated by ultraviolet irradiation using a fourth degree erythema or double-fourth degree erythema to the affected area. The surrounding tissue should of course be carefully screened. Following irradiation the site may be dressed using a proteolytic enzyme such as Trypure. Both the irradiation and the enzyme will aid the breakdown of slough. When the area is clean the aim is to stimulate rapid re-epithelialization and this may be done by the administration of heat, or a first or second degree erythema dose of ultraviolet irradiation to the wound and surrounding area.

Hidradenitis axillae

The apocrine sweat glands of the axilla are occasionally the site of a severe chronic bacterial infection which may be confused with furunculosis. The condition is more severe and may run a chronic course over 10 to 15 years, during which time there is severe scarring with possible contracture of the fibrous tissue.

The condition appears first as multiple red tender nodules which eventually break down and suppurate. Spread of infection occurs with increasing involvement of all the apocrine glands until these are ultimately destroyed.

Treatment is by local and systemic antibiotics and in order to encourage free drainage surgical interference may be necessary.

Scrupulous cleanliness of the area is essential in order to combat the superficial spread of the infection. The patient may be referred to the physiotherapist for mild short wave diathermy to the axillary region in order to encourage the free evacuation of the infected material by the application of heat. It is also important to ensure that the patient understands the need to maintain a full active range of movement in the shoulder joint to prevent contracture of the axillary tissue.

Pressure sores

A sore is a popular term for almost any lesion of the skin or mucous membrane. A local impairment of the circulation caused by sustained pressure can result in a pressure sore. The damage to the tissues is the result of a temporary reduction in the blood supply. The changes can be observed at various stages. At first the skin appears erythematous and it is important to note the colour changes as the part has a livid hue just before the skin breaks down. Once the skin has broken down it becomes an open wound which may easily become infected.

Prevention In order to prevent the occurrence of pressure sores, patients who are immobile should be encouraged to relieve pressure from weight-bearing areas at frequent intervals either by moving themselves into a different position or, if they are in bed and immobile, they should be turned frequently. They may be nursed on medical sheepskins, ripple mattresses, sorbo packs or in a Roto-rest bed. Strict hygiene should be observed and local massage over the area of pressure may be carried out.

If the area shows signs of redness over the pressure area, frequent mild thermal doses of infra-red may be given to improve the circulation. In addition, massaging the local area with an ice cube may be performed.

Skin Breakdown If the skin breaks down, a first degree erythema dose of ultraviolet using the longer wavelengths may be given to stimulate growth and increase the skin resistance. The circulation is maintained by infra-red irradiation on alternate days. If the part becomes infected then stronger erythema reactions will be required to combat the infection by making use of the bactericidal effects of ultraviolet.

Infected wounds

A wound is an injury to the body caused by physical means with disruption of the normal continuity of the body structures. An open wound is one that has a free outward opening. An open wound which has become infected may be treated with ultraviolet. The surrounding skin should be protected and a local irradiation given. The degree of erythema depends on the condition of the wound; if there is pus a fourth or double-fourth dosage is used initially, and is reduced as the infection clears. As granulation tissue appears the dosage should be reduced to a third or second degree, possibly protecting the area of granulation or using a blue uviol filter or cellophane to filter out the shorter abiotic rays. The surrounding skin may be given a first degree erythema using the Kromayer lamp at a distance or an air-cooled mercury vapour lamp.

Cleaning and Dressing the Wound   The wound will need to be cleaned before treatment and afterwards dressed with the appropriate medication using a strict aseptic technique.

Sinuses   If there is a sinus involved then a suitable quartz applicator should be used with the Kromayer to enable healing of the sinus from below upwards.

PHYSIOTHERAPY AS AN AID TO DIAGNOSIS IN SKIN CONDITIONS

Occasionally physiotherapists are asked to assist in the diagnosis of skin conditions. By using a Wood's filter in association with a Kromayer ultraviolet light source, certain types of tinea of the scalp (ringworm) can be shown as a bright blue-green fluorescence. Similarly, erythrasma gives a coral-red fluorescence. This condition usually affects the groins, toe webs and the perianal region.

Photosensitivity and photopatch testing are used in the diagnosis of conditions where the skin has become hypersensitive to light. Such conditions may arise as the result of systemic or local exposure to a sensitizing substance. There is a wide range of possible sensitizers including drugs (sulphonamides, chlorpromazine, tetracycline), soaps, antiseptics, and silver and gold salts. In other cases no direct cause for the hypersensitivity can be found. Because the tests require the use of an ultraviolet light source, physiotherapists may be asked to assist with them. A Kromayer lamp with a filter of ordinary window glass is used for the test. This eliminates rays below 320nm (3200 Å). The minimal erythema dose (MED) for the lamp without the filter is calculated using a normal skin.

Photopatch testing is carried out in the following way. Patch tests of the suspected sensitizer are applied to both sides of the back or other suitable skin surface (one side then acts as a control). The patches are removed and the skin cleaned after 24 hours. The control areas are then covered with black paper to obscure the light. The test areas are irradiated by the Kromayer lamp with the filter using the minimal erythema dose. The areas are inspected 24 hours later. A positive reaction is shown by a reproduction of the photo allergy and the sensitizing substance can then be identified. A comparison with the control side will show the degree of photosensitivity.

REFERENCES

Cole, R. S. (1970). Light induced cross-linking of DNA in the presence of a furocoumarin (psoralen). *Biochimica et Biophysica Acta*, **217**, 30.

Dall'Acqua, F., Marciani, S. and Ciavatta, L. (1971). Formation of interstrand cross-linkings in the photoreactions between furocoumarins and DNA. *Zeitschrift für Naturforschung (B)*, **26**, 561.

Pathak, M. A. and Kramer, D. M. (1969). Photosensitization of skin in vivo by furocoumarins (psoralens). *Biochimica et Biophysica Acta*, **195**, 197.

BIBLIOGRAPHY

Buxton, P. K. (1988). *ABC of Dermatology*. BMA, London.

Fry, L., Wojnarouska, F. and Shahrad, P. (1986). *Illustrated Encyclopaedia of Dermatology*. MTP Press Limited, Lancaster.

Levene, G. M. and Calman, C. D. (1988). *A Colour Atlas of Dermatology*. Wolfe Medical Publications, London.

Orton, C. (1981). *Learning to Live with Skin Disorders*. Souvenir Press Limited, London.

Vickers, C. F. H. (ed.) (1986). *Modern Management of Common Skin Diseases*. Churchill Livingstone, Edinburgh.

Weber, G. (1980). *Photochemotherapy: Information for Doctors and Patients*. Year Book Medical Publishers, London.

Wilkinson, J. D., Shaw, S. and Fenton, D. A. (1987). *Dermatology*. Churchill Livingstone, Edinburgh.

Chapter 14

Plastic Surgery

by P. J. SMITH FRCS and S. BOARDMAN MCSP

The term plastic surgery was used by the Germans at the beginning of the 20th century to describe surgery concerned with 'moulding of tissues'.

The first recorded reconstructive surgery was performed in India 600 years BC where amputation of the nose was a common punishment, and forehead skin was used to construct a new nose. Tagliococci, an Italian surgeon of the sixteenth century, reconstructed noses using an arm flap. The recorded use of free skin grafts dates from the nineteeth century when new techniques were described by Jacques Reverdin, Ollier and Thiersch in Paris and Wolfe in Glasgow. The challenge of mutilating injuries in the First World War stimulated the development of plastic surgery and it became a specialty in its own right, the pioneer in the United Kingdom (UK) being Sir Harold Gillies. During the Second World War, surgeons such as Gillies, Kilner, MacIndoe and Mowlem laid the foundation of the specialty as it is now known.

Much of the present-day plastic surgery is concerned with the replacement and reconstruction of soft tissues. This can include skin, subcutaneous tissues, nerves, tendons, blood vessels, the main object being to restore and improve function.

THE SKIN AND ITS FUNCTION

It should be remembered that skin is not just a collection of epithelial cells, but a composite organ of epidermis and dermis (Fig. 14/1). The epidermis is stratified and is made up of five layers of cells, the deepest of these, the *stratum germinatum*, being the cell-producing layer.

The dermis is made up of two layers. In the upper layer lie the capillary loops, the smallest lymphatics and nerve endings, including touch corpuscles, while the deeper layer consists largely of fibrous tissue with an interlacing of elastic fibres, and this rests directly on subcutaneous tissue. This latter consists of bundles of connective

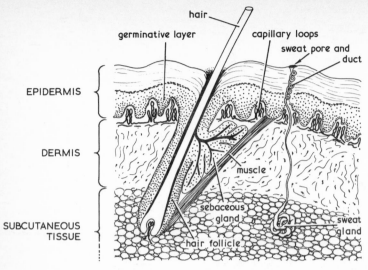

Fig. 14.1 Structure of the skin

tissue interspersed with fat cells. The glandular parts of some of the several glands and deep hair follicles lie in this area. This subcutaneous area serves to support blood vessels, lymphatics and nerves and protects underlying structures.

The skin is the largest organ of the body, representing about 16 per cent of the total weight of the normal adult. It has many functions, but when considering skin loss the two most important are protection against invasion by bacteria, and prevention of fluid and protein loss from the body.

Primary healing should be encouraged in order to avoid granulation tissue and minimize scarring. If primary healing does not take place, surgery may be required to provide skin cover. There are two methods of skin transfer:

1. Skin grafts, which are without blood supply for up to 48 hours after transfer.
2. Skin flaps, which are joined to the body by a functioning arterial and venous flow.

METHODS OF SKIN REPLACEMENT

Skin grafts (Fig. 14/2)

These may be split skin or full thickness.

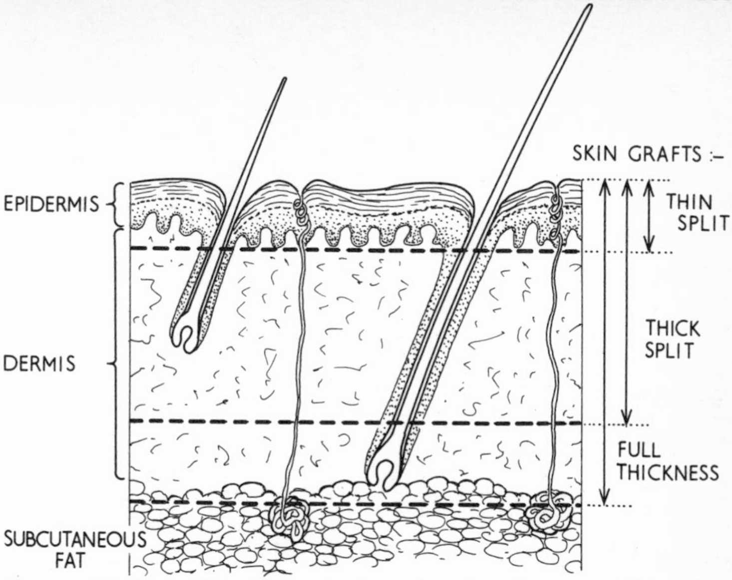

Fig. 14.2 The layers of the skin showing from where the various types of skin grafts are taken

Split Skin These can vary from the very thin to three-quarter skin thickness. They are cut with a knife or dermatome. Such grafts are used in the grafting of burns. After cutting, they are spread on Tulle Gras for ease of handling and applied to the raw areas.

The donor sites heal within 10 to 12 days. The grafted area may be nursed, exposed or with dressings, according to the wishes of the surgeon. The recipient area must always have a good blood supply and be free from necrotic tissue and infection (particularly *Haemolytic streptococcus*).

For the first 48 hours, a split skin graft survives on the exudate from the underlying granulating tissue. By 48 hours, capillaries will have grown into the graft and vascularized it. Haematoma or tangential movement of the graft will prevent this vascularization and the graft will fail.

Split skin grafts often contract considerably, and may have to be replaced or released at a later stage – Z-plasties, more split skin or full thickness grafts being added, or skin flaps used.

Full Thickness Grafts Wolfe grafts are small full thickness grafts of skin excluding fat, usually taken from the post-auricular or supra-clavicular area to repair facial defects, such as eyelids. The donor site will not regenerate and must itself be closed by a split skin graft or direct suture. Full thickness skin graft contracts less than a split skin graft and so it is the graft of choice for releasing the contracture of the eyelids which can, if not corrected, lead to corneal ulceration.

Physiotherapy following skin grafts

The aims of physiotherapy following skin grafts are:
1. To prevent chest complication.
2. To maintain mobility and function.
Pre- and postoperative breathing exercises are carried out. Should the skin grafts cover the chest wall special care must be taken when undertaking percussion techniques, in order that a shearing force and undue pressure do not damage newly applied skin.

Mobility In the early postoperative stage, joints not involved in grafting may be moved. Splints are often applied to the grafted areas to maintain a good functional position. At about four to six days movements may commence to those areas involved in the grafting, but splints are often retained at night to maintain a functional position. Once the grafts are well established, the application of a bland cream to soften scars is desirable, e.g. lanolin or hydrous ointment may be used. The area should be gently kneaded. Heavy handedness must be avoided to prevent blistering.

Split skin grafts often contract considerably. Encouragement must therefore be given to patients to continue their own massage, exercise regime and splintage, where necessary, for a few months. After six weeks should localized bands of contracture be present ultrasound may be commenced.

Many patients who have undergone skin grafting procedures are fitted with pressure garments (see Chapter 15, p.242).

Skin flaps

These normally consist of skin and subcutaneous tissue.

They take their own blood supply, and can be used to cover areas where the blood supply is poor or non-existent, as over cortical bone, cartilage, joint and bare tendon. Flaps do not contract so can be used to prevent or correct deformities. In order to maintain the viability of the flap, transfer of skin can at times only be done in stages.

Flaps may be classified according to the way in which they receive their blood supply (Fig. 14/3):
1. Random pattern flap.
2. Axial pattern flap.

RANDOM PATTERN FLAP

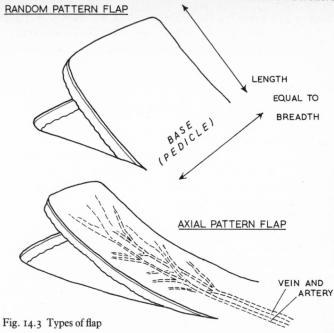

LENGTH

EQUAL TO

BREADTH

BASE
(PEDICLE)

AXIAL PATTERN FLAP

VEIN AND
ARTERY

Fig. 14.3 Types of flap

Random Pattern Flap This is dependent upon the subdermal plexus of blood vessels and therefore there are dimensional limitations to the flap.

Axial Pattern Flap This flap has a specific cutaneous artery and accompanying veins running along its axis and therefore it does not have the dimensional limitations of the random pattern flap.

Flaps may also reach the recipient area in different ways, i.e. local or distant flaps.

Local Flaps These are transferred from an area adjacent to the defect where the skin is pliable. The secondary defect is closed by either direct suture or skin graft.

Transposition flap (Fig. 14/4): This is an example of a local, random pattern flap which is often used when providing skin cover for pressure sores.

Rotation flap (Fig. 14/5): A flap which is raised as a half-circle and is frequently used to replace defects of the scalp and cheek.

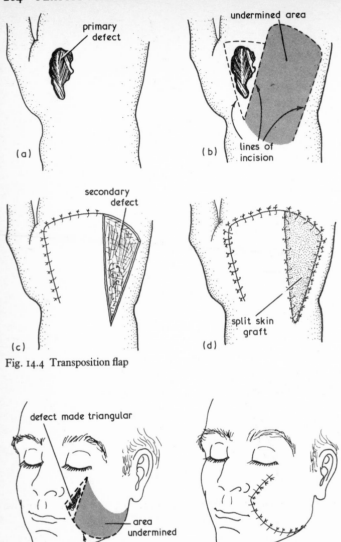

Fig. 14.4 Transposition flap

Fig. 14.5 Rotation flap

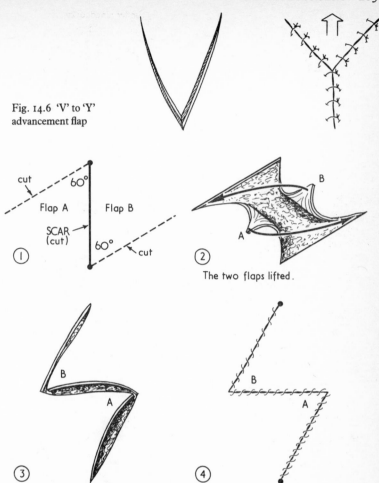

Fig. 14.6 'V' to 'Y' advancement flap

①

cut

60°

Flap A   Flap B

SCAR (cut)

60°   cut

② The two flaps lifted.

③ The two flaps rotated into position.

④ Final position; the two flaps sutured in place. NB :—
1) The length between the two dots is longer than the site of the old scar.
2) The central part of the scar is now transverse.

Fig. 14.7 The mechanics of a Z-plasty (cut one for yourself on paper)

V/Y advancement flap (Fig. 14/6): The skin is cut as a V and closed as a Y and is a method of advancing tissue to cover defects such as seen in fingertip injuries.

Z-plasty (Fig. 14/7): This is an operation whereby the direction of a scar is altered, i.e. to try and allow the scar to blend in with the surrounding tissue by, wherever possible, lying in the same direction as the skin lines. It is used to release contracture bands and revise scars.

Distant Flaps A distant flap can be applied to the defect by bringing the donor area close to the defect.

Groin flap: Where the hand is attached to the groin and the blood supply (axial) enters by the pedicle of skin. After three weeks the flap is detached and inset.

Cross-leg flap (Fig. 14/8): A flap is raised; one end is attached to the recipient site and the other remains attached to the donor site. The donor site itself is then resurfaced with a split skin graft. The position is maintained for three weeks after which the flap is detached and inset.

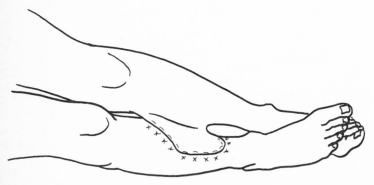

Fig. 14.8 Cross-leg flap

Some distant flaps cannot be brought adjacent to the recipient area and therefore have to be transferred by a carrier. These are often tubed and can be raised on the abdomen and carried by the wrist to their destination. The wrist is attached to the abdomen for three weeks while a blood supply is established in the flap, after which time it is detached from its base and carried to the lower leg as replacement skin (Fig. 14/9). The wrist is attached to the leg for the above-mentioned time after which it is detached and inset.

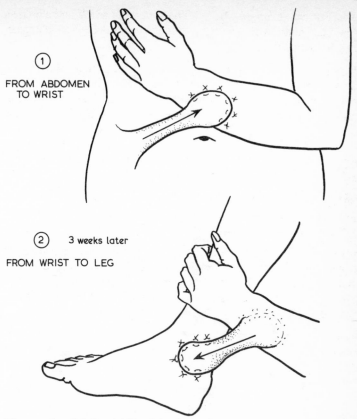

① FROM ABDOMEN
TO WRIST

② 3 weeks later

FROM WRIST TO LEG

Fig. 14.9 A pedicle flap. (1) The abdominal pedicle is raised and attached to the wrist; (2) the abdominal end of the pedicle is detached and re-attached to the ankle area

The cross-leg flap and tube pedicles have been largely superseded by free flaps due to the advent of microsurgical techniques.

Free Flap (Figs 14/10, 14/11 and 14/12) Using a microscope this flap is completely detached from the donor site and transposed directly to the recipient area; the blood vessels are dissected out (at least one large artery and a vein) and anastomosed with vessels in the recipient area.

An example of this flap is one based on the superficial circumflex iliac artery. The skin flap is raised together with the underlying artery and accompanying veins. The flap and vessels are placed over the recipient area where the vessels are anastomosed to those in the local area and the flap is sutured in place. It must be remembered

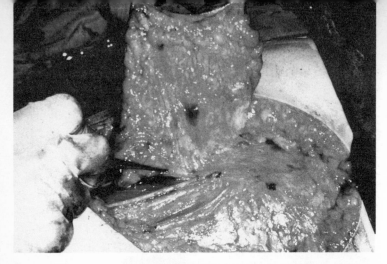

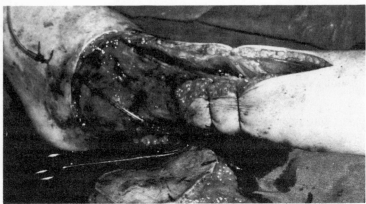

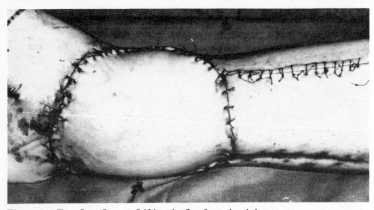

Fig. 14.10 Free flap. *Stage* 1: Lifting the flap from the abdomen
Fig. 14.11 Free flap. *Stage* 2: The area on the lower leg to be covered by the flap
Fig. 14.12 Free flap. *Stage* 3: The flap in situ

that this is a full thickness flap and therefore the donor site has to be covered by a split skin graft or, if possible, sutured directly.

Postoperatively the blood flow through the flap is monitored by a photo-electric plethysmograph. As there are no intermediate stages to this procedure hospitalization is reduced and unlike previous flaps the patient is not subjected to uncomfortable positions which often cause joint stiffness.

The length of time on bed rest is governed by the site of the flap, i.e. a patient with a flap sited in the head and neck region may be up in a chair within two to three days, whereas the patient with a flap on the lower limb may be confined to bed for 14 days.

Recent advances include myocutaneous flaps such as the latissimus dorsi and gastrocnemius flaps in which a large area of skin and underlying muscle is lifted along with one of the main supply vessels and swung into position (Fig. 14/13).

A further refinement in flap design is the fascial flap. It has been found that fascia has a good blood supply and is therefore capable of supporting skin as in an axial pattern flap and it has the advantage of providing skin cover without the bulk of the myocutaneous flap.

Physiotherapy following skin flaps

Chest physiotherapy should be carried out as for skin grafts.

Discomfort and joint stiffness occur in patients with flaps such as groin, pedicles, etc., where the recipient area is attached to the donor area. These positions are maintained for at least three weeks and can be acrobatic in nature. Such tension and consequent pain may be relieved by the application of heat or ice and massage to the muscles and joints involved. Extreme care must be taken to prevent damage to the flap by heat, as the circulation and sensation are reduced and burning and destruction may ensue. Exercises are given in the form of isometric (static) muscle contraction and, whenever possible, by movement of joints. During this period the flap may become swollen (due to its dependent position) and a low pulsed dose of ultrasound and gentle massage can be of value to alleviate this problem which could put the survival of the flap at risk. Now that free flaps are becoming common practice these acrobatic positions are no longer necessary, and although swelling often occurs joint stiffness is less of a problem.

It should be remembered that skin grafts and flaps always produce scarring and this disfigurement often creates a problem to patients. They may be anxious and apprehensive about the possibility of further operations and the eventual outcome. Therefore a great deal

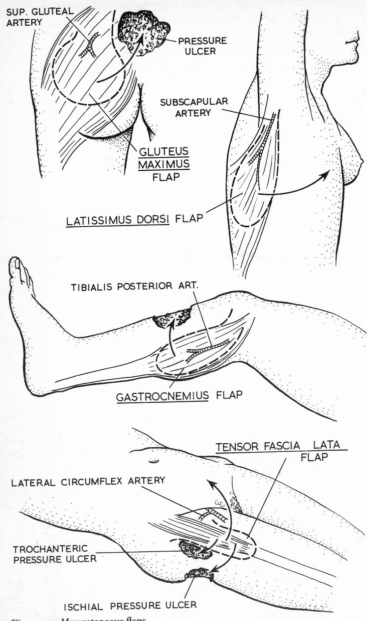

SUP. GLUTEAL ARTERY

PRESSURE ULCER

SUBSCAPULAR ARTERY

GLUTEUS MAXIMUS FLAP

LATISSIMUS DORSI FLAP

TIBIALIS POSTERIOR ART.

GASTROCNEMIUS FLAP

TENSOR FASCIA LATA FLAP

LATERAL CIRCUMFLEX ARTERY

TROCHANTERIC PRESSURE ULCER

ISCHIAL PRESSURE ULCER

Fig. 14.13 Myocutaneous flaps

of time must be spent in reassuring patients, listening to their problems and motivating them to attain the maximum function possible (see Chapter 16).

PLASTIC AND RECONSTRUCTIVE SURGERY

Plastic surgeons are called upon to treat reconstructive problems which are often complex. This specialty arose with the necessity of reconstructing large soft tissue defects following:

1. Burns.
2. Malignancy.
3. Trauma.
4. Congenital problems.

HEAD AND NECK SURGERY

This usually entails radical surgery dealing with such conditions as trauma and carcinoma of the jaw, tongue, bony and skin structures of the head and neck. The majority are tumours which arise from the mucosa and are often squamous cell carcinomas or epitheliomas. They can infiltrate local structures such as the tongue and jaw but metastasize to the regional lymph nodes. Many of these tumours require radical and wide excision thus leaving an area to be reconstructed.

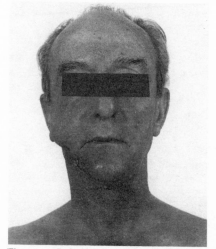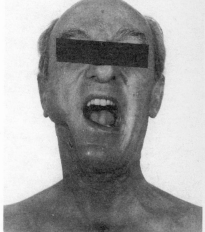

Fig. 14.14 *Left*: A patient who has undergone a right hemimandibulectomy and block dissection of lymph nodes. *Right*: The range of movement following surgery

A tumour of the floor of the mouth often invades the jaw and a hemimandibulectomy may be performed (Fig. 14/14). It is necessary to raise a flap to provide a lining for the mouth and the skin surface of the face. Previously a forehead flap was used but now a free radial forearm flap is often the flap of choice. It is not always necessary to replace the bone but if bone is required the following methods may be used at the time of the initial operation or at a later stage:

1. A free bone graft from the iliac crest.
2. A vascular bone graft from the iliac crest or a rib.
3. A titanium shell filled with cancellous bone.

A hemimandibulectomy may be accompanied by a block dissection of the cervical lymph nodes and removal of the sternomastoid muscles. A branch of the facial nerve may be sacrificed as well as the accessory nerve to the trapezium muscle both leading to some muscle weakness and pain.

Physiotherapy

These are major operations and therefore pre-operative physio-therapy must include an explanation of the procedures to be under-taken, including the possible necessity of tracheostomy, difficulty in speech, eating and general discomfort. Breathing exercises are taught. They are usually carried out in the half-lying position as flaps and grafts may be in situ and therefore the least amount of move-ment in the first few days is desirable to prevent tissue loss. Leg exercises are taught for the prevention of thrombosis.

Postoperatively, on return from theatre, the patient may have a tracheostomy and be nursed in the half-lying position. To clear the chest, breathing exercises are carried out, maintaining the half-lying position. Patients with tracheostomies receive regular suction and leg exercises are encouraged.

Special attention is paid to the flaps to prevent damage.

If the patient develops a chest problem, *treatment of this must take preference* over the reconstructive surgery; the patient may be tipped, turned and moved for postural drainage. After about seven days postoperatively shoulder girdle exercises are commenced and special attention must be paid to posture. Facial exercises can be taught and the patient should be encouraged to open and close his mouth; these movements are carried out in front of a mirror so that the mouth is opened symmetrically and function should be restored rapidly. Pro-vided the excision does not include the mandibular symphysis there should be no problem. If the symphysis is excised, there is nearly always a tendency to drooling, which makes eating and drinking both messy and difficult. Intensive exercises to the lips with finger assistance or resistance may help in the retraining.

It should be noted that radical head and neck surgery can lead to psychological problems and patients need constant reassurance and aid with communication which often includes speech therapy. Ultimately they will need help to adjust to society at large and facilities are available in the use of camouflage make-up and hairdressing.

FACIAL FRACTURES

Patients with facial fractures are admitted to a plastic surgery unit as they often have severe lacerations as a result of going through a windscreen. (Since the wearing of seat belts was made compulsory facial lacerations are seen much less frequently.) Other factors causing these injuries include direct blows, i.e. punches.

A French surgeon, Le Fort, divided facial fractures into three common areas:

1. Lower third – mandible (Le Fort I).
2. Middle third – maxilla, two zygomas, nasal and ethmoid bones (Le Fort II).
3. Upper third – frontal bone (Le Fort III).

NB The first aid treatment dealing with facial fractures must be noted. Patients should *never* be laid on their backs. The tongue should be pulled forward and loose teeth removed from the mouth as there is great danger of airway obstruction.

Fixation

As in any fractures the bones are reduced and immobilized for about five to six weeks. A mandible is fixed by interdental wiring or cap splints.

The maxilla and zygoma are often fixed by interdental wiring and external splintage (Fig. 14/15). More recently they have been plated using mini-plates and screws thus allowing for earlier jaw mobility. The nose is reduced and the septum manipulated into position. Failure to do this may lead to airway obstruction at a later date. Immobilization is maintained by (a) plaster of Paris splint; (b) two small metal plates on either side of the bridge; or (c) Orthoplast. Fractures involving the zygomas may lead to trismus, i.e. difficulty in opening the mouth. Fractures involving the floor of the orbit may

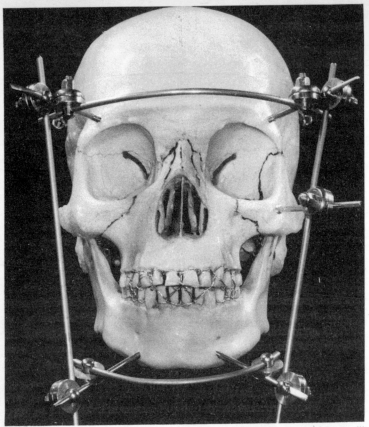

Fig. 14.15 Interdental wiring and external splintage following fractures of the maxilla and zygoma

cause the contents (eyeball) to drop down into the antrum. A silicone plastic plate is therefore inserted to maintain the correct position of the eye.

Physiotherapy

Most of these patients present as emergencies. When first seen wiring and splintage may be present and the nose may also be packed.

Breathing exercises are carried out because the patient may have a considerable amount of blood in the mouth and back of the throat which could lead to chest complications. As the teeth are wired together, difficulty may be experienced in expectorating. Suction is performed via the gap in the interdental wiring. Packing of the nose will exclude nasal suction. If trismus is still present after the splintage is removed, short-wave diathermy to the temporomandibular joint is given using low dosage.

JAW OSTEOTOMIES

These operations are performed usually for congenital abnormalities. The jaws are deformed leading to functional problems such as malocclusion of the teeth. This not only makes biting difficult but affects the cosmetic appearance.

Before undertaking these corrective operations much pre-operative preparation is necessary including special radiographs with measurements, and the making of plaster of Paris moulds by the oral surgery technicians. These can be cut and altered in order to provide a precise plan of surgery.

Mandibular osteotomy

Usually the vertical ramus of the mandible on both sides is split through an intra-oral incision allowing the mandible to be moved backwards or forwards. The fractures are held with splintage as in facial fractures for about six weeks. A bone graft from the hip or ribs may be used.

Maxillary osteotomy

This can be undertaken at many levels from the lower level (Le Fort I), to a higher level at the craniofacial junction (Le Fort III). Higher level surgery may be carried out in conjunction with a neurosurgeon and often immobilization is by external fixation.

Physiotherapy is carried out as for facial fractures.

FACIAL PALSY

Paralysis of the facial (VIIth cranial) nerve is occasionally congenital but more often acquired.

It is often one of the complications of disease of the middle and inner ear. The facial nerve can be compressed or damaged in any part of its course, but as a complication of aural disease it is in its intratemporal course that it will be affected (Fig. 14/16). During this part of the course the nerve, in the narrow bony facial canal, runs from the internal auditory meatus laterally above the labyrinth for a short distance. It makes a right-angled turn back (the genu) then runs down and back in the medial wall of the tympanic cavity and finally

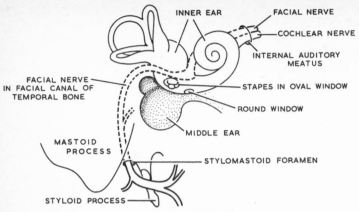

Fig. 14.16 The intratemporal course of the right facial nerve

passes vertically down in the posterior wall of the cavity surrounded by mastoid air cells. The bony wall of the canal is very thin and may actually be deficient at one or more points. Due to its position the canal and nerve may be involved both in ear diseases and in surgery with the nerve becoming inflamed, compressed or injured.

Acute infections of the middle ear can involve the sheath of the nerve, especially if an infected mastoid air cell lies just above the nerve in the absence of the bony wall of the canal.

Erosion of the bony wall of the canal is liable to occur in chronic suppurative otitis media, either by infection or a cholesteatoma.

In surgery the nerve may be damaged during the operation or by the displacement of fragments of bone. It may be compressed by haemorrhage or oedema.

In addition to involvement in diseases of the ear the nerve may also be damaged in this part of its course in fractures of the temporal bone. Idiopathic facial palsy (Bell's palsy) can also occur. The cause is unknown and there is no apparent disease of the ear; it is thought likely that vasospasm results in swelling and ischaemia and consequently compression of the nerve. Such ischaemia could be the result of exposure to draughts and cold.

Types of lesion

The lesion may be a neuropraxia due either to compression by blood or exudate, or caused by bruising. Alternatively, there may be degeneration of the nerve if compression is not relieved or the nerve is damaged during surgery. A combination of both types of lesion is possible.

Treatment A careful assessment must be made before treatment can be decided upon in order to estimate the type and level of the lesion. Such assessment includes a test of motor function, nerve conductivity tests, electromyography, and lacrimation, hearing and taste tests. Treatment is then decided upon according to the results of the above tests and the speed of onset and progression of the paralysis.

Facial paralysis developing during acute middle ear infection will usually recover completely without treatment, once the primary condition is treated. Should paralysis occur in chronic suppurative otitis media, exploration by an aural surgeon is usually considered essential. The facial canal is opened and if there are fibrosis and degeneration, the sheath of the nerve is incised, fibrous tissue removed and a nerve graft carried out. Any cutaneous nerve may be used. Recovery will be slow and may not be complete.

The onset of facial palsy immediately after aural surgery is likely to indicate that the nerve has been damaged. According to his findings the surgeon will explore at once and carry out a decompression or graft. Sometimes the nerve may be unavoidably damaged during surgery such as removal of a tumour involving the parotid gland.

A delayed paralysis following surgery will indicate either too tight packing in the ear, slight contusion of the nerve or, if the paralysis is increasing, bleeding into the facial canal. This will require either removal of the packing or exploration of the facial canal.

Idiopathic facial palsy rarely requires treatment as most patients recover within two to three weeks.

Some patients never recover and these are referred to the plastic surgeon.

Surgery The face symmetry may be improved with surgery. The most common operation used to be the fascial sling, fascia being taken from the tensor fascia lata and attached to the zygomatic arch and the zygomaticus muscle, thereby hitching up the sagging muscles.

Recently in the authors' unit a new surgical approach has been used and is undertaken in two stages.

1st stage: A gold weight is inserted into the upper eyelid and a lateral and/or medial cauthoplasty is carried out to help the patient with eyelid closure. A sural nerve graft is attached to the buccal branch of the functioning VIIth nerve and taken across the lip to the pre-auricular region of the denervated side. After six months if there is a positive Tinel demonstrated by the nerve graft the second stage of the operation is carried out.

2nd stage: Pectoralis minor is lifted and placed on the denervated side as a free muscle transfer. The artery and vein of the flap is anastomosed to the facial artery and vein and the sural nerve graft to the medial and lateral pectoral nerve which is brought with the pectoralis minor. After six months active movement has been noted in many of the patients.

Physiotherapy

Strength duration curves may be requested to determine the type of nerve lesion and the patient's progress but electromyography is used more frequently.

Movements Where there is no ability to contract the muscles the physiotherapist may carry out the movement for the patient, who is asked to 'feel' it and to attempt to hold it. As power begins to return the patient tries to join in and PNF techniques may be used. A spatula can be placed inside the cheek and the patient is asked to 'pull the cheek in' as it is pressed out by the spatula.

Infra-Red, Ice and Ultrasonic Therapy If oedema is present the above modalities may help to reduce it. The small delicate facial muscles waste quickly and can become fibrotic and contracted if recovery is delayed. Stimulation of the circulation and nutrition is therefore valuable, consequently gentle heat may be given before movement. Ice can be used but it has the disadvantage of causing rupture of tiny superficial veins, which is not desirable on the face.

Electrical Stimulation At the present time this is rarely used; occasionally if a patient cannot get the idea of the movement when paralysis has been present for some time, electrical stimulation can be used until he has acquired the 'feel' and knows what to try to do. Research is presently being carried out using a low frequency electrical neuromuscular stimulator which has been showing encouraging results in the treatment of facial palsy.

CLEFT LIP AND PALATE

Any combination of cleft lip and palate may be present:

1. Unilateral cleft lip.
2. Bilateral cleft lip.
3. Unilateral lip and palate.
4. Bilateral lip and palate.
5. Palate only.

Cleft lips are now repaired in the neonatal period and cleft palates at about three months. The cleft lip produces an immediate problem as the baby is unable to suck effectively. If it is not possible to undertake an early repair the orthodontist may construct a plate which is taped to the palate. This helps feeding and holds the alveolar segments in a good position and the lips may be strapped together using external taping.

One of the most common surgical techniques for the repair of the lip is to incise and rotate the medial side of the cleft downwards to the normal lip and advance the tissue on the lateral side of the lip to fill the defect.

Secondary surgery may be undertaken if necessary at a later stage and this is aimed at improving the lip scars and the closure of the soft palate using a pharyngoplasty. Deformities of the alveolus and teeth are dealt with by the orthodontist usually when the permanent teeth have erupted, and hearing and speech problems by the ear, nose and throat surgeon and speech therapist respectively.

Physiotherapy

As some children become undernourished, due to feeding difficulties, they are therefore more prone to chest infections thus chest physiotherapy may be necessary. This will include postural drainage, turning and vibrations, both pre- and postoperatively.

HAND RECONSTRUCTION

Plastic surgeons are involved in a wide variety of hand surgery from small areas of skin loss such as finger tip loss to the multiple and mutilating injuries which require much reconstruction (Figs 14/17 and 14/18).

It is important to understand that in major hand injuries there are three phases:

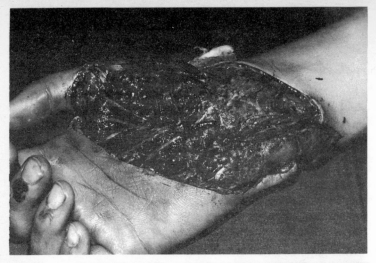

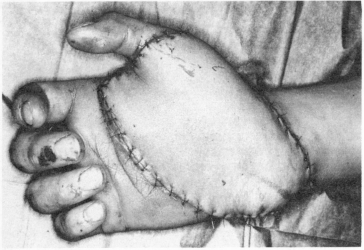

Fig. 14.17 Badly mutilated palm of hand
Fig. 14.18 Flap reconstruction of injury shown in Fig. 14.17

1. Repair of the acute injury.
2. Rehabilitation:
   (a) maturation of collagen
   (b) softening of the scar tissue
   (c) mobilization
3. Reconstruction if and when necessary.

Hand surgery and rehabilitation must aim towards producing maximum function, cosmetic appearance being of secondary importance.

One of the major problems following hand surgery is stiffness. Some causes of stiffness are (a) oedema (b) pain (c) immobilization or (d) scar tissue.

The more the above problems are reduced to a minimum, the more chance the patient has of regaining good function.

CRUSH INJURIES OF HAND

They can be most devastating and severely disabling hand injuries. Not only may there be skin loss but nerves, tendons, arteries and bones are often damaged. This leads to gross oedema, fibrosis of soft tissues and joint stiffness.

In these severe injuries toileting of the wound and excision of necrotic tissue is followed by bony fixation which is achieved using interosseus wiring with an oblique Kirschner wire, or plates and screws. The tendons, nerves, arteries and veins are then repaired and good skin cover provided. These injuries often require flap cover such as a groin or free flap; this is because split skin grafts do not take over exposed tendons and bones, and contract considerably which is undesirable in a hand.

Early postoperative care must be aimed at the reduction of swelling. Wherever possible the hand should be elevated.

Physiotherapy

Immediately after the operation physiotherapy is commenced and shoulder and elbow exercises are carried out. If a graft or flap has not been applied and tendons repaired, it may be possible to carry out hand movements in the early stage.

Oedema is controlled by elevation massage, a low dose of pulsed ultrasound, flow pulse, pressure bandage and exercises where possible.

At the earliest opportunity, active and passive exercises are commenced to each individual joint and the hand as a whole as well as accessory movement. The commencement of exercises is dependent on discussions between the surgeon and physiotherapist, taking into consideration the extent of injury and the likelihood of permanent joint stiffness which must be avoided at all costs.

When the wounds have healed a bland cream must be massaged into the scars to soften them and, if scars are adherent, ultrasound may be used and pulsed electromagnetic energy to reduce oedema.

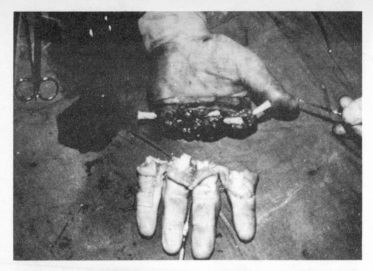

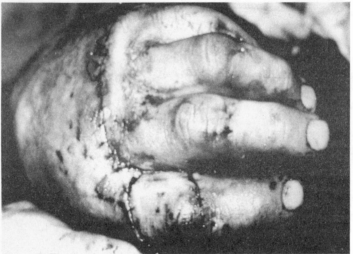

Fig. 14.19 Complete severance of fingers
Fig. 14.20 Fingers replanted

REPLANTATION

Severe injuries of the hand have in the past often led to amputation but now replantation has been made possible by the use of the microscope in surgery (Figs 14/19 and 14/20).

The term *replantation* is used only when the part is completely severed and is sewn back. *Revascularization* is the term used even if a fragment of skin or other tissue is intact with the proximal portion.

First Aid Treatment It is vital that there is little delay. The 'amputate' should be wrapped in a saline moistened swab inside a dry polythene bag and cooled in order to decrease the metabolic rate and prolong the ischaemia time. The best results are obtained if replantation is undertaken within six hours especially if the 'amputate' is large (an arm). The results deteriorate considerably after 12 hours.

Assessment for replantation

It is important that an experienced surgeon and the patient make the joint decision to replant. The best results are obtained in children and young adults who must be prepared to co-operate in the long period of rehabilitation. The nature of the tissue damage must be considered. A clean injury with minimal bone shortening is technically more possible than a crushing rotational injury where the soft tissue injury, especially vascular, is more extensive.

If replantation is technically possible future function must be considered – Will replantation give a more functional result than amputation? Important considerations are sensation and mobility allowing the incorporation of the replanted part into overall function.

The more digits that have been lost, the stronger the indications to replant, especially if the thumb and radial side of the hand is affected, as the re-establishment of pinch grip is of the utmost importance.

Operation This is a long operation and ideally two surgical teams should be used, one to prepare the 'amputate' and the other to debride the stump and identify and label the pertinent structures.

1. *Bone fixation*: The bones should be shortened as the injury will inevitably lead to shortening of all surrounding soft tissues. Rigid internal fixation using interosseus wiring with an oblique Kirschner wire or plates and screws will allow for early mobilization of adjacent joints. If amputation is near to, or through, a joint, joint arthroplasty or arthrodesis in a functional position may be the procedure of choice.

2. *Tendon repair*: The tendons are trimmed and repaired. Limited movement may be anticipated distal to the replantation site, as all the healing and subsequent scar tissue occurs in the one wound. Adherent tendon repairs often act as a functional tenodesis adding to the power of the proximal joints.

3. *Nerve repair*: If the cut is clean and the ends easily approximated the nerve is repaired at the time of injury using the microscope. Following a blunt injury a nerve graft may be necessary and this is carried out as a secondary procedure.

4. *Artery and vein repair*: At least one artery and one vein to each digit should be repaired. In a blunt or avulsion injury there may be considerable vessel damage and a reversed vein graft may be necessary to establish an adequate circulation.

5. *Skin closure*: Tight skin closure must be avoided and it may be more desirable to leave the wound open, or use a split skin graft to protect the repaired structures.

Postoperative Care   The limb should be elevated and the patient nursed in a warm environment; cold can lead to arterial spasm and thrombosis. Dressings are loose or, where practical, no dressing at all.

Devices may be set up to measure temperature and blood flow. If there is any doubt about the circulation the patient may be returned to theatre for possible insertion of a vein graft.

Physiotherapy

Movement of unaffected joints in the affected limbs should be commenced immediately to prevent unnecessary stiffness. At about five days when there is vascular stability, movements of the replanted part should begin. If the replant becomes pale or cyanosed a further period of rest may be necessary. Early passive movements of individual joints is desirable to prevent joint stiffness. Active motion may commence at about three weeks as in tendon repairs.

At a later stage, passive stretching, ultrasound and massage to stretch and soften the scar tissue will be necessary and this is usually combined with splintage.

The patient must be made aware of the dangers of anaesthesia of the skin.

Secondary reconstruction may be carried out to ensure maximum potential function. Bony non-union may require further fixation, nerve grafts to improve sensation and tendon grafts or transfers to give better joint motion.

POLLICIZATION

Tasks which require power and precision are difficult to perform in a hand without a thumb. Lack of a thumb may be congenital, due to trauma or malignancy. This is an operation devised to replace the thumb by using another digit, usually the index finger. It is transposed with intact vessels and nerves by shortening and rotating it into the desired position. The metacarpophalangeal joint of the index finger becomes the new carpometacarpal joint. The head of the second metacarpal is sutured or pushed into its new position. The hand is then immobilized in a plaster of Paris splint for three weeks.

Physiotherapy

This commences at three weeks when the plaster of Paris cast is removed. Active exercises are encouraged and it must be remembered that the new joint and skin sensation of the thumb continues to be that of the transposed digit, therefore re-education should be directed with this in mind.

TOE TO THUMB TRANSFER
(Figs 14/21, 14/22, 14/23 and 14/24)

An alternative method of thumb reconstruction is the free transference of a toe to take the place of a thumb. In the authors' unit, the second toe is used. The surgical technique is as follows:

1. Amputation of the toe at the metatarsophalangeal joint together with the dorsalis pedis artery and veins, digital nerves and tendons.
2. Fixation of bone at the level of the metacarpophalangeal joint with the use of bone grafts, wiring or pegs.
3. Anastomosis of vessels, tendons and nerves:
   1. Dorsalis pedis to radial artery
   2. Vein to cephalic vein
   3. Extensor tendon to extensor pollicis longus. Flexor digitorum profundus to flexor pollicis longus.
   4. Volar digital nerve to the digital nerve of the thumb.

Physiotherapy

At three weeks when the plaster of Paris cast is removed active exercises may commence to encourage flexion and extension of the

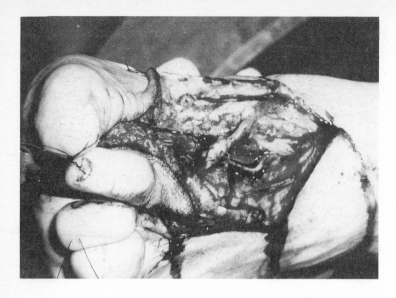

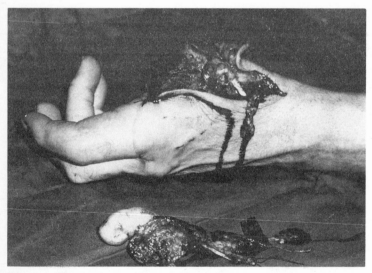

Fig. 14.22 The toe prior to suture to the thumb site

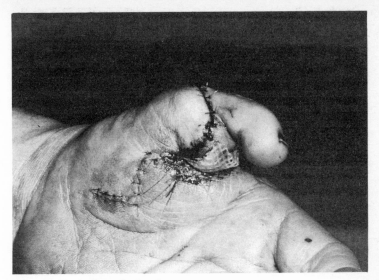

Fig. 14.23 Toe in situ as the thumb

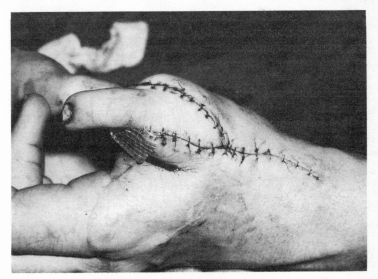

Fig. 14.24 Toe in situ as the thumb at the end of the operation

terminal joint, and apposition using the carpometacarpal joint. No movement should occur at the point of arthrodesis.

SYNDACTYLY

This is usually a congenital condition where two or more digits are joined by a skin web. Occasionally bony continuity may be present and tendons shared. The fingers are separated surgically and a skin graft may be inserted (Fig. 14/25).

Physiotherapy

Once the skin grafts have settled active movements are commenced and the patient/parent is encouraged to massage the scars in order to soften them.

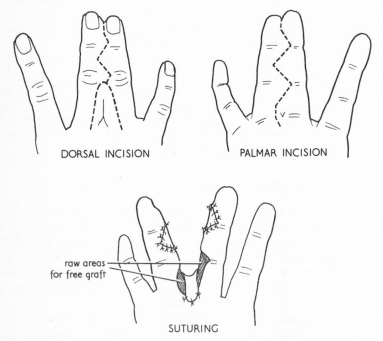

Fig. 14.25 Surgical treatment of syndactyly

PRESSURE SORES

If pressure sores fail to heal the patient may be admitted to the plastic surgery unit. They are nursed on a low air loss bed (p.196) and the wound is cleaned and dressed daily. Once the wound is clean the patient is taken to theatre. The necrotic tissue which may include bone is excised and the defect covered by skin, usually a transposition flap.

Physiotherapy

Breathing exercises are given to prevent chest infections and, wherever possible, active movements to all joints. Care must be taken to ensure that there is no stress on the flap which would endanger the circulation. It should be remembered that many of these patients have neurological conditions such as paraplegia or multiple sclerosis. It is, therefore, most important to carry out passive movements in order to prevent contractures. Total rehabilitation must be planned to suit their condition.

When the flap is stable and the circulation satisfactory, at approximately three weeks, the patient is allowed up for short periods. The length of time is gradually increased as the circulation in the flap continues to improve. A careful watch must be kept and if the flap shows signs of breaking down, the patient must be returned to bed and the pressure removed. If the patient is wheelchair-bound correct cushions to minimize the pressure should be supplied.

MALIGNANT MELANOMA

This is a malignant pigmented tumour which often presents as a dark mole. It originates in the melanocyte and may present as a completely new mole or in a pre-existing mole. It grows rapidly and later becomes irritable and occasionally bleeds. The thickness of the mole determines the prognosis. The tumour can spread via the dermal lymphatics to the lymph nodes and bloodstream and may metastasize to the liver, lungs, bone and brain.

Wide excision and skin graft has been the treatment of choice for some time. An area approximately 7cm either side and 10cm towards the proximal lymph nodes is removed and a split skin graft used to cover the defect. Many surgeons do not advocate such wide excisions in all cases, closing the wound directly. Block dissection of the proximal lymph nodes may be undertaken if they are already involved.

Physiotherapy

As this condition can affect any part of the body, physiotherapy is given accordingly.

Lower limb: The grafted area is immobilized; if a block dissection of the groin nodes has been performed the patient is nursed with the hip in flexion. Movements are given to the distal joints to maintain circulation, prevent thrombosis and stiffness in the limb. Movements are given to the other limb.

After 10 to 14 days, gentle mobilization of the hip joint is commenced and the patient is allowed to start ambulation wearing a double layer of Tubigrip to support the grafted limb.

Upper limb: If this condition occurs in the upper limb, and a block dissection of the cervical axillary nodes has been performed, postoperative breathing exercises may be necessary. Distal joints are again exercised.

Swelling may occur in either the upper or lower limb due to the interference with the lymphatic drainage. Patients must be made aware of the importance of elevation, and when necessary pressure garments and the Flowtron compression unit may be used to combat the swelling. The latter can be used by the patient at home.

LYMPHOEDEMA

This may be congenital or acquired. It is due to malfunction of the lymphatic vessels, fluid being retained in the tissue spaces. Acquired lymphoedema often follows surgery where excision of the lymph nodes has been undertaken; in the tropics filariasis can be a cause.

Treatment

Early lymphoedema can sometimes be treated by drainage procedures such as importing skin flaps with their lymphatics, omental transfers or lympho-venous shunts.

Late lymphoedema may be helped by:

1. *Thompson operation* (buried dermal flap) (Fig. 14/26): In this operation fat and lymphoedematous tissue is excised, usually from groin to ankle or wrist to axilla around half the circumference of the limb. One of the resulting two flaps is de-epithelialized and then sutured between the muscle bellies. This

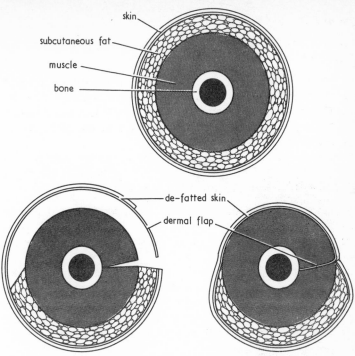

skin

subcutaneous fat

muscle

bone

de-fatted skin

dermal flap

Fig. 14.26 Thompson operation for lymphoedema (diagrammatic)

establishes a communication between the usually patent deep system of lymphatics which subsequently drains the more superficial layers. The remaining flap is sutured over the de-epithelialized area and a pressure dressing applied. The patient is nursed in bed with the leg elevated for 10 days or until the wound has healed.

2. *Charles operation*: In this operation the skin and lymphoedematous tissue is excised down to deep fascia, from knee to ankle, the skin being separated and used to cover the defect.

Physiotherapy In both cases the leg is immobilized until the wound is healed and skin grafts have become well established. After about 7 to 10 days gentle active movements are commenced. Weight-bearing is usually allowed at about 10 to 12 days with a double layer of Tubigrip being worn for support.

ULCERS AND LACERATIONS WITH SKIN NECROSIS

These conditions usually occur in older patients and those patients with impairment of blood supply or who through the use of drugs and radiotherapy develop paper thin or fibrotic skin.

Ulcers: The patient is admitted for bed rest, with elevation of the limb. Once the ulcer is clean and healthy looking, a split skin graft is applied to close the defect.

Lacerations: Skin necrosis may occur following lacerations and failure to heal after suturing. The laceration may be jagged and the surrounding tissue necrotic. Any necrotic tissue is therefore excised and a skin graft used to cover the defect.

Physiotherapy

Pre-operatively, maintenance exercises are carried out to increase circulation, prevent thrombosis, decrease oedema and prevent joint stiffness.

Postoperatively the patient will continue the maintenance exercises, but care must be taken not to disturb the skin grafts. If at five days the skin graft has only partially taken, pulsed electromagnetic energy may be used as this appears to stimulate epithelialization and can be applied through dressings. At 10 days the patient swings the leg over the side of the bed and if the circulation of the skin graft is unaffected by the dependency of the limb walking may commence with a double layer of Tubigrip for support.

COMPOUND FRACTURES

The most common fractures seen on a plastic surgery unit are compound fractures of the tibia and fibula when skin and/or bone loss are evident. Unfortunately they are often referred late and this may necessitate more complex surgery than if seen at an early date.

If there is necrotic bone present and inadequate skin cover a fracture will not unite and if infection occurs serious problems such as osteomyelitis may ensue. The injury should be seen within the first 12 hours. It is often possible to clean the wound, remove dead tissue and replace lost skin with a free flap. This means shorter hospitalization, less infection and improved healing of the under-lying fracture which is immobilized with external fixation (Fig. 14/27).

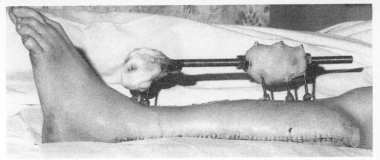

Fig. 14.27 External fixation for compound fracture of the tibia (*note*: the screws are protected by plastic)

When there is a delay in referral there is often bony infection present and therefore radical decortication insertion of a muscle flap into the guttered bone and a split skin graft to heal the wound is carried out. Once healing has occurred and the infection has cleared a flap is then applied.

In some cases a large bony defect may be present. A free vascularized fibula graft from the other leg is inserted. A portion of fibula is excised with its overlying skin, subcutaneous tissue and blood supply. The blood vessels of the graft are anastomosed to those in the recipient leg and the overlying skin provides flap cover. These patients often have an above knee plaster of Paris cylinder followed by bracing where possible for up to 12 months or more.

Physiotherapy

Exercises may be carried out on the affected limb but with particular precautions being taken not to disturb the fracture site or skin graft/flap. In patients with external fixation it may be possible to mobilize the ankle and knee and strengthen the quadriceps. Maintenance exercises are carried out as for orthopaedic conditions – sand bags, springs, etc. being used to maintain the strength of the good leg and arms.

If patients present with multiple injuries, e.g. fractured ribs, sternum or mandible, breathing exercises are necessary. As soon as skin cover has been achieved, patient are often referred back to the orthopaedic surgeon and further rehabilitation is carried out from the orthopaedic ward and later as an outpatient. Once the fracture or fibular graft is reasonably stable the patients may be allowed to weight-bear as this often encourages the formation of callus.

COSMETIC SURGERY

Rhinoplasty

This is an operation to improve the appearance or function (airways) of the nose. It is undertaken for congenital or post-traumatic deformities and often consists of:

1. Sub-mucosal resection and reconstruction of the septum with, if necessary, bone or cartilage.
2. In-fracture, i.e. the nasal bones are separated from the maxilla, thus allowing them to be mobilized and the correct position attained.

Immobilization is carried out by the use of plaster of Paris.

Face lift (rhytidectomy)

This is to eliminate wrinkles. An incision is made in front of the ears, the skin undermined, excess fat removed, a tuck taken in the fascia if necessary and then the skin pulled tight, the excess excised and the wound closed. This may be accompanied by eyelid reductions.

Dermabrasion

This is used to flatten irregularities of the skin such as are caused by acne. Sandpaper or wire brushes are used to perform the operation. It leaves a raw area which heals by the epithelium growing across from the hair follicles, sweat and sebaceous glands and heals within about 10 days. Exposure to sunlight for the following six months is discouraged as this can result in hyperpigmentation.

Port wine stains

These are congenital birth marks. They may be excised and skin grafted but this inevitably results in scarring. Many patients use camouflage make-up.

Abdominal lipectomy

This is performed to remove excess skin and fatty tissue from the abdomen and leaves a transverse lower abdominal scar. Excess fat and skin can be removed from other areas such as thighs and buttocks. A new technique which is gaining in popularity is liposuction: a metal tube is inserted into the fatty area through a small incision and attached to a high pressure vacuum suction pump thus removing fat globules.

Mammaplasty

This is carried out to reduce or augment breast tissue.

Mammary hypoplasia: This is a lack of breast tissue which may be congenital or acquired. Augmentation is achieved by the insertion of a silicone prosthesis under the breast tissue or pectoralis major.

Mammary hyperplasia: This is an increase in breast tissue which is again congenital or acquired and surgery may be carried out to remove this excess tissue. Skin, fat and breast tissue is removed from the lower half of the breast and the nipple raised to a higher level on a vascular pedicle.

Bat or prominent ears

This operation is usually performed on schoolchildren who are often teased about the condition. This is corrected by the excision of some post-auricular skin and alteration of the cartilaginous tissue of the ears is necessary.

Physiotherapy Little physiotherapy is carried out for any of the above conditions unless the patients have an underlying chest condition.

Ultrasound and pulsed electromagnetic energy may be useful to reduce oedema and haematoma and ultrasound at a later date to soften scars.

OTHER CONDITIONS

Scar revision

Disfiguring scars, i.e. those following trauma, must be allowed to mature before further surgery is contemplated. The most simple procedure is to excise and resuture. The course of scars may be altered to allow the scar to blend in with the surrounding tissue by, wherever possible, lying in the same direction as the skin lines and this is achieved by a Z-plasty. Ultrasound may be used to soften the area.

Hypospadias

This is the congenital deformity whereby the urethra opens on to the
the undersurface of the penis or perineum. The aim of surgery is to
move the opening forward to the tip of the penis. This is done by:

1. Releasing the chordae
2. Creating a gutter through which the urethra may pass and inserting a temporary catheter
3. Skin grafting around the catheter.

BIBLIOGRAPHY

Burke, F.D. (1983). Microsurgery in the upper limb. *Physiotherapy*. **69**, 10, 346–9.
Connolly, W.B. (1980). *A Colour Atlas of Hand Conditions*. Wolfe Medical and
    Scientific Publications, London.
Grabb, W.C. and Smith, J.W. (1973). *Plastic Surgery: A Concise Guide to Clinical
    Practice*, 2nd edition. Little, Brown and Co, Boston.
Jackson, I.T. and Sommerland, B.C. (eds) (1985). *Recent Advances in Plastic Surgery*
    – 3. Churchill Livingstone, Edinburgh.
Jones, B., Smith, P. and Harrison, D. (1983). Replantation (Leading article.) *British
    Medical Journal*, **287**, 1–2.
Lister, G. (1984). *The Hand: Diagnosis and Indications*, 2nd edition. Churchill
    Livingstone, Edinburgh.
McGregor, I.A. (1980). *Fundamental Techniques of Plastic Surgery and Their Surgical
    Applications*, 7th edition. Churchill Livingstone, Edinburgh.
Morgan, B. and Wright, M. (1986). *Essentials of Plastic and Reconstructive Surgery:
    with notes on clinical, nursing and general management*. Faber and Faber, London.
O'Brien, B. and Morrison, W.A. (1987). *Reconstructive Microsurgery*. Churchill
    Livingstone, Edinburgh.
Reid, C.D.A. and Tubiana, R. (eds.) (1984). *Mutilating Injuries of the Hand*, 2nd
    edition. Churchill Livingstone, Edinburgh.
Salter, M.I. (1987). *Hand Injuries: A Therapeutic Approach*. Churchill Livingstone,
    Edinburgh.
Wynn Parry, C.B. (1981). *Rehabilitation of the Hand*, 4th edition. Butterworths,
    London.

ACKNOWLEDGEMENT

Figures 14/3, 14/4, 14/5, 14/6 and 14/13 have appeared previously in *Essentials of
Plastic and Reconstructive Surgery* by Brian Morgan and Margaret Wright, and are
reproduced by permission of the authors and publisher, Faber and Faber, London.

Chapter 15

Burns

by B. MORGAN, MB, FRCS and S. BOARDMAN MCSP

Burns affect all age-groups but children and the elderly are at great risk. Similarly, psychiatric, epileptic and low income groups are particularly vulnerable. Many burns result from accidents in the home, most of which are preventable.

When heat is applied to the skin surface the results are as follows:

1. Erythema (reddening).
2. Increased capillary permeability with a loss of protein rich fluid into the surrounding tissues and from the burned surface.
3. Cell death.

The loss of fluid from the circulation is responsible for burns shock. The loss starts at the moment of burning and as Crile has stated 'the best treatment for shock is prevention', so that replacement of the fluid must commence immediately. The volume of fluid lost from the circulation is great (Fig. 15/1). It is dependent upon the surface area of burn and not the depth. The size of the patient is important and for a measure of the patient's size we conveniently use the weight.

To measure the surface area of a burn the rule of nine is used (Fig. 15/2). A formula assists the surgeon in knowing what quantity of fluid to transfuse but this is only a guide and the patient must be monitored at regular intervals to see whether he shows any signs of shock. These are:

1. A cold clammy skin and pale patient.
2. Restlessness.
3. Vomiting associated with a reduced blood supply to the viscera and alimentary tract.
4. Rapid pulse and lowered blood pressure. The blood pressure fall may not be significant because of compensatory mechanism.
5. Reduced urine output.

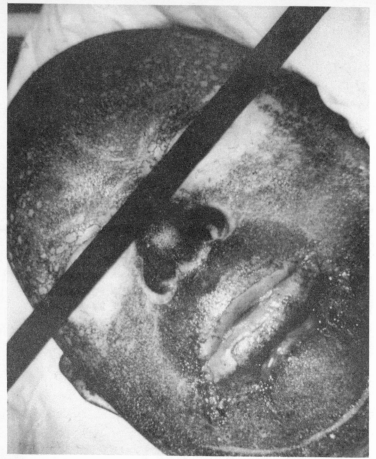

Fig. 15.1 A patient with a severely burnt face showing the gross oedema

The hourly volume of urine output is a most sensitive measure; the central venous pressure can be helpful, and centrifuged blood samples or haematocrits show haemoconcentration and raised values in burns shock.

The intravenous fluid used to replace that lost from the circulation is plasma protein fraction (PPF) or dextran. Blood may be needed if there is a 10 per cent or larger full thickness skin loss. The normal intake of fluid must be maintained either by oral administration or by additional intravenous fluids. At the end of 48 hours the fluid loss from the circulation has diminished and the danger of death from burns shock is over.

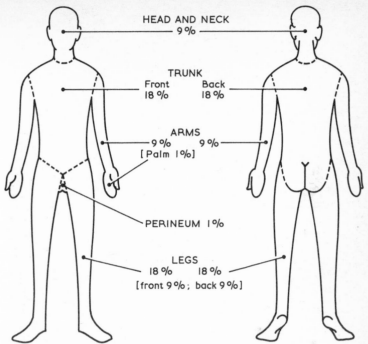

Fig. 15.2 The 'rule of nine' for assessing the extent of the burnt area

INHALATION INJURIES

The inhalation of hot gases or steam can burn the air passages but by far the greatest problem is the inhalation of toxic fumes of combustion, for instance the cyanide from polyurethane foam fires and carbon monoxide poisoning. Pulmonary oedema develops in the first 24 hours. Oxygen transfer is reduced and shunting of blood through the lungs occurs. Mild cases need an increase in the inspired oxygen but severe cases will need intubation and ventilation. The decision to intubate and/or ventilate has to be taken early; several techniques of ventilation including positive end-expiratory pressure (PEEP) are used. The oedema is slow to clear and ventilation may be needed for two weeks or more so that tracheostomy is advisable. (For a full description of techniques of ventilation the reader is referred to *Cash's Textbook of Chest, Heart and Vascular Disorders for Physiotherapists*, 4th edition.)

All extensively burned patients need to start breathing exercises within a few hours of admission. If the patient is ventilated the physiotherapist may be asked to carry out vibrations while the doctor bag-squeezes and the nurse uses suction. Suction is carried out with the greatest possible care using a no-touch technique.

After the patient has been extubated an intermittent positive pressure breathing (IPPB) machine such as the Bird or Bennett is often used. These machines are also of infinite value on patients who have an underlying chest condition present prior to the burn.

Children with burns of the face and trunk easily develop acute chest symptoms but respiratory complications often take 24 hours or more to develop.

If the patient has burns of skin over the chest but no obvious respiratory complication, care must be taken and expansion checked, but vibration and percussion are not given as further trauma to the burnt tissues may result in a superficial burn becoming full thickness. A tight eschar around the chest will necessitate an escharotomy to allow expansion and to prevent lung collapse.

THE BURN SURFACE (Fig. 15/3)

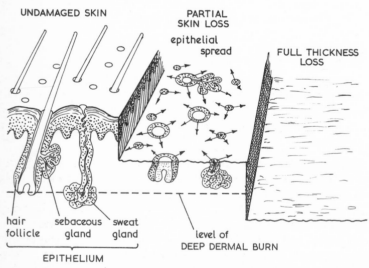

Fig. 15.3 Skin damage following different depths of burn surface

Damaged skin does not function properly. Water and heat loss is increased and, most important, infection can enter the body and the tissues. Bacteria come from the patient's own flora or from contamination from outside sources, including staff. For this reason patients are isolated. All staff including physiotherapists must ensure that their hands are carefully washed before and after treatment and protective clothing and gloves are worn in many burns units.

Partial thickness burns

The epidermis and superficial layers of the dermis only are destroyed, and the epithelium of the hair follicles, sweat and sebaceous glands spreads across the surface so that a new layer of epidermis is present in 10 to 14 days. The treatment of partial skin loss (PSL) is to prevent infection and mechanical damage and allow spontaneous healing.

Full thickness burns

The epidermis and the whole of the dermis are totally destroyed so that no regenerative islands of hair follicles, sweat and sebaceous glands can occur. Small full thickness burns heal by the epithelium growing from the margins of the burn and by the wound contracting. Large areas do not heal and need skin grafting.

Deep dermal burns

A separate group of burns is recognized where the damage, although not full thickness, is so deep that there are few hair follicles and no sweat or sebaceous glands surviving so healing is very slow and results in much scarring. These burns are best skin grafted at an early stage.

Assessment of burn depth is difficult. The depth of burn is dependent on the temperature and duration to which the area has been exposed so that the mechanism of burning is an indication of depth. An accurate account of the accident and first aid measures is important. For instance electrical burns are full thickness, whereas scalds are partial thickness. The appearance is helpful. Blistering is usually present in partial thickness burns whereas a leathery white or charred skin is seen in full thickness burns. The sensation to pin prick is lost in full thickness burns because the nerve endings have been destroyed.

If full thickness burns are circumferential around a limb the tight eschar (dead tissue) fails to allow expansion so that arteries are compressed and ischaemia of the distal part occurs. Full thickness burns of the chest, if circumferential, may limit chest expansion with dire consequences; as an emergency the eschar must be split open (escharotomy). This is a painless procedure as all the pain fibres in the skin have been destroyed.

SKIN GRAFTING

Wherever possible full thickness burns should be excised early, before they become colonized by bacteria. At or about the fourth day post-burn is the most desirable time. The burned tissue is removed until live bleeding tissue is reached. Often this is deep fascia as the blood supply to the subcutaneous fat is poor. Deep dermal burns are shaved layer by layer with a skin graft knife (tangential excision) until bleeding occurs in the dermis. Fat is not exposed.

Early grafting may not be possible if the patient is in a critical condition, if the burns are very large or if there is a mixture of full and partial thickness loss which cannot be clearly demarcated. In the last case the burns are dressed until two to three weeks after burning to allow the partial thickness burn to heal and the remaining areas are then skin grafted.

Skin grafts are taken from the unburned areas of the patient. The thighs are the best donor areas whereas the abdominal wall and the scalp are difficult sites from which to remove skin. Split skin grafts are used. The thinner the skin the better it takes but it will contract more than a thick skin graft which is a disadvantage.

Autograft This is skin taken from the patient himself. There will be no rejection by immune reaction.

Homograft This is other people's skin. It is used as a temporary cover. The skin 'takes' but will be rejected at about three weeks. The donor must be tested for HIV.

Heterograft This is skin from another species. The pig has a skin which is quite similar to human and will 'take' but is rejected at about three weeks.

Skin Culture Patients' own skin can now be cultured in the laboratory, so that sheets of skin can be produced over a three- or four-week period. However, much more research is necessary before this can be of practical value for most burns patients as the skin is of poor quality.

Meshed Skin   Shortage of autograft is a problem in large burns, but it is possible to make what little skin there is available go further by slitting holes in the sheet and expanding it up to three or four times. A special machine is used in the operating theatre for this process.

The skin graft donor areas are dressed. They heal much as a partial thickness burn does by epithelium growing across from the hair follicles, sweat and sebaceous glands. In the early stages donor areas can be very painful and the physiotherapist has to remember this when encouraging movement. The donor areas are usually healed by two weeks and can be used for further skin graft donation at about three to four weeks.

Burns dressings

A partial skin loss wound, while awaiting healing, needs protection. This is best achieved by using a dressing consisting of a non-stick layer (such as Jelonet) against the burn, with an absorbable material (gauze or cotton wool) outside this. The dressing is taken well beyond the burn wound and held firmly in place with a bandage. Infrequent dressing changes are advisable (every four or five days) as removing the dressing can damage the healing epithelium. Exudate appearing through the dressing, or what is called 'strike through', necessitates a redressing or extra packing to prevent infection entering.

Silver sulphadiazine (Flamazine) is an expensive but excellent antibacterial cream. It is particularly effective against pseudomonas infections which is a common problem in burns. The cream is spread on the burned surface and usually covered with some form of dressing. This needs changing every 48 hours. Changing dressings is a painful process and needs plentiful analgesia. Sometimes ketamine, or even general anaesthetic, is needed. A bath or shower is of great help in removing dressings that are adherent. Baths are invaluable in facilitating early movement. The patient may initially be apprehensive but exercises in the bath can be carried out more comfortably. Saline baths (commercially available 1.8% NaCl) are beneficial to the healing process (Parkhouse, personal communication). They should be at body temperature. There is however the danger of cross-infection in the burns bath but special baths and rigorous cleansing techniques can reduce the danger.

Wet dressings on immobile patients increase the risk to pressure necrosis ideally in the early stages patients with extensive burns

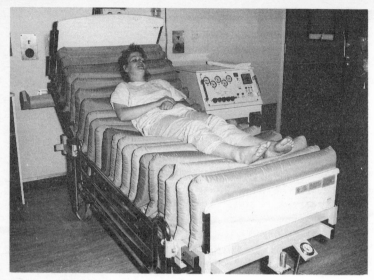

Fig. 15.4 Low airloss bed

should be nursed on a low airloss bed (Fig. 15/4) or a fluidized bead
bed. The former is an air displacement system; the bed consists of
five sections each adjusting to the body contour, the pressure of
which can be individually controlled to suit the needs of the patient.
Nursing care with this type of bed is simplified by:

1. The elimination of pressure areas.
2. The lifting and turning of the patient being reduced to a
   minimum.
3. Changing of bed linen being reduced as only a top sheet is
   required.

Physiotherapists find that the tipping mechanism is easily controlled
which is an asset in the treatment of the patient's chest. However, it
is a fact that patients have difficulty in moving themselves around
the bed and for this reason it is necessary to transfer the patient to a
hospital-type bed as soon as possible.

   In the second type of bed silicone beads which look like sand are
fluidized by passing warm air through them. The patient lies in the
fluidized beads with an even pressure on the body surface. It is not as
easy to sit the patient up.

PHYSIOTHERAPY

Positioning of the patient is most important and a close watch must be kept on this by the physiotherapist as well as the nursing staff. Burns overlying the flexor aspects of the joints give rise to contracture. These must be prevented. Splints are ideal, though with severe burns they are difficult to apply effectively. Plaster of Paris with Kramer wire, Plastazote, Polyform and Orthoplast are all used in an effort to support and maintain good functional position of joints including the cervical spine. The use of boards and splints to prevent foot drop is essential and the knees should be maintained as straight as possible. The head and neck should be supported in a mid and extended position. The hands are elevated to reduce oedema and the Bradford sling is most convenient for this (Fig. 15/5).

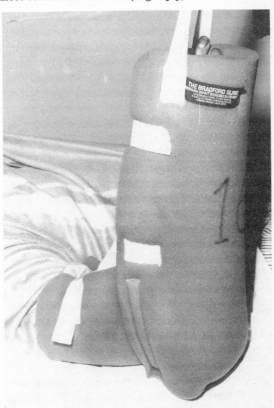

Fig. 15.5
The Bradford sling

All movements can be encouraged from the time that the patient is admitted to hospital. However, when autografts are applied the grafted areas must not be mobilized for at least five days. At that time the first dressing is carried out. However, this does not prevent the physiotherapist giving movements to ungrafted areas and it is indeed essential that they should continue them.

Patients can recommence active exercises to the grafted areas five to seven days after the grafting procedure.

A feature of burns illness is a mental surrender to apathy often aggravated by necessary isolation. Combined with this is a suppression of intellect and aesthetic interests with a withdrawal from personal relationships. The physiotherapist's daily or twice daily visits give these patients a regular and closer contact with the outside world and this in turn demands of the physiotherapist a great understanding and the ability to provide mental stimulation. In some units complete isolation is maintained only during the pre-grafting period. Then after grafting the patient is transferred to a three-or four-bedded ward where the encouragement and company of others is undoubtedly an added incentive to recovery. The treatment of burns is extremely time-consuming for the physiotherapist. When burns are extensive it is necessary to encourage specific and general mobilization: it must be remembered that these patients tire easily and should be allowed frequent rest periods. Time *must* be spent in encouragement, endeavouring to give confidence to patients who, due partly to their isolation and largely to the severity of their injuries, need maximum reassurance and come to look on their physiotherapist as a source of special contact with the rest of the medical team (see Chapter 16).

Early ambulation is desirable. If skin grafting is delayed then the patient is walked before surgery is carried out. The lower limbs are supported by firm bandaging or Tubigrip. It is advisable to swing the bandaged legs over the side of the bed before commencing weight-bearing. Following surgery, blistering of newly grafted areas can occur. For this reason weight-bearing is not commenced for seven to ten days. Standing still is not permitted, and when sitting the lower limbs should be elevated. For those with grafted legs Tubigrip, firm bandages or elastic stockings will have to be worn for six weeks to prevent oedema. Footwear may have to be adapted to cope with bandages and a heel raise may be necessary if there is calf contracture. Burns of the feet may have to be specially protected. This can be done with foam rubber or Plastazote.

The patient should attend the physiotherapy department at the earliest possible opportunity. This is often the patient's first contact with the outside world following the burn. Here, supportive therapy and great encouragement is required because the disfigurement caused by the burn is often demoralizing. Helping the patient to surmount and overcome the natural self-consciousness is something in which the physiotherapist can play a very helpful role.

HAND BURNS

Hands are common sites for burns, not only through direct involvement but also because they are so often used in a reflex action to protect the face. Burns on the dorsum of the hands are more common than those on the palmar skin which in any case is so much thicker and so usually result in partial thickness loss only. Oedema forms rapidly and is a serious threat to hand function. Elevation is of critical importance.

The burned hand takes up a poor functional position of wrist flexion, metacarpophalangeal extension and interphalangeal joint flexion. The thumb is adducted. In an unco-operative or unconscious patient the hand is splinted with the wrist extended, the metacarpophalangeal joints flexed and the interphalangeal joints extended with the thumb abducted and slightly flexed (Fig. 15/6).

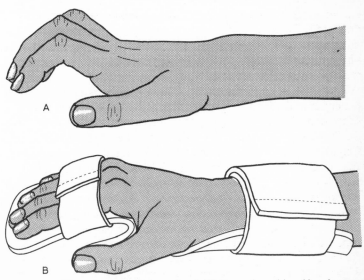

Fig. 15.6 (A) The contracture of a burnt hand. (B) Correction achieved by adequate splinting

Plastic bags

Hand burns are best treated by retaining their mobility. If the hand is placed in a plastic bag, sealed at the wrist, the moisture that collects keeps the skin and the burns supple, allowing movement with minimal pain (Fig. 15/7). The hands are elevated and regular active and passive movements under the supervision of the physiotherapist are carried out. The moist conditions support bacterial growth so antibacterial agents or silicone oil are often added to the bags. The bags need changing twice daily and for this reason hospitalization is usually advised but it is not strictly necessary. White macerated palmar skin can be a worrisome appearance for the patient who should be reassured that this is the appearance of undamaged skin. The bags are kept on until healing of the partial thickness burn is complete or until the full thickness burn is ready for skin grafting.

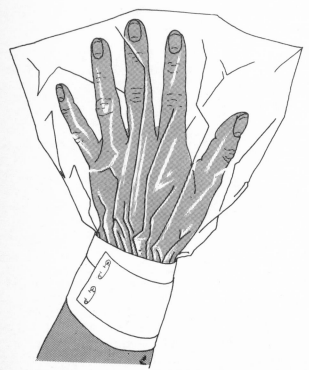

Fig. 15.7 The burnt hand enclosed in a plastic bag thus allowing exercises to be carried out

Following grafting either by early tangential or full thickness excision or by late covering of granulation tissue the grafts take two or three weeks to become stable. Although excessive movement or abrasion will detach grafts, early movement is mandatory to prevent stiffness and enable a full range of movement to be recovered. The physiotherapist needs to be active yet gentle. Silicone oil baths for the hands assist early movement of the fingers, protect the grafts and remove debris.

PREVENTION OF CONTRACTIONS

Wounds contract during healing until they are covered by epithelium. Scars and skin grafts shrink and contract particularly around joints and in the flexures of the elbow, knee and fingers but the neck and axillae are common sites too. The contracting forces of scars and skin grafts cannot be prevented by physiotherapy, active or passive movement. The best way of counteracting these contracting forces is by prolonged static splinting and often three months or longer is necessary.

Secondary correction of contractures

Despite preventive measures contractures do develop and need secondary correction. Under a general anaesthetic the contracted scar is divided and the defect filled with either a thick split skin graft or full thickness graft. These contract less than a thin split skin graft. Alternatively a flap of skin either from adjacent tissue or from a distance can be used. Flaps do not contract. They have their own blood supply and so can be placed over areas which are avascular such as bare cortical bone, open joint or exposed tendon. Flaps are needed as cover in the early stages if a bare tendon, bone or cartilage is exposed.

Hypertrophic and keloid scarring

A thin partial skin loss will heal with colour change only. The skin texture may be normal or rather papery but there is no contracture. Deep dermal or full thickness loss will heal with raised lumpy red irritating scars but go on growing for three months and then take several years to become pale and soft and may never flatten completely. This change is called *scar hypertrophy*. It can occur in adults but is common in children. Keloid scars are less common and a greater proportion of the patients have coloured skin. The initial scar

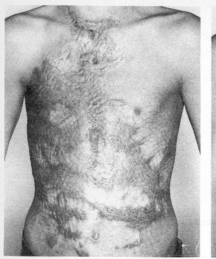 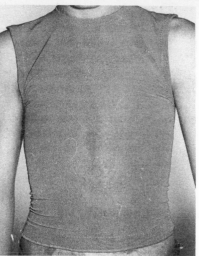

Fig. 15.8 A patient with a healed burnt and grafted chest

Fig. 15.9 The same patient as in Fig. 15.8 wearing a precisely measured pressure garment to prevent the development of hypertrophic scars

may be flat but after some weeks the scarring grows and itches and the growth extends outside the original area of injury and shows little tendency to resolution.

Pressure can prevent and treat hypertrophic scarring. Elastic garments made to measure to fit tightly over the burned area and worn day and night for 6 to 18 months are used (Figs 15/8 and 15/9). Particularly bad areas of hypertrophic scarring are covered under the garment with silicone gel sheet.

Massage with lanolin or hydrous ointment is given to soften the scar. Scars of grafts do not have entirely normal sensation. Patients must be warned about the dangers of coming into contact with direct heat, for instance hot plates, radiators, as well as against exposure to sun for at least twelve months. Infra-red lamps or wax should not be used. Warm water is of value and, particularly for the hand, silicone oil.

GENERAL MANAGEMENT

Nutrition of the patient needs careful attention. There is a vast catabolic breakdown so that muscle bulk as well as fat reserve are lost. Prevention of this and restoration of the loss needs a high protein, high calorie diet which can be given by nasogastric tube as the appetite is often suppressed. As indicated earlier, burns, for the most part, occur in the underprivileged and those at the extremes of life. There is a high incidence also of mental illness and epilepsy. The mental shock of the accident, cubicle isolation, dependence on staff and concerns about the future all add to a complex problem. Tact, understanding and sympathy yet firm handling by the physiotherapist are needed.

BIBLIOGRAPHY

Harvey Kemble, J. V. and Lamb, B. E. (1987). *Practical Burns Management*. Hodder and Stoughton, London.

Muir, I. F. K., Barclay, T. L. and Settle, J. A. D. (1987). *Burns and their Treatment*, 3rd edition. Lloyd Luke (Medical Books) Limited, London.

ACKNOWLEDGEMENT

Figures 15/3 has appeared previously in *Essentials of Plastic and Reconstructive Surgery* by Brian Morgan and Margaret Wright, and is reproduced by permission of the publisher, Faber and Faber, London.

Chapter 16

A Patient's Viewpoint of Physiotherapy Following Severe Burns

by JAMES PARTRIDGE MA (Oxon), MSc

It is now widely recognized that members of the health care team need to work together to bring about full recovery for their patients. Whatever the illness or injury suffered, doctors, nurses and para-medical staff must co-ordinate their skills so that they are of maximum value to the sick person. Such a multidisciplinary approach necessitates that team members respect and understand each other's professional abilities and that all are aware of the problems inherent in professional–patient relationships.

The delivery of effective treatment and care for the sick and injured is now the subject of a substantial literature, not just of a technical nature, but also with sociological and psychological insights brought to bear on the problem. The role of the patient has also been examined through the eyes of onlookers like anthropologists and by patients themselves. Sir Cecil Clothier's monograph *The Patient's Dilemma* challenges all in the caring professions to understand better the patient's unique position of surrender to the care and skill of others.

Important as these contributions are, however, they tend to be somewhat generalized in tone and academic in content. The student professional will find many questions left unanswered – especially about the emotional impact of injury on the patient. This was brought home to me very forcefully when I was asked to talk to a lecture room full of student nurses (at St Thomas's Hospital) about my experiences with severe burns.

I knew that many of them had already worked in a burns unit and I was rather nervous about giving them just another lecture. But very quickly it became apparent that my audience was positively bursting with bottled-up questions. Once they realized that I was willing to talk frankly, they bombarded me (very politely, of course) with questions about pain, hospitalization and recovery – How had I *felt*? and What does it feel like now? For these quite experienced student nurses this was their first and possibly only chance to articulate their personal anxieties about how they related to burns cases and to patients in general.

I hope that the presence of this chapter in an otherwise technical textbook will help physiotherapists to appreciate more fully the special circumstances and problems of being severely burned and undergoing extensive plastic surgery. My successful recovery owes much to the work of physiotherapists and I have done my best in this chapter to explain why. The art of surgery is finely displayed in operating theatres – but surgery alone will not get a patient back into active life.

LOOKING BACK

It is now 14 years since I left the plastic surgery wards of Queen Mary's Hospital, Roehampton in London. In the preceding four years I had received intensive and exhaustive treatment there for severe burns to my face, hands, legs and body sustained when a Land Rover I was driving overturned and caught fire. Now I am a dairy farmer and part-time 'A'-level economics teacher in a girls' school in Guernsey, married with three children.

The fact that I am now living at all is miraculous enough – 40 years earlier I would have had little chance in a similar accident. That I am now leading a full and exceedingly active life is just one of the many success stories that should inspire all who work with the severely burned and disfigured. Often patients lose touch with the hospital and the staff who were responsible for their treatment – as I have – and it may be tempting to put that loss of contact down to the difficulties and anxieties experienced in the aftermath of such serious injuries. Equally, no news may herald good news.

Nonetheless recovery and rehabilitation after facial and other burns is an agonizing business. I soon learnt that no amount of even the most brilliant and ingenious surgical manoeuvres can heal the deep psychological scarring that accompanies this kind of personal disaster. The physical pain and restriction of numerous operations, of thick bands of keloid scars, and of highly sensitive skin is bad enough, and can be an hourly and daily trial for years after the initial injury. But the mental process of appreciating what has happened and the life-long struggle to come to terms with disfigurement – and, most of all, of other people's reaction to it – require greater strength than the simple physical demands of recovery.

Physiotherapy in the public mind is seen as synonymous with physical exercises. Surely therefore facially damaged patients like myself do not need physiotherapy? My own experience suggests otherwise. Although my limbs definitely needed 'exercise' so did the mess which was, and is, my face. My physiotherapists duly administered the daily torture of standard exercises for bedridden cases, but they did much more than that. They became daily visitors often more able than other staff to listen. They won my respect. And, most important, they contrived to convince me that I could be mobile and strong again, both physically and mentally.

I frequently reflect on the strange irony that I am now employed in one of the most demanding physical and manual jobs. 'Single-handed farming' might seem an apt description because I have only one functional finger on my left hand. But no one can milk 40 cows without using two hands, no one can hump hay bales and push barrows of manure without two hands. I *have* two good hands. The fact is that my left hand was rescued from extinction (in other words, amputation) by hours of painstaking work by surgeons and physiotherapists – and me! Not that my physios were miracle workers; they were simply people experienced in, and dedicated to, retrieving depleted bodies and minds from the brink.

I have divided my account of my recovery into three parts: the initial stage of skin replacement after being burned, the process of plastic surgery, and the aftermath. Although I learnt some technical jargon in the course of treatment, I make no claim to know the details of operations and what follows is therefore decidedly non-technical. Indeed I am conscious that physiotherapists have developed new tools to aid their work since I was in hospital. This being so does not, however, detract from my main themes.

ACCIDENT AND HOSPITALIZATION

I was just 18 when the accident happened, a fit, sporting and not unintelligent character. My sights were fixed on going to university. I had only very rarely set foot in a hospital. 'It'll never happen to me' was my happy-go-lucky attitude to hospitals and injuries on the rare occasions when I thought about them. That illusion was suddenly shattered on a winter's night in Wales in 1970. The Land Rover I was driving was completely burned out – my four friends escaped practically unscathed but I had been lying in the blazing cab for a few fleeting seconds before I had found the energy to escape – another minute and I would have been incinerated. I thought I must be badly singed – my face seemed to be swelling fast. I supposed I ought to go to hospital for a check-up; I was conscious of people at the scene wanting to rush me to one nearby and then we went by ambulance to Chepstow hospital. I hobbled into the operating theatre there, lay down and lost consciousness, completely oblivious to the fact that I was in acute danger of kidney failure.

For the next four and a half months I was hospitalized and bed-bound. An initial medical estimate of my likely recovery time had been a cleverly optimistic three weeks. My parents and friends arrived or sent their best wishes for a speedy recovery – and I confidently believed that my 'minor burns and scalds' would not stop me taking up a job at a Canadian ski resort in the next month.

Ten days in intensive care gave me little indication of the truth. Then I was transferred to Roehampton and informed on arrival by a very affable doctor that I had 33 per cent third degree burns. Still I did not understand. The following day I was lowered into a deliciously warm saline bath. The heavy bandages on my legs and arms were removed and I started to realize: huge areas were just raw meat. A shiver of horror shot down my spine but I cheerfully laughed it off. Only later back in my bed did the devastating impact of it all hit home. I still had no idea what my face looked like – no mirrors available.

The operations soon started and I was introduced to the mysteries of plastic surgery: skin grafts, donor sites, 'strep and staph infections', keloid scarring, barrier nursing, pre-meds and post-op inspections of treated areas (sometimes undertaken after I had been injected with a drug called ketamine producing in me a series of weird and scary hallucinations). My memory of detail in the next three months is sketchy: every week I seemed to be either undergoing operations or trying to recover from one. At times infection raged and skin grafts simply slid off, but gradually the flesh returned.

I had had vague pretensions to being a reasonable athlete at school. I was certainly fit and healthy. So when a woman came in one morning soon after I had arrived at Roehampton and said she was the physiotherapist and suggested I should do a few exercises I did not anticipate any difficulties. How wrong I was! In the space of a fortnight my muscles had become flabby and depleted, my limbs were stiff and I had no strength at all. Pat, as I came to know her, had seen similar cases – 'It is bound to hurt' she would say.

It did hurt. It was agony, no more, no less. I think agony is worse than pain: I can still recall that agony, but not the pain. Sore, semi-healed, semi-raw areas are not meant to be touched, let alone moved, I thought. 'Just a little bit more . . . Well done. Again. Push . . . Good. Rest. Pull . . . OK. Rest. We'll try some more this afternoon.' These commands – or rather the coaxing – remain etched in my mind to this day. They sum up my initial response to physio-therapy which was not very favourable!

Pat, I know now, was not being sadistic. In those early days she was carefully assessing my pain threshold. By daily visits, however brief, she was observing what motivated me. We didn't talk at all about end-results; if I asked some futile question about the future, she would simply point to the progress so far. She didn't want to give me false hopes – but she said just enough to allow me to set my own private targets: 40 double knee-bends, holding a pen, playing a game of draughts left-handed, and the ultimate goal – walking.

The saturation treatment of those months left me with little energy for much else. Even the strangeness of the routine, the dreariness of the food (Complan with every meal), the frustration of seeing only people's eyes above their surgical masks, all paled into insignificance. I had no choice but to resign myself to them. Would I ever get out? The contours of the cracks on the ceiling became a dream-like landscape of hills and rivers, sun and shade. Dejection was setting in. Each day Pat came in – always keen to get me out of my apathy. And indeed the gentle moving of muscles did shake me out of my lethargy momentarily. She didn't achieve much – she probably knew from the medical staff that I was fairly weak: all my energies and body-weight were being expended on healing. I lost four stone and grew an inch just lying there for three months. But at last the patching up of raw areas was nearly complete.

At this point physiotherapy became important. And by then Pat had got to know me: the groundwork had already been done. She had bothered to come in every day. She had listened to my grumbles and often done something effective about them. She had told me much of the possibilities of plastic surgery, information which I could not obtain from other staff and which many patients never receive, and this was particularly valuable to me. Uninformed often means uninspired and this is probably especially true in the case of plastic surgery for facial damage.

Towards the end of my initial skin replacement treatment it was a physiotherapeutic aid which inadvertently opened up a whole new set of problems for me. Pat's efforts were concentrated partly on getting my legs used to being vertical again (with the support of pink elasticated bandages) and partly on straightening out the fingers on my left hand. Three of these fingers proved to be unresponsive to treatment, due to the tendons being burned through, and I eventu-ally had the fingers amputated to the first joint. Amazingly, how-ever, my middle finger had some chance of being functional. A shiny metal-coated splint was strapped to it to increase the pressure and stretch the tendons. Until then I had seen no mirror since the accident but that shiny surface allowed me my first blurred view of my horribly damaged face. Inspecting my face as closely as possible with the splint was a good preparation for the shock when I eventually plucked up courage to ask for a real mirror.

But fortunately I was soon distracted by my earnest and long frustrated desire to walk. My legs had shrivelled to matchsticks and the right thigh, being almost completely burned, had taken an age to heal. I badly wanted to walk again. The days of waiting had created such a strong ambition, one that overshadowed all other feelings – including those about the facial damage. Pat had been working on strengthening my calf and thigh muscles sufficiently and, most important, she had given me the confidence to know that I should walk again.

On the very day the world watched as Apollo astronauts walked on the moon for the second time, my recovery in a little insignificant ward in a London hospital also took a major leap forward. For the first time in four and a half months my feet touched the ground and I stumbled a few steps in a circle round my bed. Walking was the signal for me to leave the burns unit: all the skin I had lost on my face, hands, legs and body had been replaced and at last I could be discharged. My hands served very few functions, my legs allowed me to walk for 30 seconds at a time, and my face was a contorted mass of scars and inflamed skin – but at last I was out.

The elation of that moment of leaving was only slightly tinged with apprehension. The targets which I had set had all so far been achieved. I think all the hospital staff shared my joy: Pat certainly did. Although it was her job to do what she could for me, she had managed in a meaningful personal way to 'stay with me' throughout the treatment. 'Staying with me' meant visiting even when it was apparently pointless, gaining my respect and trust, realizing how to motivate me, setting realistic aims for recovery and sharing in the thrill of achievement. That list sounds like an ingredients list for successful physiotherapy and in a way it is. But what is crucial is that each patient reacts differently and that the physio has to take a personal interest and understanding in each case. Moreover, physios should understand their critical role in psychological recovery: with their whole-hearted help patients can take full advantage of the opportunities opened up by their surgical treatment.

Keloid scarring is a good illustration of this. In common with many young burns victims, I suffered greatly from keloid scarring from the outset of my treatment. Thick bands of hard intractable scars on hands and legs are extremely debilitating, and they contort the face grotesquely; the resultant pulls and stresses on neighbouring skin are excruciatingly painful. Frequently the scarring was setting in before the wounds or grafts had healed. The physio is in an awkward position here: on the one hand she can encourage movement very soon after an operation, and thereby risk damaging the recently replaced skin, in an attempt to forestall the keloiding. Alternatively she can delay exercise until healing is complete by which time it may well be too late. This dilemma was immensely frustrating for me and Pat and I spent considerable time discussing the pros and cons with the medical staff. Her willingness to get involved in the issue was perhaps the first instance of a good two-way relationship forming between us – not, I stress, a heavy emotional involvement but simply a mutual understanding and respect.

PLASTIC SURGERY

The four and a half months of skin replacement was finally completed and I was gladly discharged for a few weeks' recuperation at home. I was a changed person: the brash self-confidence of six months previously had given way to a somewhat more thoughtful but nervous disposition. I had learnt a lot about life and about myself in hospital – a totally alien environment at the start of my treatment but now one which offered considerable security and support. My joy at being discharged and at being at home again was tempered by my realization that I was totally unprepared for the outside world.

It wasn't just that I looked on the world somewhat differently. People looked at me, even stared at me, with a mixture of curiosity, pity, suspicion, sometimes with fear and anxiety. Looking at myself each morning in the mirror confirmed what I now saw in the eyes of others: my face was seriously disfigured and likely to be so for the rest of my life. The first occasion when this uncomfortable fact was vividly brought home to me was an unexpected visit to a pub with an old friend. Whereas in hospital the reactions of staff and other patients to me were, I perceived, normal and untainted by the association of disfigurement with mental abnormality, the reception I met in the pub was quite otherwise. While my friend bought drinks, I tried my best to fend off the stares, the whispering behind my back, a few hostile remarks, and the general air of curiosity that gripped all the drinkers as soon as I walked through the door. This episode not only convinced me that I should start facial reconstruction, but it also forced me into considering how I should deal with public responses to my injuries.

Two or three times a week during my period at home I went to hospital to have my dressings changed and to visit the physiotherapy department. Now that I was out of the confines of the ward new forms of exercise could be tried: weight training (at first very light indeed!) strengthened my legs and hands as well as generally tuning up other depleted muscles. I badly wanted to make big strides in fitness at this stage but soon learnt that strained and aching muscles resulted from excessive work. Slowly and patiently was the message.

My relationship with the physios was broadening out. During the skin replacement stage, Pat and her colleagues had been one of the key motivating forces in my recovery. From this point on, however, I took a much more active part in the treatment. The targets were no longer as straightforward as in the earlier phase (like walking). I was now developing more complex objectives, some to do with returning to a reasonably athletic state, others relating to mental progress. Physiotherapy was not just the general physical back-up to surgery, it became the sounding board for ideas and plans.

One major issue in those first months out of hospital was whether or not I should take up a place at university in the coming autumn. A meeting in late May with one of the surgical staff had put doubts in my mind. He wondered whether I should take a year off and get myself thoroughly ready for the ordeal. Until then I had confidently assumed that I *would* be fit enough and was inwardly preparing myself. I was thrown into turmoil. I knew that a great deal of surgery had to be done in the next few years but this suggestion seemed to be questioning my ability to follow a normal life.

Since my fitness seemed in doubt I naturally consulted Pat. Knowing me far better than did the junior surgeon, she immediately realized his mistaken approach: the surest way to halt my return to 'a normal life' was to suggest that I was physically incapable of taking up where I had left off. The accident and my injuries had to be viewed as incidental; if blown up into an insuperable barrier, my self-confidence would be further shattered. How glad I was of Pat's interest and support.

Embarking on my course of plastic surgery which was to last intermittently for three and a half years gave me the opportunity to quiz my surgeon on the chances of regaining my lost appearance. First, he said, my hands needed attention: continued physiotherapy would, with luck and hard work, gradually rejuvenate my right hand, but my left was proving unresponsive to that kind of treatment. Only the middle finger functioned efficiently. I had to decide whether I wanted the other fingers pinned straight (they were bent down towards the palm and immovable). I was sure the fingers would be even less use in that position but agreed to continue physiotherapy and reach a decision later. After one term at university I concluded that drastic action was needed: I could pick up only the lightest load with the hand as it was. What would happen, I asked Pat, if the useless bits of finger were amputated? Her experience suggested that as long as a pad of skin was surgically made to protect the knuckle stumps, the half-fingers could be very efficient. And thus it turned out.

Dealing surgically with my hand presented relatively straightforward options, and although my surgeon had never suggested finger amputation, he was pleased when I reached that conclusion on my own. I would never have believed that I could actually sign a form to have my fingers amputated, but one morning I did, and apart from the occasional phantom limb sensation early on, have never regretted it. Without the redundant ends, the fingers (or stumps) on this hand found new life. I could now pick up weights though my arm as a whole was puny. Gradually the strength returned to my fingers – many exercises were prescribed and after much painstaking work the whole hand and arm became useful instead of an awkward encumbrance.

My facial disfigurement posed an entirely different and more complex set of problems. From the outset my surgeon was at pains to stress that he could not promise miracles. Contrary to popular myth, plastic surgeons cannot stick plastic on to re-create lost looks! Every operation, he emphasized, was bound to be a gamble. A satisfactory result could not be guaranteed after one operation, or two or three or four . . . but as long as I was fit and healthy and able to withstand the physical demands of treatment he would persevere on one condition: that I *wanted* him to do so. That was a most important proviso. In the early days of plastic surgery I had no qualms: every operation seemed to take me a little closer to an acceptable facial appearance. But as time went on, after over 50 operations, my willingness and resilience were weakening. Moreover, as I learnt more about the technical possibilities and the limitations of surgery, so I realized that additional operations would achieve less and less. Thus, although I could have persisted for years, I reached saturation point. I will outline briefly what was done.

Full thickness (Wolfe) skin grafts were applied to my nose, my eyelids (upper and lower) and my top lip, the skin coming first from behind my ear and then from the inside of the upper arm. Because of the keloid pulls exerted by my chin and distorted neck, my eyelids required repeated operations to achieve a decent result. After the third of these had failed (very demoralizing after the excruciating

A PATIENT'S VIEWPOINT FOLLOWING BURNS 261

pain of having 50 or 60 little stitches all around the eye), attention shifted to my chin. This was a real patchwork quilt of grafts and scars, and after one unsuccessful attempt to salvage it with a thin skin graft, discussion started on more radical measures. As I had been using every university vacation for surgery of some kind, I could not envisage what other treatment could still be contemplated.

One afternoon in the physio department I was working off some excess energy on the weights and saying how frustrating it was not to be able to get my eyes right. A group of physios gathered and started debating the options. The difficulty I experienced – in common with many other patients – of discussing treatment options with the surgical staff was raised. I asked for a clear description of what skin flaps were and what they could achieve. I discovered that a pedicle flap could be raised elsewhere on one's body and then transferred to completely cover a scarred area. As it happened, a woman recovering from a small flap was in the department that afternoon and I was allowed to see the smooth end-product. This was not the first or last occasion when physios with experience helped me to make sense of a problem which seemed unresolvable in the confines of the ward.

My surgeon was fascinated by the whole idea: I would take a year off university, travel a bit to start with, then come in to hospital to have a pedicle flap raised and eventually spread over my chin and neck. In the event, a back pedicle was used because my stomach area was scarred. This was very convenient as there was no need for an arm attachment stage. I was extremely lucky: the 12-inch tube was healthy from the start and was moved in four stages to replace my chin very successfully. It was a long process, taking six months to complete.

My sanity remained intact principally because I could escape from the hospital regularly. With the help of physios a thick foam back support was designed which I strapped round my chest enabling me to sit with my back against a seat. This contraption allowed me to drive a car while the flap developed and became healthily established. In addition, many visitors and regular jaunts to the physio department kept my morale and fitness in trim. By July 1974, the new chin was in place and my pleasure was shared by all who had made it possible. The tensions around my eyes and nose were released and I could now rejoice in the knowledge that I looked at least tolerably socially presentable!

AFTERWARDS

The psychological impact of facial burns on the unfortunate victim is now recognized by most burns units in Britain. Psychologists and social workers are specially trained and assigned to the burns unit staff to provide in-hospital counselling and hopefully maintain contact with the burned person and his or her family in the weeks and months following discharge. This was not the case in my day and I hope that the existence of these specialists does not prevent all members of the burns and plastic surgery team from being involved in psychological rehabilitation.

Although not strictly, or solely, the province of physiotherapists, helping patients to come to terms with facial disfigurement must be very clearly on their agenda, as it must for medical, nursing and ancillary staff alike. This help requires immense sensitivity and an acute awareness of how remarks or actions might be interpreted – or misinterpreted – by the sufferer.

Facial damage from burns can leave severe scars, and the distortions, redness and blotchiness are hideous to most eyes. The victim, too, finds them grotesque and ugly. His or her self-image is ruined – and, as soon becomes apparent, it is ruined for ever. Every look in the mirror confirms this awful truth – and the eyes of others tell the same tale. One has suffered an irretrievable loss, the loss of good looks.

The picture one has of oneself is a critical factor in all relationships with others especially perhaps in dealings with the opposite sex. Any pretensions to handsomeness or beauty before being burned are completely dispelled and the victim becomes very uncertain and nervous about all social contacts. Instead of presenting a clear, 'normal' face, now it is a blemished, 'abnormal' face. For women particularly this loss of normal good looks can be so devastating that they cut themselves off completely from other people because they no longer feel they know how to face up to (literally) making relationships or even conversations.

The public eye can be very cruel. The disfigured may be stared at or avoided, people move away and occasionally jeer. Abnormal ugliness is all too frequently associated with a series of pejorative attributes. The stereotype image of the baddie in children's books and films conjures up an array of unpleasant associations so that disfiguring scars are linked with criminal and fiendish acts.

Popular culture thus influences the first reactions of people coming into contact with a burned person to produce these kinds of negative associations. More significantly, in this cosmetic age, carrying abnormal looks tends to mark one out as one of society's failures. The connection made so starkly in advertisements, soap operas and films that good looks, social status and success go hand in hand is reversed to the detriment of the disfigured.

To be more specific, my facial damage has been assumed by others to be variously the result of my mental (or even moral?) ineptitude, abnormality from birth – do I have the right to survive at all, they wonder? – or some other personal failure. I have been assumed to be rather stupid, probably illiterate, possibly mentally ill, even violent; protective parents have shielded their children from me (yet ironically it is often children who are most wonderfully naive and natural and able to ask me direct questions without embarrassment). The abnormal behaviour I have witnessed would fill a book in itself – people staring fixedly, trance-like at me; others rushing up to ask if they can help me over the road or carry my bag; and once at a restaurant a woman left her table, unable to finish her expensive meal. At the other end of the scale people seem to think I must be some sort of hero – am I a racing driver like Niki Lauda, or perhaps an RAF veteran?

While several self-help groups for the facially damaged have been established (e.g. Let's Face It; Doreen Trust, p.540), many disfigured people just try in their own way to make their presence felt and break down the public's false assumptions. To some extent the public are not just uninformed, they have been misled into thinking that cosmetic surgery is a miracle treatment that can transform battered and scarred faces back to smooth and youthful complexions. The much publicized face-lifts given to film actors and actresses create the illusion that anyone with wrinkles, scars, ugly moles or other facial blemishes can be quickly and smoothly 'reconditioned'.

Although it is many years since I received plastic surgery treatments, I am amazed how frequently people are shocked when they learn that I am not 'going in' for more surgery: it was not until I completely and positively accepted my looks that I started to organize an effective counter to this attitude. Just to resign oneself to one's looks is inadequate. One has to realize that the scars are now an integral part of 'being me'. How I reached that point of positive acceptance is not easy to describe. A combination of support from my family, friends, hospital staff and many others, and my own refusal to see the accident as the end of meaningful life probably sums up my own recovery, but other burns cases will reach that point by other routes.

Before I reached that stage, however, I think I strove to deflect any stigmatizing attitudes by an extravagant show of superficial over-confidence. Inside I was full of nervousness and acute awareness as to how I was being received by others. I recall my first days at university mostly in this light, trying manfully to deny to all around that I had anything wrong with me at all. Gradually – and it was a long process – a *modus vivendi* became established. I no longer worried about the stares, the occasional hurtful remark, the schoolgirl giggling or the awkwardness when people met me for the first time. I hope I became easier to be with, less concerned with myself and how others saw me, and more just an ordinary and an active member of society. But it took a long time and even today there are moments of anguish.

In a way the physiotherapists and the nurses who dealt with me, Pat and her colleagues, represented my first female audience and my first new friends since the accident. But more importantly, they took the trouble to understand the predicament of facial damage. As long as physios and other staff (not least the surgical staff themselves) are sensitive to the deep psychological scarring that goes with facial burns, and as long as a strong family and social network exists outside the hospital, burns victims have every chance of healing those emotional scars in time.

REFERENCES

Clothier, Sir Cecil (1988). *The Patient's Dilemma*. The Rock Carling Fellowship, The Nuffield Provincial Hospital Trust, London.

For those readers who would like to read about the techniques used for the re-fashioning of James Partridge's face the following paper will be of interest.
Evans, A. J. (1981). Cosmetic surgery of burns. *British Journal of Hospital Medicine*, June issue, 547–50.

BIBLIOGRAPHY

Partridge, J. (1990). *Changing Faces*. Penguin Books, Harmondsworth.

Chapter 17

Amputations

by C. M. C. VAN DE VEN MCSP

Amputation of a limb should be accepted as a positive form of treatment. In the case of vascular disease or diabetes, amputation will relieve the patient from a painful, useless, often infected and sometimes life-threatening extremity. This population is usually elderly and also suffering from many other medical problems.

Those who have undergone amputation as a result of trauma or malignancy are often younger. They too have to accept that amputation is a positive treatment; they will require speedy rehabilitation. Both populations, young and elderly, may require psychological help and counselling.

For whatever reason, once the amputation has been performed the amputee must be rehabilitated to a fully independent life. For some, this may mean returning to work, school or college; for others, it will mean returning home and coping with their own life in their own time.

The amputee needs time and help to overcome both the physical and psychological aspects of losing a limb. At first, the future will seem uncertain, the outcome unknown. Support and encouragement from all the multidisciplinary team, the family and friends is essential.

The multidisciplinary rehabilitation team should consist of the following: surgeon and medical staff, nursing staff, physiotherapists, occupational therapist, social worker, psychologist, dietician, general practitioner, prosthetist and the staff at the local disablement services centre (DSC). All these people must work in close co-operation with one another. Other professions may need to be involved if necessary.

Amputations of upper and lower limbs involve differences in cause and age-group; their rehabilitation will be considered separately. The ratio of lower limb to upper limb amputees is about 22:1.

LOWER LIMB AMPUTATIONS

This is the larger group of amputees and they are seen in greater number by physiotherapists.

Indications for amputation

TABLE 17/1 CAUSES OF LOWER LIMB AMPUTATIONS WITH APPROXIMATE PERCENTAGE OF CASES (DHSS, 1987)

Cause	%
Peripheral vascular disease	63.8
Diabetes	20.4
Trauma	9.0
Malignancy	3.7
Infection	1.9
Congenital deformities	0.8
Others	0.4
	100.00

From the above Table 17/1 it can be seen that peripheral vascular disease (PVD) and diabetic gangrene, both diseases associated with the elderly, account for the majority of lower limb amputations – 75 per cent of new lower limb amputees are over the age of 60. The ratio per sex is 2:1 male to female but this may be changing, possibly due to an increase in women smokers (Ham and Van de Ven, 1986). The life expectancy of amputees suffering from PVD is three to five years; 30 per cent of these amputees will lose their remaining leg within two years of the original amputation (English and Dean, 1980). These patients also have many other associated medical problems, e.g. cardiac involvement, lower exercise tolerance, arteriosclerosis of the cerebral vessels causing possible hemiplegia and diminished mental ability, poor respiratory function, reduced visual acuity, poor healing and neuropathy; possibly osteoarthritis and/or rheumatoid arthritis.

Traumatic amputations more commonly affect the younger age-groups and are mostly necessitated by road traffic accidents and industrial injuries. Malignant disease is also a reason for amputation in patients of this age-group. Amputations for congenital deformity and limb length discrepancies are usually performed on children and young adults. In these cases, surgery is best delayed until the patient is old enough to decide whether to have the amputation performed or not (Day, 1979).

Surgery and levels of amputation

Whatever the pathology predisposing to amputation, there are various factors which will influence the surgeon in the selection of level (Spence et al, 1984). As well as the pathology, surgical techniques and viability of tissue, the type of prostheses available and the patient's particular needs will be taken into account. Occupation, age and sex must also be considered.

Hemipelvectomy Amputation This amputation is performed almost solely for malignancy as a life-saving procedure, and in this instance the pathological factors are of prime importance. The surgeon has no choice but to remove the entire limb and the ilium, pubis, ischium and sacrum on that side, leaving peritoneum, muscle and fascia to contain and support the internal organs.

Hip Disarticulation This procedure is commonly performed in cases of malignancy; it may also be necessary following extensive trauma but is seldom carried out for vascular insufficiency. The limb is disarticulated at the hip joint and the bony pelvis is left intact, thus producing a good weight-bearing platform.

Mid-thigh Amputation In the patient with vascular disease, an above-knee amputation is one in which primary healing occurs more readily than the through-knee or below-knee level. However, compared with these other levels, the above-knee amputee will have more difficulty in learning to control the prosthesis and in achieving a good gait pattern. In the case of the elderly patient, the attainment of total independence will be more of a problem (Stephen et al, 1987). Proprioception from the knee joint will be lost and the patient must bear weight on the prosthesis at the ischial tuberosity. Hip flexion contractures occur very easily unless care is taken to prevent them, the short stumps tending to become flexed and abducted due particularly to the strong pull of tensor fascia lata. The longer above-knee stumps by contrast tend to become flexed and adducted, since more of the adductor group are intact and have a mechanical advantage over the pull of the short tensor fascia lata.

The above-knee stump should be of a functional length, but the surgeon must allow for about 13cm between the end of the stump and the knee axis in order to permit space for the knee control mechanism of the prosthesis. If there is a hip flexion contracture a long stump is a disadvantage – the end of the long stump magnifies the contracture and the prosthesis will be bulky and cosmetically less acceptable.

Surgeons use the myoplastic or a myodesis technique in which muscle groups are sutured together over the bone end or attached to the bone at physiological tension (Dederich, 1967). The muscles therefore retain their contractile property, circulation of the stump is improved and the stump will also be more powerful to control the prosthesis.

Amputation at Knee Joint Level This includes disarticulation of the knee, the Gritti-Stokes and supracondylar amputation.

Disarticulation of the knee: The tibia together with the fibula is disarticulated at the knee joint. The patella is retained and the patellar tendon is sutured to the anterior cruciate ligament, the hamstrings are sutured to the posterior cruciate ligament and so act as hip extensors. A strong powerful stump results with no muscle imbalance, and full end-bearing is possible on the broad expanse of the femoral condyles. Most of the proprioception of the knee joint is retained.

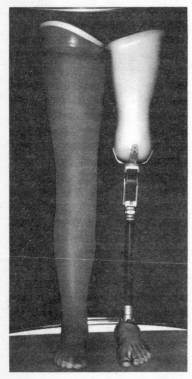

Fig. 17.1 The through-knee prosthesis. *Right*: An endoskeletal prosthesis with a polypropylene socket, a four-bar linkage knee mechanism and a quantum foot. *Left*: The same prosthesis at the definitive stage demonstrating the improved cosmesis (*Courtesy* Vessa Ltd)

Gritti-Stokes technique: The femur is sectioned transversely through the condyles and the condyles are trimmed down medially and laterally. The articular surface of the patella is shaved off and the patella positioned at the distal end of the femur. Bony union should occur and weight is taken on the patella. Primary healing is more certain than the through-knee level, but the relatively small end-bearing surface rarely permits full weight-bearing, especially if non-union between the patella and the femur occurs (Campbell and Morris, 1986).

Supracondylar amputation: The femur is divided at the level of the adductor tubercle. This then becomes a very long above-knee, necessitating ischial weight-bearing when using the prosthesis.

These levels of amputation are not suitable if a fixed flexion of the hip exists; however, the prostheses have much improved in recent years and are now more cosmetically acceptable (Fig. 17/1).

Below-knee Amputation　If at all possible, the surgeon will elect to perform a below-knee amputation. The great advantage is that the normal knee joint with its proprioception is retained and therefore balance and a good gait pattern will be more easily attained. The amputee will be able to wear a patellar tendon-bearing prosthesis (PTB) which leaves the knee function unrestricted (Fig. 17/2). The optimum level is 14cm below the tibial plateau, although a slightly shorter stump will still be suitable for a prosthesis.

The fibula is sectioned slightly more proximally than the tibia, and the end of the tibia is bevelled to avoid a prominent bone end. A myoplastic technique is used, either the Burgess or skew-flap technique (Burgess et al, 1971; Robinson et al, 1982), resulting in the advantages previously described. The majority of amputees will be successful at using a prosthesis at this level, whatever age and other medical problems present.

Symes Amputation　This involves disarticulation at the ankle joint and removal of the medial and lateral malleoli to the level of the articular surface of the tibia. This amputation is rarely carried out successfully in vascular conditions, as insufficient blood supply may result in poor healing. Good end-bearing is possible, the heel pad being sutured into position over the distal end of the tibia and fibula.

Foot Amputations　Trans- and mid-tarsal amputations result in relatively little locomotor difficulty, the main problem being that of

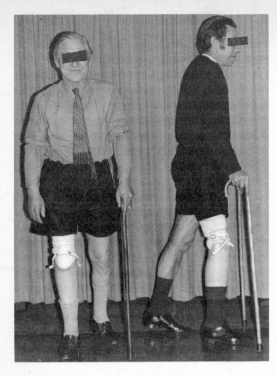

Fig. 17.2 Two patients with below-knee amputations, wearing patellar tendon-bearing prostheses. Note that control of these prostheses depends entirely upon the hip and knee joints and muscles, particularly the quadriceps and hamstrings

the provision of functional and cosmetic footwear. Other amputations, e.g. the Chopart and Lisfranc, may require special prostheses (Millstein et al, 1988)

PHYSIOTHERAPY

The physiotherapist's role in the rehabilitation of the amputee can be considered in three stages: pre-operative, postoperative (preprosthetic), and prosthetic.

Rehabilitation is one continual process, the final goal for the patient being independent while using a definitive prosthesis and the opportunity to return to normal activities, within the limitations of age and conditions.

The physiotherapist is an essential member of the multidisciplinary team and is often the link professional for carrying out the complete programme of treatment. It is usually the physiotherapist who sees the patient before amputation, early postoperatively, in the outpatient department and finally in the community. Unless one member of the team undertakes this continuity of management, communication breaks down and the total programme of care disintegrates (Ham et al, 1985).

Pre-operative programme

As soon as the surgeon has made the diagnosis and the patient knows that an amputation is necessary, a physiotherapy assessment is of key importance. This will involve both physical and social assessment.

It is important to remember that many other members of the multidisciplinary team will be endeavouring to carry out their own assessment at this time. Sensitivity and careful timing are essential, so that the patient does not become exhausted. It is also important to ensure that the patient has adequate pain control during this time.

The physical assessment should include the following:

Muscle strength and joint mobility – upper and lower limbs. Both affected and unaffected legs. Shoulder girdle. Trunk and dexterity of hands and fingers, etc.

Balance ability/posture – sitting, standing, transferring.

Functional ability – dressing and personal independence. Ability to walk.

Circulatory status – colour of skin. Sensation of hands and feet. Skin abrasions or breakdowns.

Cardio-pulmonary status – recent myocardial infarctions. Pulmonary state, etc.

Previous medical problems – previous history of surgery. Stroke, trauma, visual or hearing difficulties. Bowel and bladder problems, etc.

All this must be carefully recorded. Assessments are continuing and will be used throughout the whole programme, therefore written evidence must be available for comparison.

Social Assessment It is important to understand the patient's home and work environments, as well as his/her hobbies/leisure activities, etc. This cannot be discovered in isolation and often gradually emerges during the physical assessment. Relatives and friends must be involved during this stage and may supply valuable information. This is particularly important if the patient is ill, confused or unable to co-operate.

The physiotherapy assessment will be discussed at the regular team meetings, where all members will exchange views and findings from their own assessments.

Depending upon the patient's condition and the time permitted before amputation, a pre-operative treatment programme can be organized. This, ideally, should be in the physiotherapy department but, if necessary, in the ward. It should include:

1. Strengthening exercises for the upper trunk and upper limbs to facilitate transfers and for moving up and down the bed.
2. Strengthening and mobilizing exercises for the lower trunk, necessary for all activities, rolling, sitting up, walking.
3. Strengthening exercises for the unaffected leg for standing and transferring.
4. Exercises for the affected leg to increase the range of movement and improve stability of those joints which will remain after amputation.
5. Walking if possible. If flexion deformities are present the patient must have protective footwear on the affected leg with a heel-raise to facilitate a good heel strike and a quadriceps' contraction.
6. Maximal independence including ability to move about the bed using the unaffected leg, rolling and prone lying.
7. It is important to teach wheelchair activities even though it is hoped that the patient will ultimately achieve independence with a prosthesis. The majority of elderly patients will require a wheelchair on a permanent basis as a second method of mobility. This wheelchair should be correctly assessed by the occupational therapy or physiotherapy department.
8. There should be discussion with the patient about the possibility of 'phantom' sensation, emphasizing that this is a normal phenomenon (Mouratoglou, 1986).

Once the level of amputation has been decided, the patient may wish to see the types of prosthesis available. Sometimes it is useful to meet another experienced amputee at a similar level of surgery. This may require sensitive handling from the physiotherapist, but many patients feel the benefit from such a meeting.

Postoperative programme

The aims of treatment are:

1. Prevention of joint contractures.
2. To strengthen and mobilize the unaffected leg.
3. To strengthen and co-ordinate the muscles controlling the stump.
4. To strengthen and mobilize the trunk and retrain balance.
5. To teach the patient to regain independence in functional activities.

6. To control oedema of the stump and commence early ambulation.
7. Re-education of sensation in the healed stump.
8. Successful discharge into the community.

Chest physiotherapy will commence the first day following amputation. Most patients undergoing amputation for vascular reasons have also been extremely heavy smokers. They are generally older, often unfit and possibly confused. Chest complications are therefore not uncommon.

Great care must be taken at this stage to organize an exercise programme around the control of pain. Most amputees experience stump pain, and this may limit any treatment programme. There must be adequate pain control on a regular basis, and treatment given when pain relief is at its maximum. Knowledge of the analgesic supply must be known. Pain can be caused by a number of reasons and must be correctly assessed. It is also important to remember that postoperative pain can be directly proportional to the amount of pain present pre-operatively (Connolly, 1979). Causes may be (a) ischaemic pain due to incorrect level of amputation, (b) a non-healing stump due to infection, (c) nerve pain, which may be referred from the back or neck, (d) phantom sensation or pain. If any pain persists it should be reported to the surgeon so that further investigations can be carried out if necessary (*Blesmag*, 1983).

Prevention of Contractures Attention must be given to the position of the patient in bed. The stump should lie parallel to the unaffected leg with the joints extended. Pillows must not be placed under either the leg or stump and if the bed is soft, fracture boards should be placed beneath the mattress. Both physiotherapists and nursing staff should keep a check on the patient's position. The patient should understand its importance and be encouraged to maintain it.

Some patients will be able to progress to prone lying. The young fit amputee will achieve this easily and should be encouraged to carry this out at least for two half-hour periods each day. It is essential to maintain the correct position (Fig. 17/3). The elderly and those with severe cardiac respiratory embarrassment will be unable to tolerate or achieve this position, and should not be encouraged to try. Correct supine lying will be more suitable.

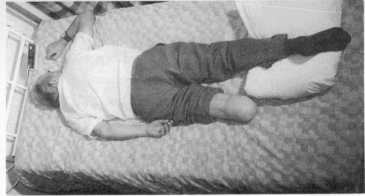

Fig. 17.3 Prone lying. Note the position of patient's head turned towards the side of the remaining leg, thus maintaining hip and knee extension of the amputated side. The remaining leg is supported to prevent damage to the foot, and a 'call button' is positioned correctly in case of distress

Providing the amputee is medically fit, transferring out of bed into a wheelchair on the first or second postoperative day should be achieved. A below-knee or through-knee level amputee is supplied with a stump board to support the stump (Ham and Whittaker, 1984). This helps to prevent contractures of the knee joint, reduces oedema and acts as a safety protection for the stump (Fig. 17/4). Amputees should not sit in a soft, static armchair.

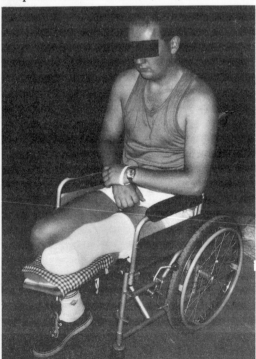

Fig. 17.4 A simple board with a covered foam support will maintain elevation and protection for a below-knee or through-knee stump. There are also commercially available stump boards. Note that this amputee is wearing a Tubifast dressing to support the tissues rather than a conventional bandage

Strengthening and Mobilizing the Unaffected Leg   Strong isometric 'holds' with the hip and knee in extension are useful in helping to retain the supportive function of the leg, and this isometric work together with resisted isotonic exercises can be started the day following operation. During the next few days, as the amputee's general condition improves, these exercises are progressed. Active and resisted exercises to the unaffected leg can also lead to 'overflow' to the stump.

Strengthening of the Stump   The amputee should move the stump independently first before the physiotherapist attempts to touch it. This applies to assisted or resisted movement. Isometric work for the stump can be started immediately. As the wound heals, manually resisted isotonic work can be given and gradually progressed. It is inadvisable, particularly when the myoplastic technique has been used, to give strong resisted work immediately, as there will be suture material in the wound and care must be taken not to pull on this.

The physiotherapist must at all times watch for any muscle imbalance and pay particular attention to the weaker groups, which will most likely be the extensors of the hip and knee and possibly the hip adductors, in fact, those muscles necessary to oppose a potential contracture. Stability of all joints of the stump will be essential in the effective control of a prosthesis.

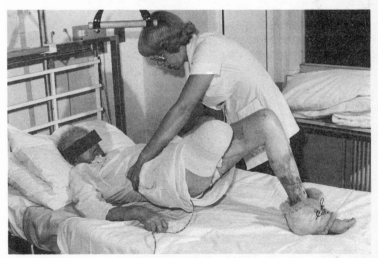

Fig. 17.5 Bridging exercises. Note the condition of the remaining leg, with protection for the ischaemic foot using a sheepskin bootee

To Strengthen and Mobilize the Trunk and Upper Limbs 'Bridging' exercises (Fig. 17/5), rolling exercises and sitting exercises (Figs 17/6, 17/7, 17/8) can be commenced during the first few days. When the amputee is able to sit on the edge of the bed, resisted sitting balance work is given (Fig. 17/9). The use of the wobble board can also improve sitting balance (Fig. 17/10).

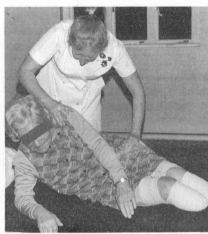

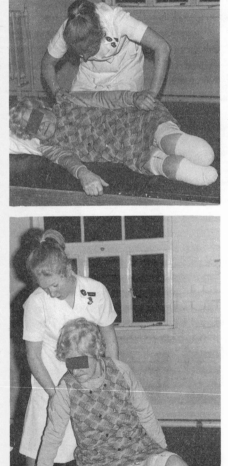

Figs 17.6, 17.7, 17.8 demonstrate a rolling to sitting sequence with guided resistance

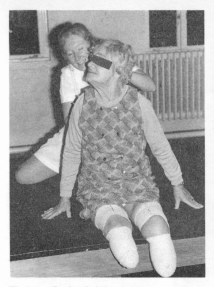 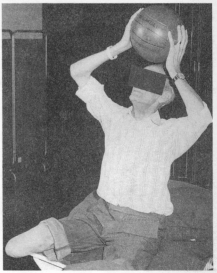

Fig. 17.9 Resisted sitting balance

Fig. 17.10 Use of the wobble board. Note pillow protection of new amputation stump, also pillows placed behind the patient as a safety precaution

Attention must be given to the upper trunk and upper limbs, and weight and pulley systems are also useful for this activity (Figs 17/11, 17/12). Dynamic stump exercises using a stool are invaluable for both general and specific stump strengthening exercises (Fig. 17/13).

Group work can be of value and fun, although elderly patients benefit more from individual treatment. Daily sessions in the physiotherapy department plus occupational therapy usually provide an adequate programme, while younger amputees may find working on the multigym both stimulating and satisfying.

Independence in Functional Activities At all times the amputee must be encouraged to be as independent as possible. At this stage the amputee should be dressed in daytime clothes. Sometimes it is necessary for the occupational therapist to give dressing practice (Fig. 17/14). Appropriate shoes should be worn on the unaffected leg: this is essential, particularly for those whose remaining leg is at risk.

Wheelchair independence must be achieved by all amputees, but particularly the elderly who may rely on this as their main method of mobility. Transfers using different methods must be practised.

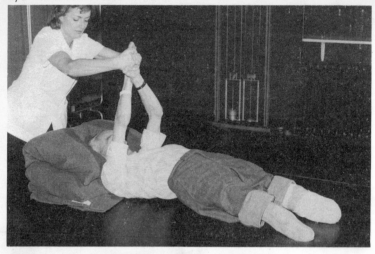

Fig. 17.11 Bilateral arm patterns: strengthening both upper limbs and trunk. Note extension of both lower limbs

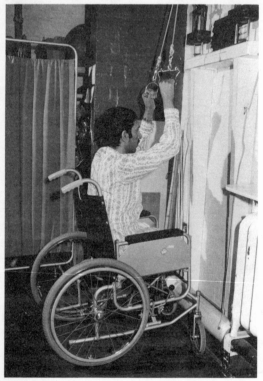

Fig. 17.12 Using weight and pulley system to strengthen upper limbs

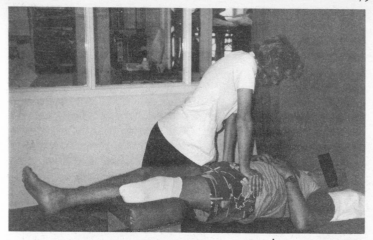

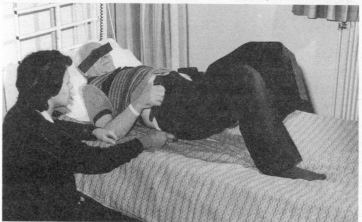

Fig. 17.13 Dynamic stump exercises. The physiotherapist is manually resisting the upward thrust of the pelvis. This facilitates and maintains strong muscle work for the hip and knee extensors

Fig. 17.14 Amputee practising dressing with the occupational therapist

The majority of amputees should attend the occupational therapy department on a regular basis to improve their new-found skills in a more functional situation, e.g. bath transfers, home and cooking activities, hobbies and leisure activities, etc.

Control of Oedema and Early Ambulation Controlling oedema is essential and it must be reduced as quickly as possible. Wound healing can be delayed by excessive oedema, and it is important that the stump assumes its ultimate size quickly, so that the limb fitting programme can begin.

There are numerous reasons for the presence of oedema and it is important that these are recognized by the physiotherapist. Oedema may result because of:

Surgical trauma
Arterial disease
Poor venous return
Diabetes
Kidney disease
Associated problems, e.g. congestive cardiac failure
Joint problems
Loss of muscle pump.

Elevation and Exercise Although bandaging and elastic socks have been the recognized method of controlling oedema historically, concern has always been expressed on the pressures exerted on fragile and somewhat disvascular tissues (Koerner, 1986). Simple methods, such as elevating the stump and teaching stump exercises, have been found to be successful and easy to carry out. The wound dressing is then held in place by Tubifast which has some form of light elastic properties in the make-up.

It is possible to elevate the foot of the bed and a stump board should be used for the below-knee and some through-knee amputees when seated in a chair (Fig. 17/4, p.274). The below-knee amputee should practise contracting the dorsi and plantar flexor muscles, and the above-knee amputees – flexor, extensor, abductor and adductor muscles.

Bandaging There has been much discussion concerning the methods of oedema control, and probably bandaging is the best known. The purpose of bandaging is to disperse the terminal oedema. Bandaging will also condition the patient to the constant all-round pressure which will be present when wearing a prosthesis. It also encourages the amputee to become used to handling the stump. Before the sutures are removed from the healed stump a crêpe bandage is used, afterwards, the Elset 'S' bandage or an elastic type bandage is applied.

Above-knee or through-knee stumps require a 4.5m (5yd), 15cm (6in) wide bandage; and the below-knee a 10cm (4in) one. Often it is necessary to halve the length to a 2m bandage for the short or thin below-knee stump. It is important to remember that the amount of

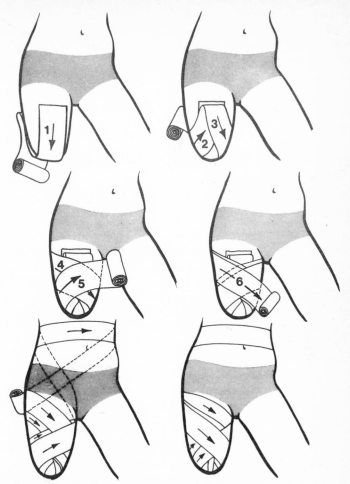

Fig. 17.15 Bandaging for an above-knee amputation (*Courtesy* Seton Ltd, Oldham)

turns is directly proportional to the pressure build-up on the stump. There are different methods of applying stump bandages (Figs 17/15, 17/16, 17/17). It is important that there is more pressure distally than proximally, and all turns are diagonal. Most methods require a fixing turn to hold the bandage in position, and both the amputee and the staff must be prepared to re-apply the bandage several times a day. It is also essential that the elasticity of the bandage is not too stretched when applying it to the stump as it may act as a tourniquet (Callen, 1981).

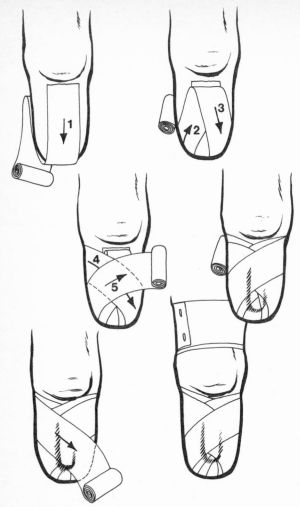

Fig. 17.16 Bandaging for a below-knee amputation (*Courtesy* Seton Ltd, Oldham)

Stump bandages should be applied regularly and great care should be taken by both the physiotherapist and the amputee when using this method of controlling oedema. The majority of amputees are suffering from vascular disease and if the pressure exerted by the bandaging exceeds arterial pressure in the extremity, pain and necrosis may occur, possibly leading to a higher level of amputation. For the younger amputee bandaging is often both comfortable and supportive.

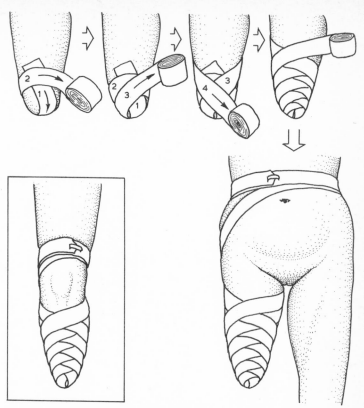

Fig. 17.17 Alternative method of bandaging

Shrinker Socks   There are several commercial elastic socks available through the DSCs, made for below-knee and above-knee amputees. The stump has to be measured and the correct sock is then supplied. They should only be used on a mature and fully healed stump (Manella, 1981). Elderly vascular amputees should be observed for half-an-hour while wearing the sock to ensure that circulation is not compromised. These socks should not be worn at night.

Rigid Dressing – Plaster of Paris   This has been a popular method of controlling oedema and helping towards early ambulation in the past. In some centres amputees have their rigid dressings changed after a number of days for a second rigid dressing, while for others bandaging is then continued after the first plaster of Paris dressing (Mueller, 1982).

Occasionally, instead of using the plaster of Paris just as a rigid dressing, it can be used as an early weight-bearing method. A prosthetic shin and foot, or length of tube, are put at the distal end of the plaster and the patient learns to walk partially weight-bearing in the parallel bars or using elbow crutches. It does, however, require a very closely co-ordinated team of specialists, and the patient needs to be in the care of a specialist unit. Vastus medialis and vastus lateralis muscles may require extra strengthening after the removal of the plaster of Paris.

Intermittent Pressure Machines   There are several machines used which supply a varying and intermittent pressure, resulting in an overall pumping action of the stump. They are commercially available; among the types are the Hemaflow and Jobst pumps. Many can be used at home.

Pneumatic Post-amputation Mobility Aid (PPAM Aid)   This not only helps to reduce oedema but is a valuable early mobility aid (Redhead et al, 1978).

The equipment consists of an outer plastic inflatable sleeve, a small inner plastic bag which is invaginated on itself, a metal frame with rocker base and a pump unit with gauge (Fig. 17/18). The pumping effect by the inflatable bags reduces the oedema as the amputee walks partial weight-bearing in parallel bars. Progression to

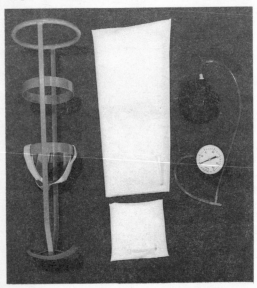

Fig. 17.18 The component parts of the PPAM Aid

elbow crutches is possible for some (Fig. 17/19). The PPAM Aid is not worn outside the rehabilitation department. It is not made and fitted for each individual amputee and can be used as early as five to seven days postoperatively, with the consent of the consultant.

It is important, particularly for the elderly, to encourage standing and walking as early as possible. In this way balance and postural reactions are maintained and improved, and the walking pattern retained. It can be used as an assessment tool to observe if the amputee will have the ability to balance and walk, before progressing to a prosthesis. This is particularly useful in the case of the hemiplegic patient. Some bilateral below-knee amputees can also use the PPAM Aid if they were able to walk using a PTB as a unilateral

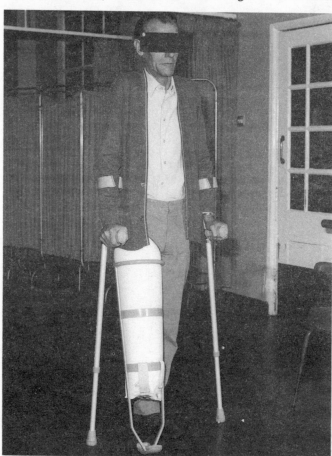

Fig. 17.19 Patient walking partial weight-bearing on PPAM Aid

amputee. The PPAM Aid can be used for above-knee, through-knee and below-knee amputations. Two PPAM Aids should never be used simultaneously.

There are other methods of early ambulation available. Some companies are manufacturing simple modular walking aids, such as the Femurette for above-knee amputees and the Tulip limb for below-knee amputees (Fig. 17/20).

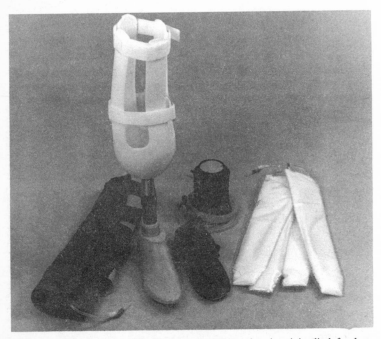

Fig. 17.20 The Tulip limb. A commercially available early gait training limb for the below-knee amputee (*Courtesy* R. Taylor & Son (Orthopaedic) Ltd)

Re-education of the Healed Stump Once there is healing the patient should be encouraged to handle and percuss the stump. This helps to reduce the sensitivity of the tissue, reduces phantom sensation and the patient becomes used to pressure. Exercises such as kneeling and weight-bearing through the stump also help (Fig. 17/21).

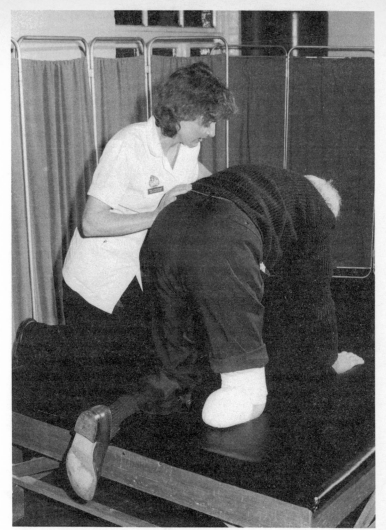

Fig. 17.21 Stabilizations with the patient in a kneeling position on a hard bed

Discharge into the Community The timing of discharge will depend upon local decisions: some amputees will leave the hospital after an appointment has been made at the DSC or some will wait until after the first visit to the DSC. A few will remain as in-patients until the first prosthesis is delivered and learn to walk, at which point they will be discharged.

To achieve a successful return home, especially for the elderly, close contact with local organizations and local services may be necessary. The younger amputee may need support and help in returning to work, school or college. The community physiotherapy service will be of great assistance in some of these difficulties. The majority of amputees will need to visit their homes before discharge, and in the case of a bilateral amputee several visits home are necessary, particularly when wheelchairs will be necessary.

Referral to the Disablement Services Centre (DSC) The amputee should be referred by letter or appropriate referral form to the local DSC a few days postoperatively. This will give the centre time to organize an appointment. The amputee will be seen by both the doctor and the prosthetist. The hospital notes and various assessments made on behalf of the multidisciplinary team must accompany the amputee. Generally, measurement and casting for the first temporary prosthesis will take place provided the amputee is considered suitable to be given a prosthesis. At this first visit some amputees are not ready for measurement but subsequent visits can always be arranged.

A temporary prosthesis will take a few days to make. If the amputee has been discharged home during this period, active exercise must be maintained. Often the community physiotherapy service will assist with this programme of treatment.

Prosthetic stage

As soon as the amputee takes delivery of the temporary prosthesis, arrangements are made to continue rehabilitation, either in the physiotherapy department of the referring hospital or in the department at the DSC. The amputee must learn not only to walk safely with a good gait pattern but also to be able to put on the prosthesis independently, to stand up from a chair, climb stairs, walk up and down a slope, on rough ground and possibly manage public transport.

Before teaching an amputee to use a prosthesis, the physiotherapist must understand the basic concepts of normal human gait. This is a product of many complex interactions between internal and external forces acting on the body. The gait cycle consists of a swing phase and a stance phase and occurs between one heel contact and the next heel contact of the same leg. The centre of gravity during the gait cycle displaces vertically and laterally. This contributes to balance control and energy efficiency and also affects the width of the walking base (Hughes and Jacobs, 1979).

Treatment plan

Each amputee is different, and must be assessed individually and treated accordingly; the following are treatment plans based on two different amputee groups:

A. The elderly amputee – generally suffering from peripheral vascular disease and diabetes.

Aims:
– To attain an optimal gait pattern, taking into consideration other physical limitations.
– To maintain safety.
– To improve functional ability.
– To ensure a steady progress.
– To supply correct walking equipment.

B. The young amputee generally caused by trauma and malignancy.

Aims:
– To attain an optimal gait pattern.
– To progress quickly.
– To return to normal functional activities, including recreational interests.

The amputee should attend gait rehabilitation on a daily basis so as to maintain continuity in the use of a prosthesis. Rehabilitation should commence in the parallel bars, which give security and safety, enabling the amputee to concentrate in using the prosthesis and maintaining a reasonable gait pattern. Adequate balance must be achieved prior to ambulation. Reduced proprioceptive input on the amputated side necessitates excellent balance ability on the remaining leg. This may be difficult particularly for the elderly amputee with vascular problems in the remaining leg. Lesions on the remaining foot must be dressed and sufficiently protected by adequate footwear.

Before commencing a prosthetic session, the physiotherapist must teach the amputee the mechanics and safety aspects of the prosthesis.

Standing exercises will help the amputee feel, move and position the prosthesis. Gradually, experience will be gained on the limitation imposed by the prosthesis – learning how to recover balance in all directions must be achieved.

Progressing to step positions and practising the prosthetic swing and stance phase will help the amputee to master the prosthetic gait pattern in a safe and energy efficient manner (Waters et al, 1976).

Without balance, both on the remaining leg and the prosthesis, walking using a prosthesis will be impossible.

Obviously the walking pattern will depend upon the strength and mobility and overall physical condition of the amputee, and also the type of prosthesis supplied. The physiotherapist should have the knowledge and experience to assess and teach so that the most functional use is made of the prosthesis. If the prosthesis is of no functional value then its use will be minimal and it may well be rejected.

Once a reasonable gait pattern has been achieved safely in the parallel bars, progression to walking sticks is encouraged. Occasionally the more frail may have to use tetrapods or a frame. Although these aids give more support this action is often worth delaying. Once such equipment is supplied and becomes familiar, progressing to sticks becomes difficult later and it is impossible to attain a good gait pattern using a frame. Generally, an amputee should not be permitted to use elbow crutches as little weight will be taken through the prosthesis and the amputee will never become a natural limb wearer.

Amputees must be able to 'don and doff' their prosthesis independently – obviously the methods will vary according to the level of amputation and the type of prosthesis. A prosthetic socket can be compared with a shoe in that it must be comfortable and fit well; all sockets are constructed to accommodate the anatomical contours of the stump and must be 'donned' accordingly. Stump socks, if used, must be wrinkle free.

The through-hip amputee will need to stand to 'don' a prosthesis, the above-knee amputee can sit but will need to stand for final adjustments. The through-knee amputee needs to stand to ensure correct weight-bearing while the below-knee amputee can carry out this action in a sitting position.

Fastenings and suspensions can be adapted for individual limitations, e.g. Velcro fastening and D-ring.

Stairs, kerbs and slopes must be achieved independently. Those with a below-knee level of amputation will find these easier than those amputees with the higher levels. Initially, for all amputees, the sound leg steps up and the prosthesis follows. When stepping down the prosthesis leads.

Slopes are more difficult for the amputee. The remaining leg steps up and the procedure is reversed when the amputee walks down the slope. Some steep slopes are best approached by ascending and descending sideways.

Most amputees worry about falling; they must be reassured that if they fall they can get up again. This is difficult and needs repeated practice. Many different methods are used. Amputees are usually taught to roll towards the sound side, using momentum together with hand support, to reach the kneeling position; then holding on to furniture or using an aid, standing can be achieved.

Many will need help in using transport, buses, cars and bicycles – these should be practised with physiotherapy support.

All amputees must practise walking outside on different surfaces. Grass, paving stones and pebbles are exceptionally difficult to cope with, especially for those with above-knee prostheses. Nowadays the variety of prostheses available, especially for the above-knee and through-knee amputee, has improved and there are several safety knee mechanisms for those who are walking with a free-knee gait pattern (Fig. 17/22). The physiotherapist must be aware of these components and ensure that the amputee has the one most suitable for the particular activities required. Suspensions have also altered, rigid pelvic bands are still supplied for above-knee levels but many more silesian-type suspensions are used.

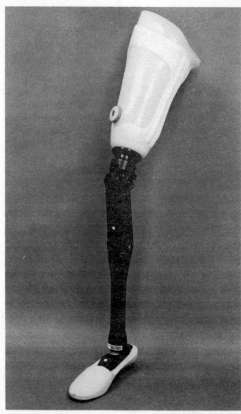

Fig. 17.22 An endoskeletal prosthesis for the above-knee amputee with a self-suspending polypropylene ISNY-type socket, a stabilized knee mechanism and a multiflex foot (*Courtesy* C.A. Blatchford & Sons)

THE BILATERAL AMPUTEE (lower limb)

Unilateral amputees suffering from PVD should be regarded as potential bilateral amputees within two to three years. Occasionally, as a result of trauma, it will be necessary to amputate both lower limbs immediately.

Bilateral amputees need balance, strength, co-ordination and determination to succeed in functional prosthetic use. Major lifestyle changes will have to be accepted. The outcome of successful gait training with two prostheses will depend on the level of amputation and the amputee's present physical condition. Generally the following rules for prosthetic rehabilitation will apply:

- Bilateral below-knee amputees are capable of walking in prostheses.
- The amputee with a combination of a below-knee amputation and one at a higher level may possibly walk.
- The bilateral above- or through-knee amputee is unlikely to walk unless extremely fit and young.

Energy expenditure increases considerably when walking with two prostheses and this must be taken into consideration when the amputee and physiotherapist are setting realistic goals. All bilateral amputees must have a wheelchair for an alternative method of mobility, and some high level amputees may wish to use cosmetic prostheses when wheelchair ambulant. All wheelchair activities must be taught – transfers, manoeuvrability and sitting balance.

Before embarking on a programme of prosthetic rehabilitation, several goals must be achieved, such as independence in dressing, sitting balance and independent transfers. Those amputees with contractures will have enormous difficulties coping with prostheses.

Prosthetic rehabilitation will commence using the parallel bars; the bilateral above-knee amputee will be reduced in height and will start with short rocker pylons with extension rockers. The amputee's level of centre of gravity is therefore reduced, making balance easier (Fig. 17/23). The amputee will be weight-bearing through both tuberosities and in effect is walking on two stilts. The gait pattern for both the above- and through-knee amputee will start with a stiff knee pattern, having a wide base giving more stability. The steps will be of a shorter length, with a slower walking speed. Few of these amputees return to their 'normal' height. Some bilateral above- or through-knee amputees progress to a free-knee gait pattern, if they are very young and fit.

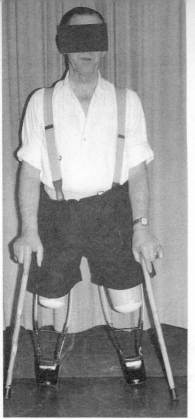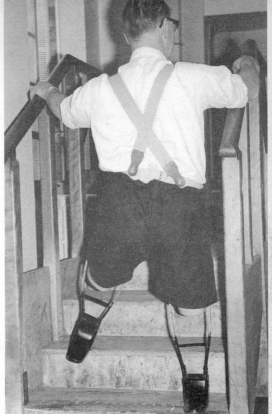

Fig. 17.23 (*left*) Double above-knee amputee on short rocker pylons. Note the need for the wide base

Fig. 17.24 (*right*) Climbing stairs – the rocker is placed on the edge of the step and the patient extends the hip on that side as he pulls with his hands on the rails

Bilateral below-knee amputees usually commence with two patellar tendon-bearing prostheses, and may not have to be reduced in height. Their gait pattern should remain normal but will be usually slower than the unilateral amputee.

As the amputee progresses, a variety of walking aids will be tried, the bilateral below-knee will normally manage sticks, whereas the above-knee may need tetrapods. A frame is not stable for the bilateral amputee and should be avoided. Many amputees tend to fall backwards when trying to lift the frame.

Like the unilateral amputee, the bilateral amputee has to succeed in the activities of daily living, such as 'donning and doffing', getting up from chairs, coping with stairs, slopes, etc. (Fig. 17/24). These are all time and energy consuming and many do not achieve these activities (Van de Ven, 1981).

All amputees, at whatever level and whether unilateral or bilateral, must have visits home at various stages during the rehabilitation programme. Bilateral amputees may require more than one visit and emphasis must be on both prosthetic mobility and wheelchair mobility.

UPPER LIMB AMPUTATIONS

This small group of amputees results from:

Trauma: Mostly industrial injuries or road accidents.
Disease: Mostly malignancy resulting in high-level amputation; vascular disease is very rare.

A large number of those requiring upper limb prostheses are the congenitally limb deficient.

Most upper limb amputees are young, of employable age and male. The psychological shock of losing a hand cannot be under-estimated; the hand not only fulfils many functional tasks but is also an important tool through which to experience the environment. It is also an important means of non-verbal communication – expressing affection, anger, etc. An artificial limb will, to a limited extent, replace the functional tasks of the hand but cannot replace the other more subtle aspects of the hand. The physiotherapist can do much in helping the patient come to terms with the loss as she will be involved early in the rehabilitation process (Van Lunteren et al, 1983).

Level of amputation

The factors to be considered are similar to those already discussed in the lower limb section. In addition, if a patient is unlikely to be a prosthetic limb wearer then as much length of the limb as possible should be preserved. If a prosthesis is likely to be worn then mid-forearm or mid-upper arm amputation enables the most functionally and cosmetically acceptable prosthesis to be fitted.

Physiotherapy

Pre-operative The physiotherapist may have an opportunity to treat the patient pre-operatively. As with the lower-limb amputee a physical and social assessment should be carried out. The patient's attitude to the amputation and how he sees the future is a very important aspect of his rehabilitation and should be taken into consideration.

Postoperative   The aims of treatment are:

- To strengthen muscles controlling the stump.
- To maintain full range of movement in the shoulder girdle and all remaining joints.
- To strengthen and mobilize the unaffected arm.
- To strengthen and mobilize trunk.
- To prevent contractures.
- To control oedema of the stump.
- To maintain good posture.
- To re-educate sensation of the stump.

On the day following amputation, exercises to the shoulder girdle and the unaffected arm are commenced. The patient will depend upon good mobility of this region for the control of his prosthesis. Some traumatic above-elbow amputees also have brachial plexus damage and this must be taken into consideration.

Patients should be encouraged to look at, and touch, their stump as soon as possible. Discussion about any phantom sensation they may have will be helpful.

The stump must remain in a good position and this should be supervised by both nurses and physiotherapists. The contracture most likely to develop in the above-elbow amputee is that of flexion, adduction and medial rotation at the shoulder. The contracture most likely to occur in the below-elbow amputee is that of flexion at the elbow. A constant check on the posture of the patient is necessary to ensure a level shoulder and good position of the head and neck.

A few days following amputation, active exercises for the muscles controlling the stump can be started and gradually progressed to strong resisted exercises when the sutures are removed. Once the sutures have been removed (usually on the 14th day) stump bandaging may be commenced in the same way as for a lower limb amputee. Care must be taken to obtain more pressure distally, preventing a tourniquet effect, and the range of movement of the remaining joints must be retained.

The patient should be encouraged to use his stump as much as possible. Co-operation with the occupational therapist at this stage will be useful. A leather gauntlet can be made into which cutlery can be fitted, thus enabling the patient to eat bilaterally. The occupational therapist will also be able to advise on methods of dressing, washing, etc.

The patient is likely to be discharged from hospital five to seven days postoperatively and should continue to be seen as an outpatient. He should be referred to a DSC as soon as possible to enable him to discuss his needs with the medical officer, prosthetist and occupational therapist, to see different prostheses and to meet other arm amputees. A cast can be taken when the stump is healed and the oedema controlled – approximately six to eight weeks postoperatively.

Prosthetic stage

Training with the prosthesis is usually carried out by an occupational therapist, the emphasis being placed on the training in functional skills towards personal independence, employment and leisure activities.

Upper limb prostheses are made in three weights – heavy working, light working and dress. The choice of type of prosthesis will be determined by the length of the stump, and the needs of the patient. Working arms are controlled by the patient's body power via straps that pass posteriorly across his scapulae to the opposite axilla. The above-elbow amputee activates elbow flexion and the terminal device by protraction of the scapulae and forward flexion of the shoulder joint (Fig. 17/25). The below-elbow amputee activates the terminal

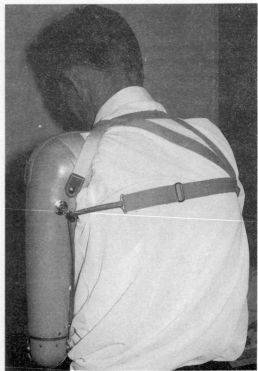

Fig. 17.25 Posterior view of an above-elbow prosthesis showing leather operating cord (inferior) attached to the appendages. Protraction of the scapula to operate terminal device

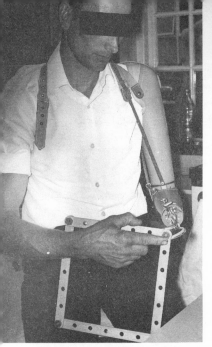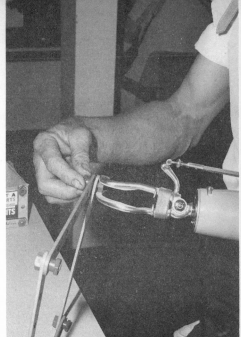

Fig. 17.26 Anterior view showing the strap to operate elbow lock

Fig. 17.27 Close-up of split hook

device by slight forward flexion of the shoulder and extension of the elbow. All arm prostheses are supplied with a cosmetic hand, but for practical activities numerous terminal devices are available, the most common being the split hook (Figs 17/26, 17/27).

The occupational therapist will assess the patient to decide what devices will be needed to enable him to be independent and capable of work; these will then be supplied and suitable training in their use given (Crosthwaite Eyre, 1979). The length of training varies from patient to patient. It starts with operation of the terminal device, usually a split hook, first in unilateral activities followed by simple bilateral tasks progressing to more complicated tasks which the patient is likely to encounter in his work, home or leisure. Most patients return to their former work but some require retraining – this should be considered early in the rehabilitation process. There are upper-limb amputees in many fields of work.

After 6–12 months the patient may be assessed for an electrically powered prosthesis. There are two types:

a. *Myo-electric control*: Especially for below-elbow amputees. This is operated by two electrodes positioned closely against the skin – as the flexor or extensor muscles bulk contracts, the electromyographic

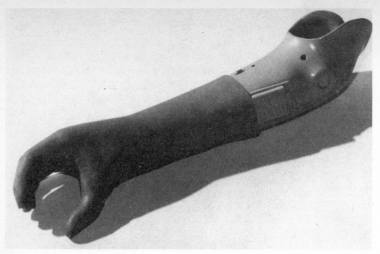

Fig. 17.28 Myo-electric below-elbow prosthesis

(EMG) signals are picked up and amplified and this triggers the hand to open or close thus enabling the patient to have a functioning hand without a harness (Fig. 17/28). However, the arm is heavier and the grip less precise than that of the split hook (Agnew, 1981).

b. *Servo control*: Mostly for above-elbow and through-shoulder amputees. This is operated in a similar way to the body-powered prosthesis but requires only one centimetre of excursion to achieve full opening of the hand. This is of benefit to many who find the split hook difficult to operate.

BILATERAL AMPUTEE (upper limb)

These amputees will require more assistance adjusting to their loss. They must be encouraged to be as independent as possible as soon as practical; an occupational therapist should be involved early to make gauntlets, supply aids and teach methods of achieving independence. Most bilateral amputees manage very well with prostheses and many are employed.

THE LIMB DEFICIENT CHILD

The cause of limb deficiency in most cases is unknown. The most common deficiency is a terminal arrest at the mid-forearm level, presenting as a below-elbow amputation. These children are unlikely to require physiotherapy. They should be seen at a DSC as soon as possible so that the parents can have an opportunity to discuss their child's care with the medical officer, occupational therapist and prosthetist; they can see types of prostheses and meet other families.

Most of these children will receive a cosmetic prosthesis at six months, a body-powered functional prosthesis at 18 months and be assessed for the myo-electric prosthesis at 3½–4½ years (Mendez, 1985). The prosthesis will be the non-dominant assistance to their sound hand.

Children with lower-limb deficiencies may require physiotherapy treatment, e.g. proximal focco femoral deficiency or absent tibia. Some will need a raised shoe, others may benefit from an extension prosthesis, a few may require a Symes amputation. Referral to a DSC allows the parents and therapist to discuss the different options.

A few children have several limbs affected. These families require much support and encouragement. Most of these children manage in normal schools. Many become fully independent although this depends on the number and severity of limbs affected, the child's personality, the home environment and the input of professionals involved in their care. These children have to make the most of what they have – they require excellent balance and strong mobile trunks. Prostheses should be made available to them although many will manage better without. There are often numerous professionals involved in these children's care and sometimes it will be the physio-therapist who acts as the co-ordinator of the team which will include school, home, DSC and hospital.

THE FUTURE

Prosthetic design is continually changing and improving. There is more emphasis on the supply of endoskeletal prostheses enhancing the advantages of modular systems and greater flexibility. Computerization in socket design and manufacture is now in use in some areas (Klasson, 1988). Different methods of fabrication using high technology also exist and are being investigated further (Davies et al, 1985). However, the more traditional exoskeletal prostheses will still have an important part to play particularly for the amputee with special needs (Booker et al, 1988).

Management and services systems for the amputee in the United Kingdom have changed, particularly in England since publication of the McColl Report (McColl, 1986). Provision of prostheses and wheelchairs is now the responsibility of the Disablement Services Authority (DSA). This is a special health authority which has been created to transfer the service to Regional and District Health Authorities within the National Health Service by 1991.

In Scotland the Prosthetic Service is operated by the Area Health Boards through six centres, two in Glasgow and one each in Edinburgh, Dundee, Aberdeen and Inverness. Medical, nursing and therapy staff who care for the patients are employed directly by the local Health Board. Prosthetic fitting and assembly is carried out by commercial contractors who also employ (most of) the prosthetists and all the prosthetic technicians.

All this represents a continual change. It is envisaged that the service for amputees will improve and with the new prostheses available then prosthetic enhancement will be achieved.

REFERENCES

Agnew, P.J. (1981). Functional effectiveness of a myo-electric prosthesis compared with a functional split-hook prosthesis: a single subject experiment. *Prosthetics and Orthotics International*, 5, 92–6.

Blesmag (1983). Spring edition. British Limbless Ex-servicemen's Association. London.

Booker, H. and Smith, S. (1988). The A/K, B/K revisited. *Physiotherapy*, 74, 8, 366–8.

Burgess, E.M., Romans, R.L., Zettle, J.H. and Shrock, R.D. (1971). Amputations of the leg for peripheral vascular insufficiency. *Journal of Bone and Joint Surgery*, 53A, 874–9.

Callen, S. (1981). A modern method of stump bandaging. *Physiotherapy*, 67, 5, 137–9.

Campbell, W.B. and Morris, P.J. (1986). A prospective randomized comparison of healing in Gritti-Stokes and through-knee amputation. *Annals of the Royal College of Surgeons of England*, 68, 1–4.

Connolly, J. (1979). Phantom and stump pain following operation. *Physiotherapy*, 65, 1, 13–14.

Crosthwaite Eyre, N. (1979). Rehabilitation of the upper limb amputee. *Physiotherapy*, 65, 1, 9–12.

Davies, R.M., Lawrance, R.B., Routledge, P.E. and Knox, W. (1985). The Rapidform process for automated thermoplastic socket production. *Prosthetics and Orthotics International*, 9, 27–30.

Day, H.J.B. (1979) Congenital lower limb deformities and extension prostheses. *Physiotherapy*, 65, 1, 3.

Dederich, R. (1967). Technique of myoplastic amputations. *Annals of the Royal College of Surgeons of England*, 40, 222–7.

DHSS (1987). *Amputation Statistics for England, Wales and N. Ireland, 1986*. Statistics and Research Division, Norcross, Blackpool FY5 3TA

English, A.W.G. and Gregory Dean, A.A. (1980). The artificial limb service. *Health Trends*, 12, 77–82.

Ham, R.O., Thornberry, D.J., Regan, F.J. et al (1985). Rehabilitation of the vascular amputee: one method evaluated. *Physiotherapy Practice*, 1, 6–13.

Ham, R.O. and Van de Ven, C.M.C. (1986). The management of the lower limb amputee in England and Wales today. *Physiotherapy Practice*, 2, 94–100.

Ham, R.O. and Whittaker, N. (1984). The King's amputee stump board – a new design. *Physiotherapy*, **70**, 8, 300.

Hughes, J. and Jacobs, N. (1979). Normal human locomotion. *Prosthetics and Orthotics International*, **3**, 4, 12.

Klasson, B. (1988). Computer aided design, computer aided manufacture and other computer aids in prosthetics and orthotics. *Prosthetics and Orthotics International*, **9**, 3, 11.

Koerner, I. (1976). To bandage or not to bandage. That is the question. *Physiotherapy Canada*, **28**, 2, 75–8.

McColl, I. (1986). *Review of Artificial Limb and Appliance Centres*. HMSO, London.

Manella, K.J. (1981). Comparing the effectiveness of elastic bandages and shrinker socks for extremity amputees. *Physical Therapy*, **61**, 334–7.

Mendez, M.A. (1985). Evaluation of a myo-electric hand prosthesis for children with a single below-elbow absence. *Prosthetics and Orthotics International*, **9**, 3, 137–40.

Millstein, S.G., McGowan, S.A. and Hunter, C.A. (1988). Traumatic partial foot amputation in adults: a long term review. *Journal of Bone and Joint Surgery*, **70B**, 251–4.

Mouratoglou, V.M. (1986). Amputees and phantom limb pain: a literature review. *Physiotherapy Practice*, **2**, 177–85.

Mueller, M.J. (1982). Comparison of removable rigid dressings and elastic bandages in pre-prosthetic management of patients with BK amputations. *Physical Therapy*, **62**, 10, 1438–41.

Redhead, R.G., Davis, B.C., Robinson, K.P. and Vitali, M. (1978). Post-amputation pneumatic walking aid. *British Journal of Surgery*, **65**, 9, 611–12.

Robinson, K.P., Hoile, R. and Coddington, T. (1982). Skew-flap myoplastic below-knee amputation: a preliminary report. *British Journal of Surgery*, **69**, 554–7.

Spence, V.A., McCollum, P.T., Walker, W.F. and Murdoch, G. (1984). Assessment of tissue viability in relation to the selection of amputation level. *Prosthetics and Orthotics International*, **8**, 67–75.

Stephen, P.T., Hunter, J. and Aitken, R.C.B. (1987). Mobility survey of lower limb amputees. *Clinical Rehabilitation*, **1**, 181–6.

Van Lunteren, A., Van Lunteren-Gerritsen, G.H.M., Stassen, H.G. and Zuithoff, M.J. (1983). A field evaluation of arm prostheses for unilateral amputees. *Prosthetics and Orthotics International*, **7**, 3, 141–51.

Van de Ven, C.M.C. (1981). An investigation into the management of bilateral leg amputees. *British Medical Journal*, **283**, 707–10.

Waters, R.L., Perry, J., Antonelli, O. and Histon, H. (1976). Energy cost of walking of amputees: the influence of level of amputation. *Journal of Bone and Joint Surgery*, **58A**, 42–6.

BIBLIOGRAPHY

Atkins, D. (1989). *Comprehensive Management of the Upper Limb Amputee*. Springer Verlag, New York.

Bannerjee, S. (1982). *Rehabilitation Management of Amputees*. Williams and Wilkins, Baltimore.

Bloom, A. and Ireland, J. (1980). *A Colour Atlas of Diabetes*. Wolfe Medical Publications, London.

Engstrom, B. and Van de Ven, C.M.C. (1986). *Physiotherapy for Amputees – the Roehampton Approach*. Churchill Livingstone, Edinburgh.

Faris, I. (1983). *The Management of the Diabetic Foot*. Churchill Livingstone, Edinburgh.

Galley, P.M. and Forster, A.L. (1987). *Human Movement: An Introductory Text for Physiotherapy Students*, 2nd edition. Churchill Livingstone, Edinburgh.

Goodwill, J.C. and Chamberlain, M.A. (eds) (1988). *Rehabilitation of the Physically Disabled Adult*. Croom Helm, London.

Horton, R.E. (1980). *Vascular Surgery*. Hodder and Stoughton, London.

Kegel, B. (1986). *Journal of Rehabilitation. Research and Development*. Clinical Supplement No 1. Veterans Administration, USA.

Levy, W.S. (1983). *Skin Problems for the Amputee*. Warren H. Green Inc, St Louis, USA.

Mary Marlborough Lodge (1988). *Equipment for the Disabled. Wheelchairs*. Oxford Health Authority.

Mensch, E. (1987). *Physical Therapy Management of Lower Extremity Amputation*. Heinemann Medical Books, London.

Murdoch, G. (1988). *Amputation Surgery and Lower Limb Prosthetics*. Blackwell Scientific Publications Limited, Oxford.

Pelosi, T. and Gleeson, M. (1988). *Illustrated Transfer Techniques for Disabled People*. Churchill Livingstone, Melbourne.

RADAR (1986). *Wheelchairs and their Use. A Guide to Choosing a Wheelchair*. RADAR, London.

Robertson, E.S. (1980). *Rehabilitation of Arm Amputees and Limb Deficient Children*. Baillière Tindall, London.

Rose, G.K., Butler, P. and Stallard, J. (1982). *Gait: Principles, Biomechanics and Assessment*. ORLAU Publishing, Oswestry, Shropshire.

Saunders, G.T. (1986). *Lower Limb Amputations. A Guide to Rehabilitation*. F.A. Davis Co, Philadelphia, USA.

Troup, I.M. and Wood, M.A. (1982). *Total Care of the Lower Limb Amputee*. Pitman Medical, London.

Vitali, M., Robinson, K.P., Andrews, B.G. and Harris, E.E. (eds) (1986). *Amputations and Prostheses*. Baillière Tindall, London.

Walker, W.F. (1980). *A Colour Atlas of Peripheral Vascular Disease*. Wolfe Medical Publications, London.

ACKNOWLEDGEMENTS

The author thanks the following for help in the revision of this chapter:

Mrs Penny Buttenshaw MCSP, Superintendent physiotherapist, Disablement Services Centre, Roehampton and Mrs Jane Dolman MCSP, Senior physiotherapist, Queen Mary's University Hospital, Roehampton for professional advice.

Miss Fiona Carnegie BAOT, Senior occupational therapist, Disablement Services Centre, Roehampton for revising the section on upper limb management.

Mrs M.E. Condie MCSP, Strathclyde University, for supplying information on the management of Scottish services.

Mrs D. Browning for typing and secretarial assistance.

Chapter 18

Cranial Surgery
by M. LIGHTBODY MCSP

Brain lesions may cause motor and sensory defects but may be accompanied by other severe disorders, for example of sight, hearing, intellect, speech and personality. Psychological disturbance, requiring full understanding and suitable management, may accompany both brain and spinal cord lesions. Early diagnosis of brain lesions and prompt admission to a neurosurgical unit is essential to ensure maximum benefit: delay may cause irreparable damage and permanent disability.

Although research continues to increase understanding of the central nervous system in terms of anatomy, physiology and function, much remains to be discovered. Increasing knowledge of brain areas, pathways, connections, spinal cord tracts and functions has opened up new fields in surgical neurology. Improved investigative and operative equipment and techniques, anaesthesia, antibiotics and other drugs continue to reduce operating time, and reduce to a minimum postoperative complications and morbidity.

Teamwork is essential for the fullest rehabilitation of patients. Interchange of knowledge between members of the rehabilitation team allows a full understanding of the particular problems of each patient. Encouragement, patience, and perseverance are of paramount importance during the rehabilitation period which begins immediately the patient enters hospital.

ANATOMY AND PHYSIOLOGY

For the purposes of description, the brain can be divided into two hemispheres and the brainstem. It must be remembered that the entire mechanism is extremely complex; no one part works as a separate entity, and the response of the brain is the result of the integrated action of its various systems. The anatomical units are not necessarily the functional units. For example, the extra-pyramidal system and the reticular formation appear to have specific functions and yet are comprised of widely spread grey and white matter; the distribution of the blood supply divides the brain into areas different from the anatomical lobes.

The effects of lesions at some strategic sites throughout the brain are given in the following brief guide.

Cerebrum (Figs 18/1 and 18/2)

The cerebrum is the largest part of the brain, and consists of two hemispheres connected by bundles of nerve fibres, the corpus callosum. The surface of each hemisphere covered by layers of cells constitutes the cerebral cortex. This represents the highest centre of function and can be roughly mapped into areas, each concerned with a specific function. To facilitate reference each hemisphere is divided into four lobes, frontal, temporal, parietal and occipital. The right hemisphere controls the left side of the body, and the left

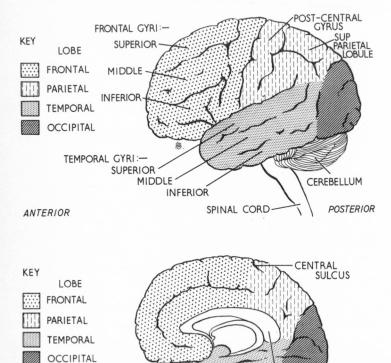

Fig. 18.1 Lateral aspect of the brain

Fig. 18.2 Sagittal section of the brain

hemisphere controls the right side of the body and usually speech function, depending on the 'handedness' of the person.

Frontal Lobe (Figs 18/1 and 18/3)

Area	Function	Effect of a lesion
(A) Motor area (which gives rise to the cerebrospinal tracts)	Controls voluntary movement of the opposite half of the body which is represented on the cortex in an upside down position (Fig. 18/4)	Flaccid paralysis. A lesion between the hemispheres produces paraplegia
(B) Pre-motor area	Localization of motor function	*Spastic paralysis Psychological changes
(C)	Controls movements of the eyes	The eyes turn to the side of the lesion and cannot be moved to the opposite side
(D)	Motor control of larynx, tongue, and lips to enable movements of articulation	Inability to articulate
(E) 'Silent area'	Believed to control abstract thinking, foresight, mature judgement, tactfulness	Lack of a sense of responsibility in personal affairs

*The effects of a lesion in the pre-motor area vary with the rate of onset; a lesion which occurs suddenly, such as a head injury or a haemorrhage, will result in a flaccid paralysis initially, spasm gradually developing over a variable period of time. A lesion which has a slow mode of onset, such as a slowly growing neoplasm, will produce spasm in the early stages.

Temporal Lobe (Figs 18/1 and 18/3)

Area	Function	Effect of a lesion
(F and G)	Hearing and association of sound	Inability to localize the direction of sound
(H) Auditory speech area	Understanding of the spoken word	Inability to understand what is said

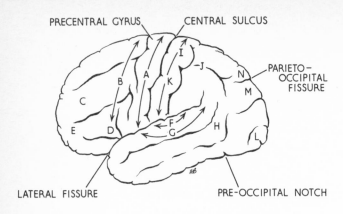

PRECENTRAL GYRUS   CENTRAL SULCUS

PARIETO−OCCIPITAL FISSURE

LATERAL FISSURE   PRE-OCCIPITAL NOTCH

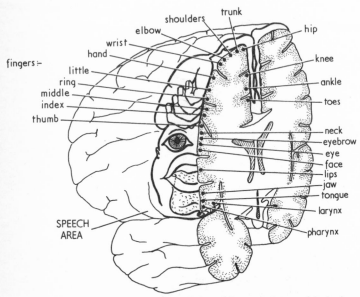

shoulders   trunk

elbow   hip

wrist

hand

fingers :−

little

ring

middle

index

thumb

knee

ankle

toes

neck
eyebrow
eye
face
lips
jaw
tongue

larynx

SPEECH AREA

pharynx

Fig. 18.3 Diagrammatic representation of some of the cortical areas of the brain

Fig. 18.4 The motor homunculus superimposed on the pre-central gyrus illustrates the proportions and positions of body representations in the motor cortex. For the post-central gyrus there is a similar representation for sensation

Other areas on the medial aspect of the temporal lobe are associated with the sense of smell and taste. The optic radiations sweep through the temporal lobe to reach the occipital lobe and these may also be damaged by a lesion of the temporal lobe giving rise to a quadrantic field defect (Fig. 18/5).

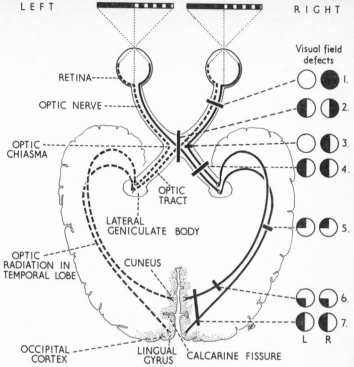

Fig. 18.5 The effects of injury in the visual pathway. (1) Complete blindness in one eye. (2) Bi-temporal hemianopia. (3) Complete nasal hemianopia right eye. (4) Left homonymous hemianopia. (5 and 6) Quadrantic defects. (7) Complete left homonymous hemianopia

Parietal Lobe (Figs 18/1 and 18/3)

Area	Function	Effect of a lesion
(I, J and K)	Sensory receptive areas for light touch, two-point discrimination, joint position sense and pressure	Corresponding sensory loss giving rise to a 'neglect phenomenon'. 'Body image' loss is associated with lesions of the non-dominant hemisphere

Visual defects arising from lesions in the parietal area may be highly complex and the patient unaware of them. Sensory loss gives a severe disability, which is out of proportion to any associated voluntary power loss.

Occipital Lobe (Figs 18/1 and 18/3)

Area	Function	Effect of a lesion
(L)	Receptive area for visual impressions	Loss of vision in some areas of the visual fields (Fig. 18/5)
(M and N)	Recognition and interpretation of visual stimuli	Inability to recognize things visually

Brainstem

All nerve fibres to and from the cerebral cortex converge towards the brainstem forming the corona radiata, and on entering the diencephalon they become the internal capsule (Fig. 18/6). When the cerebral cortex is removed the remainder, or central core, is termed the brainstem. Its components from above downwards are: the diencephalon; the basal ganglia; the mesencephalon or midbrain; the pons; and the medulla oblongata.

The nuclei of the cranial nerves are scattered throughout this area.

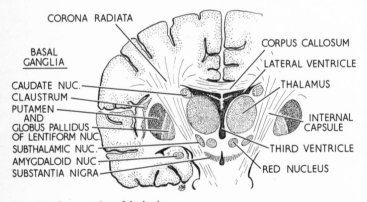

Fig. 18.6 Cross-section of the brain

Basal ganglia and extra-pyramidal system

Broadly speaking the basal ganglia include the corpus striatum, amygdala, claustrum, substantia nigra and subthalamic nuclei. The corpus striatum consists of the caudate nucleus and the lenticular nucleus, the latter being composed of the putamen and the globus pallidus.

The extra-pyramidal system includes parts of the cerebral cortex, thalamic nuclei connected with the striatum, corpus striatum, sub-thalamus, rubral and reticular systems and its functions are concerned with associated movements, postural adjustments and autonomic integration. Lesions may result in voluntary movement being obscured or abolished and replaced with involuntary movements.

Lesions of the extra-pyramidal system can produce either hyperkinetic or hypokinetic disorders.

Midbrain, pons and medulla oblongata

The midbrain, pons and medulla oblongata also act as a funnel for tracts passing from higher levels downwards to the spinal cord and for sensory tracts from the spinal cord passing upwards to higher centres. In view of it being a relatively small area, any lesion can give rise to widespread effects. Involvement of any of the following are likely.

Cerebellar function may be affected due to interference of the efferent and afferent pathways passing through the brainstem.

Sensation of all types may be affected as the fasciculi gracilis and cuneatus terminate in nuclei in the medulla oblongata. Nerve fibres then arise from these nuclei, cross the mid-line and continue upwards to the thalamus in the medial lemniscus. The spinothalamic tracts which cross in the spinal cord pass directly upwards through the brainstem.

Loss of motor function occurs if the cerebrospinal tracts are damaged. These pass downwards from the internal capsule to decussate at the lower end of the medulla oblongata.

The conscious level can be depressed if there is damage to the reticular formation which is scattered throughout the brainstem.

Vomiting and disturbed respiratory rate can occur with pressure on the vomiting and respiratory centres in the medulla oblongata.

Cranial nerve nuclear lesions may result with characteristic palsies.

Cranial Nerves (Fig. 18/7)

Cranial nerve	Function	Effect of a lesion
I. Olfactory	Sense of smell	Loss of sense of smell
II. Optic	Vision	Various visual field defects (Fig. 18/5) Visual acuity affected

III. Oculomotor	Innervates medial, superior, inferior recti and inferior oblique muscle and voluntary fibres of levator palpebrae superioris. Carries autonomic fibres to pupil	Outward deviation of the eye, ptosis, dilation of the pupil
IV. Trochlear	Motor supply to the superior oblique eye muscle	Inability to turn the eye downwards and outwards
V. Trigeminal	(a) Motor division to temporalis, masseter, internal and external pterygoid muscles (b) Sensory division: touch, pain and temperature sensation of the face including the cornea on the same side of the body	(a) Deviation of the chin towards the paralysed side when the mouth is open (b) Loss of touch, pain and temperature sensation and of the corneal reflex
VI. Abducent	Innervates the external rectus muscle	Internal squint and therefore diplopia
VII. Facial	Motor supply to facial muscles on the same side of the body	Paralysis of facial muscles
VIII. Acoustic	Sensory supply to semicircular canals Hearing	Vertigo. Nystagmus. Deafness
IX. Glossopharyngeal	Motor to the pharynx Taste: posterior one-third of the tongue	Loss of gag reflex. Loss of taste in the appropriate area
X. Vagus	Motor to pharynx Sympathetic and parasympathetic to heart and viscera	Difficulty with swallowing. Regurgitation of food and fluids
XI. Accessory	The cranial part of the nerve joins the vagus nerve	
XII. Hypoglossal	Motor nerve of the tongue	Paralysis of the side of the tongue corresponding to the lesion, thus it deviates to the paralysed side when protruded

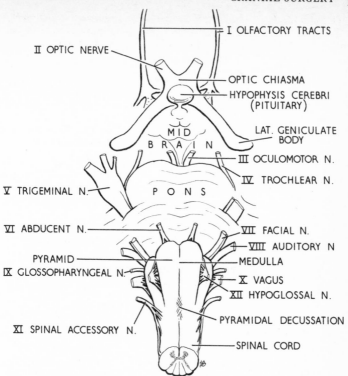

Fig. 18.7 The brainstem and cranial nerves (viewed from below)

Cerebellum (Fig. 18/8)

The cerebellum lies in the posterior cranial fossa of the skull connected to the pons and medulla oblongata by the cerebellar peduncles. The surface is corrugated and consists of cells forming the cerebellar cortex. It is divided into two cerebellar hemispheres which join near the mid-line with a narrow middle portion called the vermis.

Although the whole of the cerebellum is highly integrated and disease often results in diffuse damage, the signs and symptoms of cerebellar lesions can be summarized as follows:

1. Vermis lesions causing truncal ataxia, tendency to fall back and to one side depending on side of lesion.
2. Cerebellar hemisphere lesions causing limb ataxia, hypotonia, static or postural tremor and nystagmus.

Circulation of the brain

The four major vessels which supply the brain, the right and left vertebral and internal carotid arteries, form an anastomosis at the base of the brain, called the circle of Willis (see Fig. 18/13(c) p. 332). From this arterial complex many branches are given off, to be distributed to the brainstem, cerebellum and cerebrum. Interference with the circulation in any of these branches will cause characteristic deficits, depending on the parts of the brain deprived of blood supply.

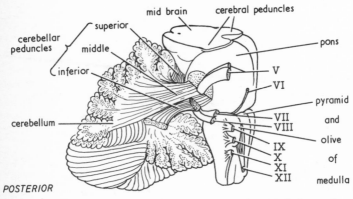

Fig. 18.8 Right antero-lateral view of the dissected cerebellar hemisphere and peduncles showing the lower cranial nerves

The ventricular system

The ventricular system consists of four fluid-filled cavities within the brain. There is a right and left lateral ventricle, and a third and fourth ventricle in the mid-line. Cerebrospinal fluid (CSF) is produced in the choroid plexuses of the ventricles and circulates within the system to the fourth ventricle where it escapes through the foramina of Luschka and Magendie, into the subarachnoid space (Fig. 18/9). CSF flows all around the brain and spinal cord, bathing it and cushioning it against jarring forces.

Obstruction of the system leads to hydrocephalus, raised intracranial pressure and eventually neurological deficits as the underlying structures are compressed or distorted.

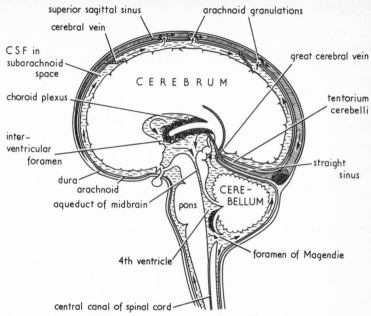

Fig. 18.9 Circulation of the cerebrospinal fluid

EXAMINATIONS AND INVESTIGATIONS

Before surgery can be considered, extensive examinations and investigations may need to be carried out to localize the lesion and decide upon its nature and likely prognosis.

Examinations

A history of the patient's present illness, previous illnesses and any relevant family illness is noted, as are social circumstances, occupation, drinking and smoking habits. Whenever possible this information is obtained directly from the patient, but if the patient's level of consciousness or language function is disturbed it will have to be obtained from other sources such as spouse, parents or friends. If the patient has a history of unconscious episodes, such as epileptic attacks, a description of these attacks from an observer may provide useful information.

The patient undergoes a general examination but special attention is devoted to the central nervous system; each cranial nerve is tested, reflexes, motor power and all types of sensation are carefully checked. Full assessment of the central nervous system may be complicated by lack of co-operation, but adequate information is usually obtained to establish a diagnosis.

Assessment by the physiotherapist

Detailed and precise pre-operative assessment is ideal but this may be difficult if the patient requires immediate surgery, or if the conscious level affects co-operation.

The assessment will give a baseline from which further improvement or deterioration can be measured. A postoperative deterioration may be the result of removal of brain tissue during the course of surgery, but, more important, it may be one of the signs of onset of postoperative complications, such as haemorrhage or thrombosis.

The assessment by the physiotherapist requires an accurate evaluation of:

1. Voluntary movement and muscle power, as this is useful both for diagnosis and future treatment.
2. The range of movement which may be correlated with any incidental findings of importance, for example previous underlying orthopaedic pathology.
3. Muscle tone, which may be either hypo-, normo- or hyper-tonic. Changes in muscle tonus may be subtle but they are important indications of the patient's progress. Awareness of the state of muscle tone is an integral part of treatment. Muscle tone may be described as the resistance to stretch, and can be judged by palpation of the muscle belly, the resistance felt to velocity, sensitive passive movements, tendon responses, observation of active movements and posture.
4. Equilibrium and righting reactions.
5. The sensorium and mental status of the patient.
6. Sensory modalities particularly cutaneous, deep and proprioceptive responses.
7. The functional ability of the patient to determine the level and quality of his independence. (Chapters 6, 7, *Cash's Textbook of Neurology for Physiotherapists*, 4th ed., describe the assessment of patients with a neurological disorder.)
8. The early assessment of the patient's respiratory function is desirable but will depend upon his physical state and the degree of urgency for operation.

Special investigations

These procedures should not restrict treatment although some aspects may need modifying.

Lumbar Puncture A needle is inserted into the subarachnoid space between the third and fourth lumbar spinous processes; the pressure of the cerebrospinal fluid is determined and a sample of fluid taken for diagnostic purposes. Following lumbar puncture the patient is advised to be flat in bed for six hours, and active physiotherapy can be given in any of the lying positions. A severe headache may develop after a lumbar puncture. This can be relieved by elevating the foot of the bed for 24–48 hours.

The indication for a lumbar puncture is to examine the CSF in patients with meningeal irritation.

Radiographs Plain films of the skull are not usually necessary, but if indicated they can be supplemented by special views of various areas. A general radiographic examination may be indicated and a chest radiograph is always taken.

X-ray Computed Tomography (CT scan) This technique has revolutionized the field of investigation. The patient's head is centred in a gantry containing an x-ray tube on one side, and banks of detectors on the opposite side. The gantry moves around the patient's head and the x-ray beam is measured by the detectors before entering, and on leaving, the head. The detectors are so arranged that tomographic cuts are obtained. All this information is processed by a computer and displayed on a TV screen as a cross-sectional picture of the head from which the operator can visualize the internal structure of the brain and identify certain abnormalities which may be present.

Cerebral Angiography This procedure is used mainly in the investigation of patients with cerebrovascular disease and suspected intracranial haemorrhage. The site of arterial stenosis or occlusion is easily seen. In spontaneous intracranial haemorrhage the site of an aneurysm or arteriovenous anomaly can only be determined by angiography. Postoperative angiography is a useful means of checking the efficiency of surgical treatment of aneurysms and anomalies.

Transfemoral catheterization and selective catheterization of the carotid and vertebral arteries are carried out with injection of contrast medium into these vessels which allows the display of major cerebral arteries.

Following angiography the patient is nursed flat for 24 hours, then allowed to sit up and get out of bed if no headache is present.

Magnetic Resonance Imaging (MRI)   MRI is increasingly used as it is more sensitive in detecting abnormalities in brain substance, such as areas of demyelination and oedema.

Electro-encephalography The electro-encephalograph (EEG) amplifies and records the electrical activity of the brain. It has been replaced by CT scan, but is used as an aid to the diagnosis of epilepsy and location of a focus.

Monitoring Intracranial Pressure A monitoring system can be used to measure intracranial pressure over a period of approximately 48 hours. The information gained allows fuller assessment of the patient's condition and his further management. This means of measuring intracranial pressure over a period of time has been extremely useful in the management of certain head injury patients whose condition has remained static for no apparent reason. The monitoring can show up huge variations in pressure over a long period, which go undetected with random measurements, and can indicate the need for a 'shunt' to reduce intracranial pressure, with a resultant improvement in the patient's condition.

Because the patient is connected to a delicate piece of apparatus, he is necessarily kept lying quietly in bed for the duration of the monitoring. Physiotherapy can be continued. Moving or turning the patient, and coughing or straining, will dramatically alter the CSF pressure, and hence the recording needle may swing violently. It is necessary to note both type and time of physiotherapy so that when the results are analysed these changes in pressure are interpreted correctly.

GENERAL SIGNS AND SYMPTOMS OF CEREBRAL LESIONS

Raised intracranial pressure

Intracranial pressure depends on the volume of the skull contents. In a child under the age of 18 months, any slow abnormal increase in volume will result in a disproportionate increase in the size of the head. In individuals over the age of 18 months there is no increase in the size of the head, thus the effects of raised intracranial pressure will produce a disturbance of cerebral function more rapidly. Increased volume may be caused by a space-occupying lesion, such as a tumour or abscess, a blockage in the cerebrospinal fluid pathways or by haemorrhage from an aneurysm. With raised intracranial pressure the soft-walled veins become compressed, giving rise to oedema and subsequent lack of oxygen to the brain tissue, and although the symptoms vary in degree, the classical picture of raised pressure is a combination of the following features.

Drowsiness Drowsiness is the earliest and most important sign of raised intracranial pressure. The brain can adapt to very slowly increasing pressure and the patient may become gradually demented with little else to show. Rapidly increasing pressure will produce drowsiness and it becomes progressively more difficult to rouse the patient. Unconsciousness and death can follow in a short time.

Headache In the early stages of raised intracranial pressure, headache may be paroxysmal occurring during the night and early morning. With continued increase in pressure it becomes continuous and is intensified by exertion, coughing or stooping. The pressure headache is usually bilateral and becomes worse when the patient is lying down and is relieved when sitting up. Other causes of head pain are irritation of parts of the meninges, involvement of the Vth, IXth and Xth cranial nerve trunks, referred pain from disorders of the eyes, sinuses, teeth and upper cervical spine, and tension headaches due to muscle spasm.

Papilloedema This is oedema of the optic discs which can cause enlargement of the blind spot and subsequent deterioration of visual acuity and complete blindness.

Vomiting This occurs when the headache is most severe and tends to be projectile in nature.

Pulse and Blood Pressure Acute and sub-acute rises in pressure cause a slowing of the pulse rate, but if pressure continues to rise the pulse rate becomes very rapid. A rapid increase in intracranial pressure causes a rise in the blood pressure, but a chronic rise does not affect it, and in some lesions below the tentorium cerebelli the blood pressure is below normal.

Respiratory Rate   This is not affected by a slow rise in pressure but a sufficiently rapid increase in pressure, which produces a loss of consciousness, usually results in slow deep respirations. This may change after a period and become irregular, of the Cheyne-Stokes type.

Epileptic Convulsions   Generalized fits may occur but it is not clear whether these are caused by the raised intracranial pressure or by the actual lesion itself.

Meningeal irritation

Meningeal irritation is characterized by headache and, perhaps, neck and backache and pain down the back of the legs. Associated vomiting and photophobia are almost the rule. The signs are those of limitation of neck flexion together with limitation of straight leg raising. Causes of meningeal irritation are subarachnoid bleeding, meningitis or pus in the CSF.

Eye symptoms

Eye symptoms are often present with a brain lesion and they can directly affect a patient's capabilities during his rehabilitation. Among those most commonly found are:

Damage to the optic nerve, optic chiasm or optic tracts will cause field defects (Fig. 18/5).
Damage to the IIIrd cranial nerve can cause a ptosis, an inability to open the eye.
Nystagmus: This is frequently present in cerebellar or brainstem lesions and is an involuntary jerky movement of the eyes.
Diplopia or double vision: This is present if there is any imbalance of the eye muscles and may be overcome by covering alternate eyes on alternate days until the imbalance adjusts itself.

Ear symptoms

Deafness may be caused by tumours of the VIIIth cranial nerve such as acoustic neuromas; these tumours may give rise to vertigo.

Speech disorders

These have already been briefly mentioned and are mainly associated with lesions of the temporal lobe on the dominant side.

Level of consciousness

Numerous factors can be responsible for alteration in the level of consciousness but essentially they are any cause of raised intracranial pressure:

1. Haemorrhage which can be either extradural, subdural, subarachnoid, or intracerebral.
2. Infection as in the case of meningitis and encephalitis.
3. Space-occupying masses causing increased intracranial pressure and compression of the brainstem.
4. Operational trauma.
5. Postoperative complications such as oedema or haemorrhage.
6. Certain types of trauma produce a craniocerebral injury.

Any known disturbance of hearing, vision or speech function must always be taken into account, and the patient given every opportunity to be able to respond.

General attitudes of the patient should be noted also:

1. A patient who lies curled up, turned away from the light, and does not like being interfered with, who is irritable to varying degrees and who may be confused or even delirious, might be showing signs of cerebral irritation.
2. When the neck is held stiffly into extension, and the patient resists flexion sometimes accompanied by retraction of the head, it may be due to irritation from subarachnoid haemorrhage, meningitis or raised intracranial pressure.
3. Trunk and limb rigidity or stiffness may be signs of involvement of the base of the brain. The spine and lower limbs are held in total extension, the forearms pronated, elbows extended and the wrists and fingers flexed. This posture is usually described as decerebrate rigidity.

Other localizing signs may include: ataxia; cranial nerve palsies; and reflex changes.

ASSESSMENT OF CONSCIOUSNESS

The conscious level is the most important observation made. Various ill-defined stages have been used to formulate different scales of consciousness in the past but these stages may mean different things to different people. An accurate scale where there can be little divergence is needed. One such scale is the Glasgow Coma Scale

(Teasdale and Jennett, 1974). This assesses the patient's motor activity, verbal performance and eye-opening responses (Table 18 I).

TABLE 18 I NEUROLOGICAL OBSERVATION CHART FOR ASSESSMENT OF CONSCIOUSNESS (BASED ON THE GLASGOW COMA SCALE)

Time	0–24h	22.00	24.00	02.00	04.00	06.00
Eye opening	Spontaneous					
	To speech	x —— x		x (peak at 02.00)	x —— x	
	To pain					
	None					
Best verbal response	Orientated					
	Confused					
	Inappropriate	x —— x —— x			x —— x	
	Incomprehensible					
	None					
Best motor response	Obeying					
	Localizing	x —— x —— x			x —— x	
	Flexing					
	Extending					
	None					

Motor activity, if not in response to commands, can be assessed by the response to painful stimuli. The response may be either 'localizing', e.g. if the hand moves towards the stimuli, or 'flexor' or 'extensor' to indicate the direction of the movement. There may be no response. If one limb or one side is clearly worse than the other side, this is regarded as evidence of focal damage.

Verbal responses can indicate either full orientation and awareness of self and surroundings or confusion, inappropriate speech or incomprehensible speech.

Eye opening responses indicate whether the arousal mechanisms in the brainstem are active. The eyes may open in response to speech, to pain, or spontaneously.

CRANIAL SURGERY

Table 18 II summarizes the conditions for which surgery may be necessary. It is not proposed to describe in detail specific surgical procedures: the Bibliography on page 343 includes textbooks to which reference may be made for a description of the actual surgical techniques.

TABLE 18 II   NEUROLOGICAL CONDITIONS FOR WHICH SURGERY MAY BE APPLIED

Condition	Adult	Paediatric and juvenile
Cerebral trauma	Head injuries	Head injuries
Neoplastic lesions	Cerebral – primary – metastatic Tumours from related structures, e.g. meninges; cranial nerves; pituitary fossa Cerebellar	Cerebral – primary Tumours from related structures, e.g. choroid plexus or ventricle Cerebellar
Cerebrovascular disease Haemorrhage Ischaemic lesions	Intracranial aneurysms Spontaneous subdural or extradural haemorrhage Angiomatous malformations Carotid stenosis	 Angiomatous malformations
Hydrocephalus	Secondary (e.g. with space-occupying lesions) Aqueduct stenosis	Congenital Secondary – tumours – spina bifida

Spina bifida		Spina bifida cystica
		  meningocele
		  myelomeningocele
		Encephalocele

Dyskinesia	Parkinsonism	Cerebral palsy
		  spastic hemiplegia
		  choreoathetosis

Epilepsy	Intractable Focal pathology EEG focus	Primary focus associated, for example, with Sturge-Weber syndrome
Cerebral infections	Abscess	Abscess
Repair of skull defects	Cranioplasty	Craniosynostosis
Miscellaneous	Intractable pain, e.g. trigeminal neuralgia	

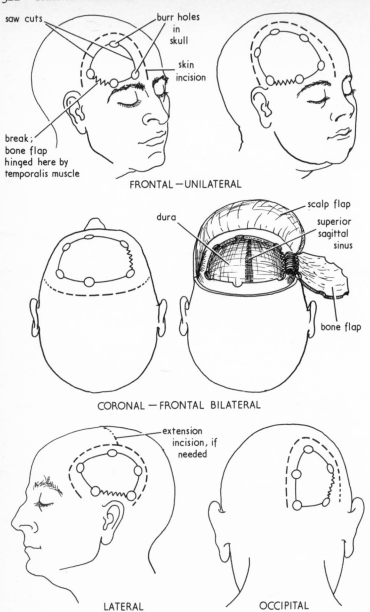

Fig. 18.10 Some supratentorial surgical approaches

GENERAL POINTS RELATING TO SURGICAL PROCEDURES

Most operations are performed under general anaesthesia and may take a considerable period of time to complete. During the course of surgery a bone flap may be turned back, but this is usually replaced at the end of the operation. Figures 18/10 and 18/11 illustrate some of the surgical approaches.

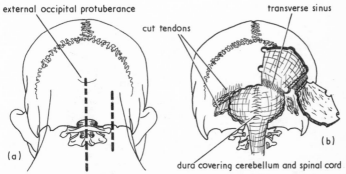

Fig. 18.11 Surgical approaches to the posterior fossa. (a) Mid-line or paramedian incision. (b) Craniectomy with an additional occipital bone flap when more exposure is necessary. The posterior arches of C1 and C2 have also been removed

Postoperative treatment

On returning from the operating theatre the patient may have a pressure bandage on the head if there is oozing from the wound. Eyes are very vulnerable to swelling and do so as a result of operational trauma. The position of the patient on the operating table may also be a contributory factor, hence for the first two or three postoperative days the patient may be unable to open either eye.

Intravenous infusion begun during the operation may be continued for one or two days; then, if the ability to swallow is affected, the patient is artifically fed via a nasogastric or naso-oesophageal tube.

A urinary catheter may be in situ. A restless, confused patient may try to remove head bandages, drains and intravenous infusions so hands may have to be restrained by padding and bandages. Reassurance and/or pain relief may be all that is necessary to settle the patient down.

During the first few postoperative days intensive nursing care is required, the patient's condition being carefully observed and charted. Deterioration can occur very rapidly due to postoperative complications, thus any change must be reported immediately as it can be a matter of life and death. Surgical resection of brain tissue may account for neurological deficits.

Bone Flap   This may be removed if the brain is very swollen during operation or if the skull is splintered as a result of a head injury. When bone has been removed the patient may not be nursed on the affected side but can be turned for procedures as long as no pressure is exerted on the head. Replacement of this flap is advisable once oedema has subsided, as the patient tends to suffer from headache, dizziness when stooping and is afraid of damage from a bump to the area. Following head injury, or invasion by tumour, the bone may be so badly damaged it has to be discarded, and the defect is then filled with plastic material.

The young active patient who is once more ambulant may be provided with a protective metal plate inside a cap, or a crash helmet to prevent further trauma, until the defect is repaired.

Ventricular Drainage   The patient may return from theatre with ventricular drainage if there are signs of inadequate cerebrospinal fluid circulation at operation. A catheter is introduced into a lateral ventricle by means of a burr hole in the skull and the cerebrospinal fluid drained into a bag; the height of the bag is set at a level determined by medical staff, usually 10–20cm above the ventricle. Care should be taken when treating the patient to ensure that the level of the head is not altered in relation to the bag as this alters the drainage pressure.

Lumbar Drainage   This may be set up several days postoperatively if there are signs of continued raised intracranial pressure. The needle is placed as for a lumbar puncture and tubing connects it to a drainage bag. If the drainage is to be continuous the patient is nursed in side lying, well supported by pillows. Turning is done by lifting the patient from side to front, to his other side.

Complications

Apart from the complications arising from brain damage the following may also arise:

Cerebrospinal fluid may leak following the original operation, which may require further surgical repair.

Postoperative oedema, thrombosis or haemorrhage from cerebral blood vessels, or arterial spasm occurs in a small number of patients.

Pulmonary embolus and thrombus formation elsewhere.

Epilepsy may develop after a variable period of time.

Infection at the operation site is serious, particularly if the dura has been opened, as it can lead to meningitis and encephalitis.

Respiratory complications are fairly common.

PHYSIOTHERAPY

The general principles of physiotherapy in cranial surgery are virtually the same as for other surgical procedures.

1. Prevent respiratory complications.
2. Assess any problems and neurological deficits, and treat where appropriate.
3. Prevent the development of contractures and pressure sores.

Guidelines for treating specific conditions will be described as indicated.

General

Rather special anaesthetic conditions are required for neurosurgery (Greenbaum, 1976) and although techniques are continually improving, some operations may still take several hours and the patient is subjected to long periods of anaesthesia. Breathing exercises are taught and the patient is asked to practise them before operation and as soon as he is sufficiently awake afterwards. A check must be made that the patient can cough and he should demonstrate that he is able to cough effectively, as a shallow throat cough is quite ineffective in clearing secretions. Patients who are known smokers should be advised to stop before operation.

The patient should also be reminded to move his legs frequently (particularly the feet and ankles) after the operation to prevent venous stasis and consequent deep vein thrombosis. Assistance with movements may be necessary – the physiotherapist should show the nursing staff how to help movement when they carry out nursing procedures provided no undesirable changes in muscle tone are provoked.

Postoperative assessment of voluntary movement, power, muscle tone, sensation, degree of ataxia, balance and gait is carried out appropriately as the condition of the patient allows.

Respiratory complications

Postoperative complications such as cerebral oedema and haematoma formation may directly affect respiration. The cough reflex may be lost or diminished to an ineffective level, and the ability to swallow affected. The physiotherapist must be on the alert for those problems, as patients with coughing and swallowing difficulties are at risk from aspiration of food and fluids. Feeding by nasogastric tube is preferred until swallowing is established.

Treatment and prevention of chest complications may have to be carried out within limitations imposed by the patient's condition as follows:

1. Postural drainage may be contra-indicated immediately after operation as it may cause a raised intracranial pressure.
2. Blood pressure fluctuations occur in certain positions, so avoid sitting the patient up too rapidly or turning quickly.
3. The patient may have a diminished cough reflex or facial weakness and therefore have difficulty in expectoration.
4. A disturbed conscious level may make co-operation difficult. Deep breathing should be encouraged, and manual pressure on the chest wall as the patient breathes out is useful. Instruction to cough can be accompanied by pressure on the chest as this is attempted. Demonstration of coughing may help the dysphasic patient.

Suction If there is a depressed conscious level or an ineffective cough suction may be necessary to clear secretions. It may be helpful if there are two people when treatment with suction is required: the nurse can use the suction while the physiotherapist assists the patient with breathing and attempts to cough.

Involvement of the lower cranial nerves (IX–XII) may increase the difficulties of maintaining an open airway. Patients who are unable to maintain their own airway for any reason will require intubation either orally or nasally. If clinical signs and blood gas analysis indicate poor oxygenation artificial mechanical ventilation may be necessary. If it is thought that the airway is at risk for a lengthy period a tracheostomy may be necessary.

Facilitation Techniques Some respiratory facilitation techniques suitable for the unconscious adult patient have been described by Bethune (1975). These include stimulating a co-contraction of the abdominal muscles, pressure on upper and lower thoracic vertebrae, stretch of isolated intercostal muscles, moderate manual pressure on the ribs, stretch of the anterior chest wall by lifting the posterior basal area of the supine patient, and peri-oral stimulation by firm pressure applied on the top lip.

INTRACRANIAL TUMOURS

Intracranial tumours may be primary or secondary. Secondary tumours are usually blood-borne metastases and derive from neoplasms of the bronchus, breast and kidney as well as from thyroid carcinomas, malignant melanomas and a variety of less common primary lesions. Primary intracranial neoplasms may be derived from the brain itself (cerebral hemispheres and the cerebellum), the meninges (meningiomas), cranial nerves, the pituitary gland, the pineal body and blood vessels.

Intrinsic tumours of the cerebral hemispheres (the glioma series) are locally invasive and thus considered malignant. The degree of malignancy depends on their rate of growth and histological character. Total removal of these tumours is seldom possible because of their infiltration of the brain tissue.

Meningiomas are generally benign and do not often invade the brain but present problems in view of their size and extreme vascularity. Total removal is often feasible.

The location of a tumour is the important factor irrespective of its pathology because it may involve the vital centres, thus directly threatening life, or limiting surgical accessibility.

Signs and Symptoms Some degree of raised intracranial pressure usually exists. Focal signs develop pointing to the site of the tumour.

Investigations These include skull and chest radiographs, CT scan and, possibly, angiography.

Surgical treatment

In order to attempt removal an operation (craniotomy) is necessary and, where possible, the tumour is removed totally, or as near totally as possible. If it is not possible to remove the tumour a biopsy will be taken to enable a diagnosis to be established. Tumours may recur following incomplete removal. Occasionally a bone flap may be removed to effect a decompression. Radio-sensitive tumours may be given a course of radiotherapy and cytotoxic (anti-tumour) drugs may also be given.

Surgical removal of intrinsic tumours of the dominant fronto-temporal or temporo-parietal areas is rarely attempted as this may lead to severe hemiplegia and dysphasia. Intrinsic brainstem tumours are rare and direct surgical intervention not possible.

Physiotherapy A patient without operative complications is encouraged to get up on the day following surgery. Hemiparesis or hemiplegia is treated accordingly. Where the prognosis is known to be poor, all steps must be taken to ensure maximum independence without recourse to sophisticated techniques (Downie, 1978).

Cerebellar tumours

The majority of cerebellar tumours arise in or near the mid-line and may extend into one or both cerebellar hemispheres. These tumours are most likely to be medulloblastomas or cystic astrocytomas in young children; haemangioblastomas in young adults or metastases in older age-groups.

Signs and Symptoms These differ considerably depending on the site of the tumour. The following occur in varying degrees: raised intracranial pressure, usually due to obstructive hydrocephalus; and focal signs: cerebellar, brainstem or cranial nerves, e.g. ataxia, probably most marked in walking, giddiness, nystagmus.

Surgical treatment

It may be necessary to treat hydrocephalus before approaching the lesion itself. This is achieved by 'shunting' (p.336). To excise this type of tumour a different approach is necessary. A mid-line incision is made and the occipital bone covering the cerebellum is removed (craniectomy); the posterior arch of C1 is also removed because part of the cerebellum has often herniated through the foramen magnum by pressure from the tumour (see Fig. 18/11(b)).

Physiotherapy A patient with a cerebellar lesion fatigues quickly. He will probably have a history of vomiting for a variable period of time before operation, leading to debility and dehydration. Shorter treatment sessions more often allow enough time for rest, and prevents the overtiring which reduces functions.

Tumours of the cerebello-pontine angle

A sub-section of posterior fossa tumours worthy of special mention are those occurring in the cerebello-pontine angle (Fig. 18/12). Surgery to these requires a more lateral approach. Several types of tumour occur in this confined and critical area, and any space-

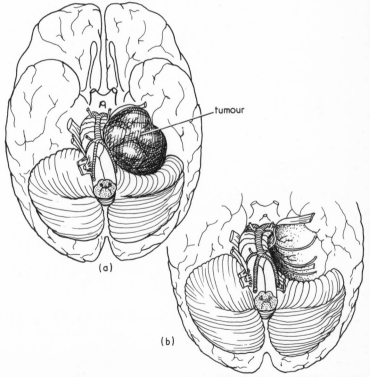

Fig. 18.12 (a) Tumour of the left cerebello-pontine angle (viewed from above). (b) The tumour bed showing distortion of the brainstem and nerves

occupying lesion will gradually compress the nearby structures and result in deficits related to the appropriate cranial nerves, as well as producing a rise in intracranial pressure and long tract signs.

Signs and Symptoms   These may include: deafness, tinnitus and vertigo; facial weakness from compression of the VIIth nerve; loss of corneal reflex, loss of pain and temperature sensations with compression of the Vth nerve; ataxia of limbs on the side of tumour occurring with compression of the cerebellar hemisphere and cerebellar peduncles; and spasticity and dementia (with large lesions, the latter due to raised intracranial pressure).

The most common lesion to occur is the acoustic Schwannoma (neuroma) which arises from the VIIIth nerve. These are probably the most difficult group of tumours to remove, especially if large.

Surgical treatment

Some tumours in this area can be completely removed but large tumours, particularly those adherent to the brainstem, may prove more difficult to excise and the lower cranial nerves may be damaged.

Postoperative Treatment   The patient may have swallowing difficulties and poor cough reflex; this requires the same care as for a cerebellar tumour. If there is a VIIth nerve palsy the patient will be unable to close his eye. The nurse devotes special care to the eye and a tarsorrhaphy (partial suturing together of the upper and lower lid) may be necessary to prevent damage to the cornea and infection.

Physiotherapy   Physiotherapy is as for cerebellar tumours but special attention is frequently required to re-train oro-facial dysfunction. This is best done by a co-ordinated programme arranged between the speech therapist, physiotherapist and nursing staff. It can be a frustrating and humilating experience for a patient to find he is unable to feed himself, to manipulate the food in his mouth and that he dribbles and drools. If he cannot control liquids adequately and coughs and splutters, he feels he is choking with every mouthful. Some of these difficulties can be overcome by ensuring correct head position, by facilitating a co-contraction of the tongue and cheeks and selecting food of appropriate consistency. Water is difficult as the patient is unable to control it with his slow and inaccurate movements. Lumpy or chunky foodstuffs are inappropriate initially and generally the most satisfactory consistency is that of ice-cream, purées and yoghurt. Slowly and carefully the patient progresses both to more-liquid and more-solid food as he learns to cope with the difficulty.

Damage to Facial Nerve When the facial nerve cannot be preserved intact during surgery an attempt may be made to re-innervate the distal portion of the cut nerve. This can be achieved by an anastomosis with either the spinal accessory or hypoglossal nerves. Cross-facial nerve anastomosis to innervate both sides from one nerve is sometimes considered.

The spinal accessory nerve can be split to allow relative preservation of the shoulder girdle innervation, whereas using the hypoglossal nerve will cause some tongue paralysis. If facial-accessory anastomosis is used, particularly attention is paid by the physiotherapist to shoulder girdle re-education.

SUBARACHNOID HAEMORRHAGE

Intracranial aneurysms

Intracranial aneurysms are balloon-like dilatations occurring at the bifurcation of vessels of the circle of Willis (Fig. 18/13). The precipitating cause is thought to be a congenital defect in the wall of the blood vessel. Aneurysms are also associated with arteriosclerosis and hypertension. Their size varies from a pea to a plum and multiple aneurysms may be present. Age-groups most affected are those between 30 and 50 years.

Rupture of an aneurysm is the most common cause of spontaneous subarachnoid haemorrhage.

Signs and Symptoms These depend on the severity and site of bleeding. A minor leak from an aneurysm gives sudden severe (usually occipital) headache, which then radiates up over the head and settles in a generalized headache and neck stiffness. Severe haemorrhage will cause increased intracranial pressure and decreased level of consciousness with neurological deficits depending on degree of damage from haemorrhage.

Investigations These are: lumbar puncture to establish the presence of blood in the CSF, and to exclude bacterial meningitis; CT scan to estimate position of haematoma formation; and angiography to determine the site of aneurysm.

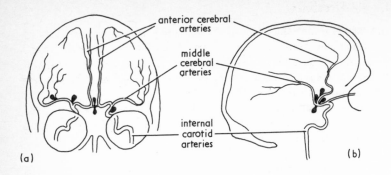

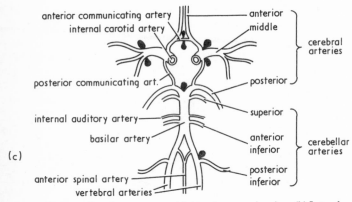

Fig. 18.13 Common sites for aneurysms. (a) Anterior-posterior view. (b) Lateral view. (c) Vessels of the circle of Willis

Pre-operative treatment

As soon as subarachnoid haemorrhage is diagnosed precautionary measures are taken to prevent a fatal re-bleed before surgery. This risk can be reduced by keeping the patient on strict bed rest and as flat as possible; some neurosurgeons suggest that patients should be allowed to get out of bed for toilet purposes as this raises the intracranial pressure less than straining when lying down. Hypertension is controlled by using beta-blockers/diuretics, care being taken to avoid precipitous falls in blood pressure.

If headache remains severe an analgesic that does not depress respiration (e.g. codeine phosphate) is prescribed. Nausea and vomiting are controlled by anti-emetics.

Surgical treatment

Surgery is undertaken only if the patient is conscious and showing improvement from any neurological deficit arising from the initial bleed. This is usually 7–10 days post-bleed. Postoperative vasospasm of the vessels around the aneurysm site is a danger and there is less likelihood of this if surgery is delayed.

The aneurysm is usully occluded by placing a clip across the neck of the aneurysm, or by a clip and wrapping the aneurysm in cotton wool and glue or muscle.

Complications Further bleeding may occur while the surgeon is attempting to obliterate the aneurysm. Traction upon blood vessels in the field of surgery can cause ischaemia of the area of brain which they supply. Oedema, thrombosis and vasospasm may follow surgery. These postoperative complications can be manifest within a few hours of surgery and can completely alter the neurological state and, therefore, outcome.

Physiotherapy This is similar to treatment following uncomplicated surgery for tumour. Once the aneurysm is clipped it is safe and will not re-bleed. Deficits are dealt with accordingly.

INTRACRANIAL ANGIOMATOUS MALFORMATIONS (ARTERIOVENOUS ANOMALIES)

These malformations are congenital abnormalities of vascular development; they occur on the surface of the brain or within brain tissue deriving a good blood supply from one or both hemispheres and are usually found in the younger age-groups including children.

The blood vessels of the malformation show degeneration of their walls, and direct communication between arteries and veins in some areas. If the malformation is small no diversion of blood from the capillary bed occurs, but a large one robs the brain of its blood supply.

Signs and Symptoms These are variable but the following may occur: headaches of a migrainous character; focal epilepsy; subarachnoid haemorrhage; intracerebral haemorrhage which may produce focal signs such as mono- or hemiparesis together with a sensory or visual loss.

Investigations Angiography and CT scan will determine the site of the lesion. EEG may be used for investigating epilepsy.

Surgical treatment

A direct intracranial approach is made and the lesion excised if it lies superficially. A deep-seated hemisphere lesion is untreatable by surgery. Sometimes complex lesions may be treated by the occlusion of the feeding vessels.

Physiotherapy This follows the same course as that for an aneurysm (p.333).

CAROTID ARTERY STENOSIS

Discussion of occlusive cerebrovascular disease can be confusing because of the terminology used. Jennett (1983) has described it as follows: 'Stenosis implies narrowing only, occlusion a complete block, while thrombosis describes a pathological state which may sometimes be the cause of an occlusion but is more often a consequence of obstruction. Ischaemia refers to inadequate perfusion of an area of brain with functional failure; only if it is sufficiently severe and prolonged does infarction develop. Carotico-vertebral insufficiency is a useful term for symptomatic extra-cranial obstructive vascular disease.'

Atheroma is the most usual cause of stenosis of the common and internal carotid arteries, and thrombus formation may complete the occlusion. The site of the narrowing is most frequently at the origin of the internal carotid artery, and the severity is variable.

The deprived hemisphere is dependent upon the collateral circulation derived through the circle of Willis for its blood supply.

If the major problem is caused by multiple emboli shooting off from the site of the thrombus, then anticoagulants may be used with great care.

Signs and Symptoms A wide variety of symptoms and modes of onset can be produced by carotid artery occlusion.

Hemiplegia: This may be profound and occur suddenly, with loss of consciousness. There may be hemiparesis progressing to hemiplegia. There may be transient motor weakness ('stuttering') usually affecting one extremity.

Dysphasia, sensory loss, eye symptoms: These are associated in some degree with the loss of voluntary power.

Headache: Occasionally present behind the eye.

Investigations A CT scan will differentiate between an infarct and haemorrhage. Angiography will reveal any stenosis or occlusion.

Surgical treatment

In carefully selected cases surgery is of value. Contra-indications are gross arteriosclerotic involvement of other cerebral vessels, and loss of consciousness with the onset of symptoms, which carries a poor prognosis.

Surgical measures aim to restore the normal blood flow and prevent further emboli to the blood vessels of the brain causing ischaemia and infarction.

Endarterectomy: The atheromatous portion of the artery and any thrombus is removed, by opening the artery and then resuturing it.

Physiotherapy A patient with stable neurological signs after uncomplicated surgery may be mobilized early.

Immediate measures are required for the re-education of hemiplegic limbs. Bearing in mind the likely sensory loss and visual field defects the patient must be reminded constantly of the affected limbs. Patients with deficits remain on bed rest longer and are mobilized at a slower pace.

HYDROCEPHALUS

Hydrocephalus in adults may be secondary to a mass lesion particularly in the posterior fossa, third ventricle or midbrain where a tumour may block the flow of CSF through the ventricular system (obstructive hydrocephalus); or following a subarachnoid haemorrhage or meningitis when adhesions occur in the subarachnoid space and prevent CSF circulating over the brain (communicating hydrocephalus).

Aqueduct stenosis may produce a slowly developing hydrocephalus in which an acute episode may be precipitated by a mild head injury.

The commonest underlying causes of hydrocephalus in the neonatal period are birth trauma and meningitis. Congenital malformations such as a narrowed aqueduct and spina bifida are found in about one-quarter of cases (Jennett, 1983).

Surgical treatment

Treatment is often by 'shunting'. CSF is drained from the lateral ventricle via a tube and valve system into the internal jugular vein, thence to the right atrium (ventriculo-atrial) or to the peritoneum via subcutaneous neck and trunk tubing (ventriculo-peritoneal).

Physiotherapy Patients are nursed flat in bed for two to three days and are gradually sat up over the next two days. More severe cases are nursed head down for one or two days and may take five to six days to be upright. There is danger of a subdural haematoma forming as the result of traction on the veins in the subdural space if the patient is sat up too rapidly. Once up, the patient can be steadily mobilized. Further operative procedures may be necessary where tumour is involved.

CEREBRAL ABSCESS

A brain abscess develops either in the cerebral hemisphere or cerebellum according to how pus enters the brain. Approximately half of them arise from local spread (usually ear, mastoid and otitis media and air sinuses) and half by bloodstream spread. The inflammation around the pus causes considerable oedema so patients are drowsy and have headache but rather less obvious focal signs. Cerebral abscess still carries high mortality due to speed of development, and epileptic fits are common sequelae.

Surgical treatment

Treatment is vigorous. Pus is aspirated through burr holes, and large doses of antibiotics are administered intravenously. If repeated aspiration does not clear the pus then it will be necessary to turn a bone flap to effect this.

Physiotherapy Treatment is as for craniotomy for tumour. In cases where there is markedly raised ICP, the conscious level will be decreased and careful attention is paid to the chest, limbs and positioning. Any neurological deficit is treated accordingly.

MOVEMENT DISORDERS

The treatment of movement disorders falls within the realm of functional neurosurgery. It includes the use of stereotaxic surgery which is a means of making discrete lesions in selected parts within the brain without recourse to open operation.

The most successful use of stereotaxy has been that of treating parkinsonian tremor. Other conditions sometimes treated by stereotaxic surgery include intractable pain and some psychiatric conditions.

Particularly in patients with parkinsonian tremor, careful selection of cases in which surgery is contemplated is necessary as many of these patients are elderly and frail.

Investigation and Assessment CT scan or MRI, video recordings and neurophysiological measurements of the tremor are carried out. The patient is fully assessed by the physiotherapist, speech therapist and occupational therapist.

Surgical treatment

The procedure requires fixing to the skull a special frame capable of holding the apparatus used to make the lesion. Contrast medium may be introduced into the ventricles via a burr hole and radiographs taken. Measurements on the radiographs are taken relating the outlined structures to the target area. More recently CT guided methods have been increasingly employed. The target point is selected and co-ordinates, computed on the CT software, then related to the stereotaxic frame and an electrode is introduced to this target point. The trajectory of the electrode is checked by a recording from the nervous tissue during advancement of the electrode. For destructive lesions a radio-frequency current is passed and the lesion made at the electrode tip. The size of the lesion is regulated by the electrode size and tip temperature. Usually the lesion is only about 5mm×3mm (Hitchcock, 1978).

In the classical operation for parkinsonian tremor, an electrode is stereotactically guided through a frontal burr hole to the ventrolateral nucleus of the thalamus (Fig. 18/14). A lesion in the globus pallidus will reduce rigidity, although nowadays this is largely treated by drug therapy.

Specific lesions made in the thalamic or dentate nuclei are used for the abolition or reduction of disorders such as dystonias, dyskinesias and spasticity. Occasionally psychiatric conditions benefit from discrete surgical lesions such as amygdalotomy and cingulectomy.

Physiotherapy A patient whose main symptom is rigidity may have difficulty coughing therefore chest care is important. Bilateral

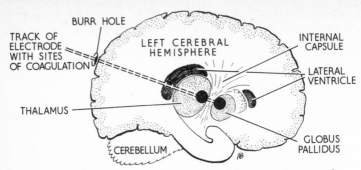

Fig. 18.14 Position of a burr hole and electrode track in stereotaxic surgery for parkinsonianism

lesions may produce speech and swallowing problems. Functional re-education may be required. After a loss of severe tremor stabilizing exercises help regain functional use of the limbs, particularly the arms. Full range joint mobility is rapidly regained when symptoms have been relieved.

EPILEPSY

Epilepsy can be described as a paroxysmal transitory disturbance of the functions of the brain which develops suddenly, ceases spontaneously, with a strong tendency to recurrence. Many varieties of epileptic attack exist depending upon the site of origin, extent of spread and the nature of the disturbance of function.

Causes Epilepsy may be caused by: a local lesion in the brain, such as tumour or abscess; complications of head injury; hereditary predisposition; and unknown causes.

Investigations EEG recordings of the electrical activity of the brain can help to pinpoint the cause of epilepsy. If a focus can be determined, its nature can be investigated by other means. Other appropriate procedures will be selected according to the particular history and clinical features of the patient.

Surgical treatment

Surgery is of value to a patient who has epilepsy as the presenting feature of a brain lesion, or a definite focus which gives rise to his epileptic attack. Surgical procedures vary with the type of lesion to be excised. Temporal lobe epilepsy may be treated by lobectomy. Cortical excisions, hemispherectomy and callosal section are also performed.

Physiotherapy Rehabilitation follows general principles with deficits being treated accordingly.

INTRACTABLE PAIN

There have been considerable advances in the treatment of intractable pain over the past decade due largely to the establishment of several regional centres for pain relief which are able to combine the services of physicians, surgeons, anaesthetists and radiotherapists to provide comprehensive treatment.

Intractable pain describes chronic severe pain which may persist after the primary lesion has been treated and cannot always be totally relieved even by constant narcotic therapy. This becomes progressively less effective and there is a danger of addiction to the drugs used. Figure 18/15 shows some pain pathways.

Pain is difficult to quantify and has different characteristics depending on its origin. Innumerable factors can influence it; some of the most important being the patient's personality, intelligence and emotional maturity. Careful clinical and psychological assessments are thus essential before surgical measures are undertaken to relieve pain. Figure 18/16 shows some of the surgical procedures used in pain alleviation.

Pain is of malignant or benign aetiology. Carcinomas outside the nervous system are frequently the cause of malignant intractable pain. Among the benign causes are herpes zoster, scar tissue, amputation stump neuromas, phantom limb pain and some cord lesions.

A general principle of surgical treatment is to start with the smallest effective procedure working up to large ones if necessary, and wherever possible to start peripherally in the nervous system and work centrally. Surgery can be directed at peripheral nerves and nerve roots, spinal cord and the brain, and may involve open operations or percutaneous procedures. Many such operations involve making small electrical lesions at various points within the nervous system or local administration of drugs using catheters placed in the epidural space.

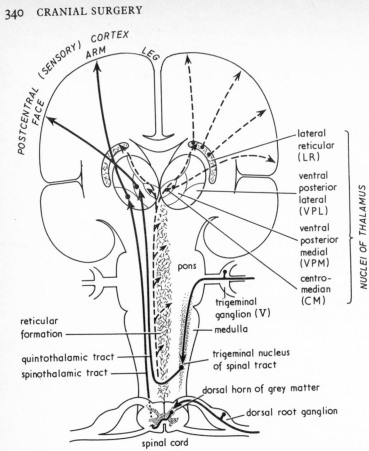

POSTCENTRAL (SENSORY) CORTEX
FACE ARM LEG

lateral
reticular
(LR)

ventral
posterior
lateral
(VPL)

ventral
posterior
medial
(VPM)

centro-
median
(CM)

NUCLEI OF THALAMUS

pons

trigeminal
ganglion (V)

reticular
formation

medulla

quintothalamic tract

trigeminal nucleus
of spinal tract

spinothalamic tract

dorsal horn of grey matter

dorsal root ganglion

spinal cord

Fig. 18.15 Projections of some pain pathways. The centromedian nucleus (CM) and the ventro-postero-medial nucleus (VPM) of the thalamus are sites for stereotaxic interruption of central pain pathways. Interruption of the trigeminal nerve tract at spinal or pontine levels or at the trigeminal ganglion are possible sites for treating facial pain

Surgical treatment

Local Surgery A local procedure to excise a neuroma or a form of percutaneous or transcutaneous electrical stimulation may be all that is necessary to effect relief.

Posterior Rhizotomy The appropriate posterior spinal nerve roots are sectioned between the spinal cord and the posterior spinal ganglion on the same side of the body that the intractable pain is felt.

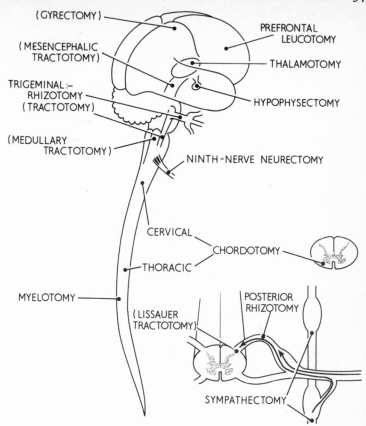

Fig. 18.16 Some surgical procedures used to alleviate pain

Due to the overlap of the sensory supply from one dermatome to another, it is necessary to section at least two sensory roots above and below the area in which pain is localized by the patient. This operation has been used for post-herpetic pain and painful scars, but after a period of time the intractable pain has a tendency to recur. It is of no use for limb pain, as it destroys muscle and joint sensation which would give rise to a severe disability.

Dorsal Root Entry Zone   This procedure involves operations on the root entry zone of the spinal cord (see Further Advances, p.343).

Cordotomy   Fibres of the lateral spinothalamic tract are divided on the opposite side of the body to that on which the pain is experienced.

To achieve a permanent result the procedure must be done at least several segments higher than the localization of pain to allow for the fact that fibres carrying pain and temperature sensations enter the spinal cord and ascend for several segments before crossing the mid-line to join the lateral spinothalamic tract, and that no matter how deep the incision made at operation the level of sensory loss always descends during the first postoperative week.

Spinothalamic cordotomy is used to relieve pain for malignant disease especially affecting the pelvic region. It has poor results for upper limb pain and de-afferentation pain (i.e. pain in an already numb area).

Bilateral cordotomy may be necessary for bilateral symptoms but this can produce weakness below the level of the surgical lesion. Bladder and bowel function may be disturbed. High cervical cordotomy can damage the innervation to the diaphragm and intercostal muscles producing ipsilateral paralysis.

Stereotaxic cordotomy can bring greater accuracy in making a lesion in open cord surgery. Percutaneous cordotomy is an alternative to open procedures: it only requires local anaesthesia and there is no painful wound. However, precise localization of the lesion can be more difficult.

Myelotomy This is essentially a mid-line lesion in the cord involving the pain fibres that cross in the mid-line. It is used for bilateral leg pain but runs the risk of producing sphincter dysfunction.

Thalamotomy Thalamotomy is used for de-afferentation pains and for other types of pain where cordotomy is inappropriate or has failed. Destructive lesions are made stereotactically without causing significant sensory loss.

Physiotherapy The patient is encouraged to get up on the second day post-surgery. Chest care is important if there is diaphragm and intercostal muscle paralysis. Static muscle contractions start two or three days after surgery progressing to active extension exercises after a week. Following high cervical cordotomy gentle neck mobilization can start five or so days post-surgery.

It is important to teach the patient to look after any area of pain and temperature loss and he should be reminded to test the temperature of water with the sound side before immersing the affected side.

Further advances

Cordotomy and many peripheral procedures are of little value in treating de-afferentation pain (e.g. phantom limb pain) or pain occurring in the upper limbs. Some recent advances are stereotactic methods of stimulation of the peri-aqueductal grey matter (for general mid-line and bilateral limb pains) and chronic thalamic stimulation for certain forms of de-afferentation pain. Lesions can be made at the dorsal root entry zone (DREZ) of the spinal cord for pain in limbs. This procedure involves making small electrical lesions at open operation at the point of entry of the pain fibres from the sensory roots into the spinal cord, thereby avoiding loss of touch and proprioception which would render the limbs useless.

REFERENCES

Bethune, D. D. (1975). Neurophysiological facilitation of respiration in the unconscious adult patient. *Physiotherapy Canada*, **27**, 5, 241.

Downie, P. A. (1978). *Cancer Rehabilitation: An Introduction for Physiotherapists and the Allied Professions*, pp.78–9. Faber and Faber, London.

Greenbaum, R. (1976). General anaesthesia for neurosurgery. *British Journal of Anaesthesia*, **48**, 773.

Hitchcock, E. R. (1978). Stereotactic surgery for cerebral palsy. *Nursing Times*, **79**, 50, 2064.

Jennett, B. and Galbraith, S. (1983). *An Introduction to Neurosurgery*, 4th edition. Heinemann Medical Books, London.

Teasdale, C. and Jennett, B. (1974). An assessment scale of coma and impaired consciousness: a practical scale. *Lancet* (July 13).

BIBLIOGRAPHY

Barr, M. L. and Kiernan, J. A. (1988). *The Human Nervous System*, 5th edition. Harper and Row, Philadelphia.

Bobath, B. (1978). *Adult Hemiplegia: Evaluation and Treatment*, 2nd edition. William Heinemann Medical Books Limited, London.

Bobath, B. (1985). *Abnormal Postural Reflex Caused by Brain Lesions*, 3rd edition. William Heinemann Medical Books Limited, London.

Carr, J. H. and Shepherd, R. B. (1980). *Physiotherapy in Disorders of the Brain*. William Heinemann Medical Books Limited, London.

Carr, J. H. and Shepherd, R. B. (1987). *Movement Science: Foundations for Physical Therapy in Stroke Rehabilitation*. William Heinemann Medical Books Limited, London.

Davies, P. M. (1985). *Steps to Follow*. Springer-Verlag, Berlin.

Downie, P. A. (ed.) (1987). *Cash's Textbook of Neurology for Physiotherapists*, 4th edition. Faber and Faber, London.

Harrison, M. J. G. (1987). *Neurological Skills: A Guide to Examination and Management in Neurology*. Butterworths, London.

Lindsay, K. W., Bone, I. and Callander, R. (1987). *Neurology and Neurosurgery Illustrated*. Churchill Livingstone, Edinburgh.

Miller, J. D. (ed.) (1987). *Northfield's Surgery of the Central Nervous System*, 2nd edition. Blackwell Scientific Publications Limited, Oxford.

Ross Russell, R. W. and Wiles, C. M. (1985). *Neurology*. William Heinemann Medical Books Limited, London.

Walsh, K. W. (1987). *Neuropsychology – A Clinical Approach*, 2nd edition. Churchill Livingstone, Edinburgh.

Walton, J. N. (ed.) (1985). *Brain's Diseases of the Nervous System*, 9th edition. Oxford University Press, Oxford.

ACKNOWLEDGEMENT

The author extends her thanks to Mr C. B. T. Adams MA, MChir, FRCS and Mr Peter Teddy DPhil, FRCS, consultant neurosurgeons at the Radcliffe Infirmary, Oxford, for their help and advice in the revising of this chapter.

Chapter 19

Acute Head Injuries

by M. LIGHTBODY MCSP

The role of the physiotherapist in the treatment of patients with severe head injury is vital in the acute stage of their management and in their rehabilitation. Head injuries may be either open or closed.

Open These injuries mean that the skin and skull have been penetrated by a missile or sharp object, also possibly causing penetration through the dura into the brain, i.e. a compound (through the skin) depressed fracture of the skull.

Closed These are the most common form of head injury and may cause a linear skull fracture or no fracture at all, but of more importance is the effect on the brain. The real damage results from the brain being suddenly shaken within the skull by a sudden acceleration (such as a blow to the back of the head) or deceleration (the moving head comes in contact with a fixed object). This causes, at its mildest, concussion, but more severe damage causes serious brain injury or even death.

The subsequent management of head injury will largely depend on:
Diagnosis – how severe is the injury?
Assessment – what is the conscious level?
Detection of complications – e.g. blood gas deterioration.

When the patient first arrives in the casualty department, the admitting doctor must take an accurate history, from witnesses if the patient is unable to communicate. This should include: type of accident; an assessment of level of consciousness at the time of injury and any deterioration or improvement; any respiratory or bleeding problems; any evidence of fitting; and, if possible, any relevant past medical history should be obtained as this may influence the management of the head injury.

Assessment

The immediate assessment concerns the respiratory state, the conscious level and the cardiovascular state. The result of this assessment will dictate priorities of treatment. It will be followed by a thorough neurological and general examination.

Respiratory State   Respiratory distress and, therefore, inadequate ventilation may be caused by:

1. *Obstruction of the airway*: The airway may be partially or completely blocked by inhalation of vomit or blood; the tongue flopping against the back of the throat; jaw fractures; false teeth or other foreign bodies inhaled at the time of the accident.
2. *Depression of the respiratory centre*: The brain injury may damage the respiratory centre in the brainstem affecting control of rate and rhythm of respiration.
3. *Associated injuries*: Primary damage to the chest wall and lung tissue can lead to further respiratory disturbance requiring immediate attention.

Conscious Level   This is the most important observation. It is best described in terms of speech or movement with or without stimulation, and a scale of response measured in these terms is used. This gives an overall impression and an accurate picture can be made over time by different observers without wide variation in meaning (e.g. Glasgow Coma Scale, p. 319).

Any alteration in response can be seen easily if the observations are plotted on a graph.

Cardiovascular State   Hypotension will lead to reduced cerebral perfusion and neurological deterioration.

Neurological Examination   Neurological examination will include: level of consciousness; pupil reaction; pulse, blood pressure, respiratory state; and movement of limbs (lateralizing and focal signs). From the examination an assessment of severity of the injury can be made. The Glasgow Coma Scale is a method of putting a numerical figure on the severity of the injury. Some attempt at prognosis can be made using the Glasgow Outcome Scale (Jennett and Bond, 1975).

Investigations   Skull and chest radiographs are mandatory. A CT scan and cervical spine radiographs may be indicated in more severe injuries. Blood chemistry relevant to surgery, and investigations relevant to other suspected injuries are also necessary.

Skull fractures

Linear: Most skull fractures are linear and undisplaced. They may radiate to the base of the skull and through foramina damaging blood vessels and cranial nerves.

Depressed: An area of bone is displaced on to or through underlying dura and brain with the possibility of damage to these structures. They may require surgical elevation.

Compound depressed: These fractures invariably require exploration and elevation.

Associated injuries

Many patients with a head injury have additional injuries. These injuries may be relatively minor and can await attention, or they may demand as urgent attention as the head injury itself. For example, chest injuries causing hypoxia and hypercarbia may further aggravate cerebral oedema. Abdominal bleeding from damaged viscera may cause hypotension reducing cerebral perfusion. Fracture-dislocation of the cervical spine may be caused by hyperextension movement when damage is to the front of the skull and face. Fractures of the face, ribs, pelvis and long bones may be present.

Priorities of treatment have to be decided upon.

MECHANISM OF BRAIN DAMAGE

The primary brain damage sustained in a head injury is not in itself treatable but subsequent deterioration due to secondary damage may be prevented and reversed in some cases. Treatment is aimed at preventing and minimizing these secondary effects.

Secondary causes of damage

Raised Intracranial Pressure (ICP) There are various reasons for an increase in ICP and these include: haematoma formation (extradural, subdural or intracerebral); cerebral oedema, and hydrocephalus. The ICP is also modified by changes in blood gases.

The skull is essentially a closed box lined by dura containing CSF (10 per cent) brain (80 per cent) and blood (10 per cent). If any of these increase in volume then the pressure will increase. The brain, given time, can adapt to very slowly increasing pressure and produces signs and symptoms at a later stage. However, rapidly increasing pressure with profuse shearing within the brain tissue will eventually cause brainstem compression because the cerebellum is forced down into the foramen magnum. The clinical effects of this process are increased drowsiness, unconsciousness and, once coning has occurred, death.

Haematoma Formation

Extradural haematoma (EDH): An EDH usually develops within 12 hours of the injury. A skull fracture is almost always present in adults. This causes tearing of blood vessels in the dura, particularly the middle meningeal artery.

Subdural haematoma (SDH): Acute SDH is generally associated with severe head injury and profound underlying brain damage. It is thus often only part of the total brain injury and not always the most important component. The size may not relate to the severity of brain damage.

Intracerebral haematoma (ICH): This may be present and like an acute SDH, is only part of the total brain injury.

Cerebral Oedema Just as any other damaged tissue swells when injured so cerebral oedema may occur and will produce a rise in ICP. It may have a delayed onset and give rise to problems some days later.

Hydrocephalus (see p. 335)

Blood Gas Changes Hypercarbia gives rise to an increase in cerebral blood flow (CBF) and this will accentuate any existing tendency to an increase in ICP. Profound systemic hypoxia secondary to lung problems will also accentuate oedema formation in a damaged brain where blood supply may be impaired.

Infection If the scalp overlying a depressed fracture is torn a route for infection is created. Meningitis and cerebral abscess may result.

CSF Rhinorrhoea and Otorrhoea Fractures involving the base of the skull may create a fistula between the subarachnoid space and nasal cavity or middle ear. This is a further route for infection.

Fat Embolism   Fat embolism is associated with severe trauma, especially extensive long bone fractures. The mechanism of production of 'fat embolism' is not clear. It may be due to fat globules from the fracture site entering the bloodstream and when lodged in the lung reduce gas exchange leading to hypoxia and confusion.

Epilepsy   Epilepsy may follow a head injury and it may occur at any time. It reflects brain bruising or, occasionally, a developing haematoma.

Management of secondary causes of damage

Raised ICP   The management of raised ICP is determined by the cause.

Haematoma formation: prompt removal of an EDH by craniotomy can produce complete recovery. An acute SDH may be evacuated through burr holes or craniotomy but tends to carry a poor prognosis.

Cerebral oedema: Attempts are made to reduce the swelling. These include the use of mannitol and other diuretic drugs and intermittent positive pressure ventilation (IPPV).

Blood gas changes: Hypercarbia may result from inadequate spontaneous ventilation raising carbon dioxide levels and consequently increasing ICP by cerebral vasodilation. Hypoxia from underventilation due to obstruction, aspiration or brainstem damage can have a significant effect on ICP and may further aggravate damage and neurological deterioration, thus a vicious circle is set up. IPPV is almost certainly required.

Infection   Thorough surgical exploration is mandatory to elevate a depressed fracture and clean scalp wounds to minimize the risk of infection.

CSF Rhinorrhoea and Otorrhoea   Surgical intervention to close any communication between the subarachnoid space and nasal cavity or middle ear may be required.

Fat Embolus   Main treatment is the appropriate management of the respiratory problem.

PATIENT CARE

Management of the unconscious patient

The unconscious patient is best nursed in an intensive therapy unit (ITU) as these units maintain the high levels of care required by these patients.

Patients who are managing to maintain their own airways and adequate oxygenation are unlikely to require intubation and mechanical ventilation. They are nursed in a position which allows the head to be raised at 30 degrees and in side lying to prevent inhalation of secretions. Regular turning will prevent consolidation and collapse and the breakdown of pressure areas. Problems may arise with positioning and turning if there are associated injuries which require splinting, such as plaster casts or traction, although these can usually be minimized. A tube is passed via the nose or mouth to allow appropriate nutrition to be given.

Neurological observations are carried out frequently so that immediate action may be taken if any deterioration is noted.

Chest Care   This is best carried out to coincide with turns and before bolus feeds. A continuous feed should be switched off. The chest is vibrated on the expiratory phase of breathing. Tipping the patient with his head down is not advised due to the risk of elevating ICP. When suction is required to remove secretions, procedures via the nose are contra-indicated if CSF rhinorrhoea is present: this indicates a CSF leakage through a skull fracture with a risk, therefore, of ascending infection. The frequency of treatment depends on the individual patient, but even if there are no obvious lung problems treatment is given to prevent the unnecessary complications of retained secretions.

Patients with known or suspected raised ICP need careful handling and will be attached to ICP monitoring equipment. This differs from the monitoring described previously in that rises in ICP must be treated immediately, as opposed to looking for trends over a period of time.

General Care   An unconscious patient must be treated as a whole person and not as a series of joints and muscles. As consciousness returns the clinical features resulting from the head injury are evident but the predominant problem, spasticity, will be evident early on. Handling these patients is often made more difficult from spasticity with the release of primitive neuromuscular activity such as reflex patterns. Techniques to preserve mobility and inhibit primitive responses are employed as far as possible. These, combined with careful positioning after treatment sessions and every turn, should help reduce the problems to which hypertonicity leads at a later stage. *Never* assume that these patients are unaware of what is happening around them. Talking to them, telling them what you are doing and why, asking them to try and help, provide important stimuli from other sensory pathways alongside the stimuli from movement and handling.

Management of the severely head injured patient

Hypoxia causing further brain damage is an important cause of neurological deterioration. Cerebral hypoxia may be produced by: airway obstruction from inhalation of blood or vomit or head position; depression of the respiratory drive; associated chest injury, infection or pulmonary oedema; and fits.

If the patient is unable to maintain his own airway a cuffed endotracheal (ET) tube is passed. This may be sufficient to obtain adequate oxygenation and remove any retained secretions to stop any further deterioration. When it is evident that the respiratory effort is inadequate, artificial ventilation (IPPV) is required.

Chest Care Techniques of shaking and vibration are best used while the patient is being ventilated by bag squeezing, i.e. off the ventilator. Careful suction via the ET tube should clear secretions.

Chest Care of Patients with Rising/Raised ICP This deserves special mention.

The brain is able to compensate to some degree while its structures are being distorted and displaced. The compensatory mechanisms will eventually reach a level where a small rise in intracranial volume may cause a dramatic rise in ICP (Fig. 19/1). This rise may well be precipitated by various procedures such as postural drainage, shaking, bag squeezing, prolonged suction and coughing.

It is important to keep the chest clear of secretions as patchy collapse with sub-clinical hypoxia and hypercarbia is probably more damaging to the brain than any other factor. Therefore, it is important that if the stage of decompensation is being reached the patient must be protected during chest physiotherapy; effective treatment can be carried out without provoking large increases in ICP. This can be achieved by sedation, analgesia and muscle paralysis.

Patients having controlled IPPV usually need continuous sedation

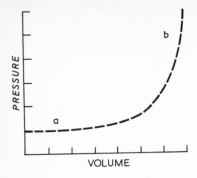

Fig. 19.1 The relationship between a small *volume* rise and the resultant dramatic pressure rise: a = stage of compensation; b = stage of decompensation

using anaesthetic agents and analgesics. A bolus dose of sedation is given prior to physiotherapy and, once stable conditions have been established, the techniques mentioned previously are employed and the ICP recording observed for significant changes. Total treatment time is a crucial factor and should be kept to a minimum, shorter sessions, more often, being preferable. Suction, in particular, is a relatively dangerous procedure because of its effect on ICP (Garradd and Bullock, 1986).

There are other indications for the use of IPPV including repeated fitting, spontaneous hyperventilation, cyanosis and under-ventilation and associated pathology, e.g. chest injury. An acute head injury requiring significant intracranial operative procedures may need a period of ventilation after surgery.

The duration of controlled IPPV is 12–24 hours in patients ventilated purely because of intracranial operative procedures and in those who show signs of rapid improvement. For the majority, two to three days of controlled IPPV is indicated while in those with signs of advanced intracranial compression a much longer period of ventilation may be implemented.

LATER MANAGEMENT AND COMPLICATIONS

The variety of physical problems evident after head injury may present in combination with sensory and emotional features.

Physical and motor problems include spasticity and rigidity, and ataxia. Sensory disturbance will involve perceptual problems including vision and hearing, apraxia and agnosia. Emotional and intellectual disturbance will involve memory and behavioural disorders.

Unless there are reasons to delay the start of an active rehabilitation programme (e.g. associated injuries such as limb fractures, chest injuries) patients should be introduced to changes of position out of bed and movement early on. Aim for normal sitting posture, avoiding tipping chairs.

The tilt table can be used for periods of standing in the very early stages in conjunction with standing with necessary assistance and standing transfers. Lack of head control can impede progress to activities in sitting and standing.

The gymnastic ball has specific qualities which can be used to gain mobility, stability and postural control. Increased tone in the lower limbs that requires more than manual techniques to inhibit and maintain range of movement may benefit from the application of below-knee weight-bearing plasters. This is a skilled task and care must be taken to obtain correct alignment of foot and ankle.

There is a role, too, for the physiotherapist in the re-education and facilitation of normal swallowing mechanisms working alongside the speech therapist.

Vigorous management of patients in the acute stage will be of little value if proper and adequate rehabilitation is not undertaken following the initial recovery. Rehabilitation is a team effort and co-operation among all disciplines can only lead to improved care and the best possible outcome for the patient.

REFERENCES

Garradd, J. and Bullock, M. (1986). The effect of respiratory therapy on intracranial pressure in ventilated neurosurgical patients. *Australian Journal of Physiotherapy*, **32**, 2, 107.

Jennett, B. and Bond, M. (1975). Assessment of outcome after severe brain damage. *Lancet*, **1**, 480.

BIBLIOGRAPHY

Camkin, T. V. and Turner, J. M. (1986). *Neurosurgical Anaesthesia and Intensive Care*, 2nd edition. Butterworths, London.

Evans, C. D. (ed.) (1981). *Rehabilitation after Severe Head Injury*. Churchill Livingstone, Edinburgh.

Fussey, I. and Giles, G. M. (eds) (1988). *Rehabilitation of the Severely Brain Injured Adult: A Practical Approach*. Croom Helm, London.

Hugo, M. (1987). Alleviating the effects of care on the intracranial pressure (ICP) of head injured patients by manipulating nursing care activities. *Intensive Care Nursing*, **3**, 78.

Jennett, B. (1976). Resource allocation to the severely brain damaged. *Archives of Neurology*, **33**, 595.

Jennett, B., Snoek, J., Bond, M. and Brooks, N. (1981). Disability after severe head injury: observations on the use of the Glasgow Outcome Scale. *Journal of Neurology, Neurosurgery and Psychiatry*, **44**, 285.

Jennett, B. and Teasdale, G. (1981). *Management of Head Injury*. (Contemporary Neurology Series.) F. A. Davis Co, Philadelphia, USA.

Parsons, L. C. and Shogan, J. S. O. (1984). The effects of the endotracheal tube functioning/manual hyperventilation procedures on patients with severe closed head injuries. *Heart and Lung*, **13**, 4, 372.

Shalit, M. N. and Umansky, F. (1977). Effect of routine bedside procedures on intracranial pressure. *Israel Journal of Medical Science*, **13**, 9, 881.

ACKNOWLEDGEMENT

The author expresses her thanks to Dr J. H. Kerr DM, FFARCS, consultant anaesthetist, the Radcliffe Infirmary, Oxford, for his help and advice in the revising of this chapter.

Chapter 20

Introduction to Paediatrics

by C. BUNGAY MCSP

Working with children is exciting, challenging and enriching. Therapists entering this field of physiotherapy will need to be prepared to adapt the techniques that they have learned in relationship to adults to the ever-changing needs of the growing child. The physiotherapist will inevitably work within the context of the child and his family and have opportunity to work with that child in a range of situations extending into home, pre-school groups, education and leisure activities. Because of the complex needs of the total child and his family, the physiotherapist may work with many other disciplines including medical, nursing, social work, educational and care staff, psychological and psychiatric teams as well as speech and occupational therapists. To work effectively and efficiently the paediatric therapist must, in addition to her physiotherapy skills, have a clear understanding of the developmental processes of childhood, the range of provision that is available to all children and the network of support that is available to families with sick or disabled children.

It is clear from the list above that the number of people who could make a contribution to a child's treatment and management is considerable; to make the best use of these resources and reduce confusion to the recipient families it is essential that the workers involved work in a co-ordinated manner. In many areas and under different groupings people work in teams, sharing skills and planning the input to the individual child and family. The physiotherapist working in such teams must be able to communicate her observations, assessments and treatment plans to the child, his parents and other members of the team. She must know how and when she can directly contribute to the child's treatment and when it would be more appropriate to share her knowledge, skills and techniques with another worker. She may in turn be able to learn skills from other team members and broaden her range of working practice.

WHAT IS CHILDHOOD? (Fig. 20/1)

Childhood may be described as the journey from the total dependency of the new-born infant to the mature young adult who is able
to function as an independent person within the society in which he
lives. There are numerous parameters to this development includ_ng
motor, cognitive, linguistic, emotional and psycho-social areas.
Illness, deprivation or disability may profoundly disrupt these
processes.

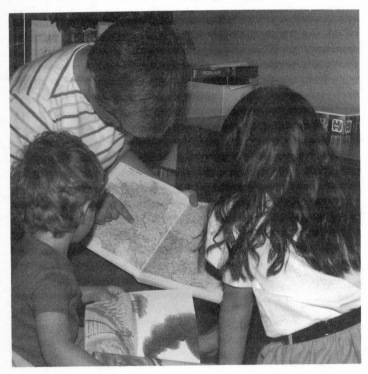

Fig. 20.1 What is childhood?

A child is not a miniature adult. He has different emotional and
physical needs at every phase of his maturation. This is easy to
recognize when thinking of the different needs of a neonate and a
baby of six months, but more subtle when thinking about the
differences between, for example, a two- and three-year-old. The
growth in the level of understanding and concentration alone
between these two ages is enormous. The therapist who expects

active co-operation and attention to a treatment schedule for 30 minutes with a boisterous two-year-old will be sadly disillusioned. The child will be angry, frustrated and bored. The chances of that family returning for treatment, however important, are very low! It is essential that therapists learn to appreciate the subtly changing needs of the developing child and accept the challenge of working with him in a way that is appropriate and relevant.

Children relate to treatment in ways that are, at least on face value, different from adults. They take time to establish trust in the person working with them and confidence in their new surroundings. Communication with the child is likely to be more honest and less inhibited by the 'risk of upsetting the therapist'. If Mr Smith doesn't see the point of an activity he is likely to work on at least for a while 'because the therapist must know best'. Not so little Johnny. He will either cry with frustration or simply say 'No'! The wise therapist will plan her treatment so that whatever her long-term objectives there are short-term goals that Johnny will understand and feel are rewarding. Sometimes these rewards may not relate directly to his treatment. They may be a promised game or activity to follow a treatment session. The time scale must be one that is within the understanding of the child and the reward consistent and reliable. It should also be remembered that parents need rewards as well as their children. They too need attainable goals and constant feedback as to how they are achieving these.

Family life (Fig. 20/2)

All children need to grow within the nurturing care of a family of their own. They need to establish a warm, reliable and caring bond with parent figures. Most commonly this is within the family unit at home. The classic model will consist of mother, father and siblings living within the family home. At varying distances and with differing levels of involvement there may be grandparents, aunties, uncles, cousins and close friends. This latter group is sometimes referred to as the 'extended family'. The child who is the patient functions within this network. His needs must be balanced with the needs of the whole. If a child is sick or more permanently disabled, it is very natural that the parents' concern rests with the most vulnerable member of the family. It is important that therapists, as part of the team caring for the child, help the parents to maintain a view of the whole family and their needs. Siblings in particular may in their turn become very vulnerable. They too are growing up, in this case alongside their sick or disabled sibling. They may be too young to understand what this is about, but they will be fully aware of the lack of available time and energy to meet their own needs. They may even feel that attention is being withdrawn as a punishment. When working with the family it is important to enable the parents, siblings and extended family to participate in the treatment and rehabilitation of the child. It is however important that the 'patient' takes his place *within* the family and is not always the focus of attention.

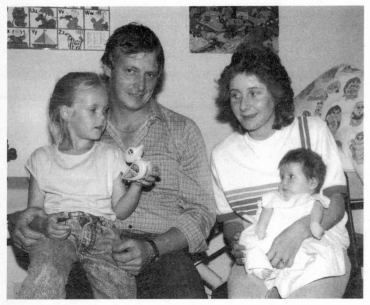

Fig. 20.2 Family life

Growing up

Before looking at child development in some detail, let us consider the background in which this is happening.

Each family unit functions within a society reflecting ethnic, religious and social influences. Any physiotherapist must be aware of the cultural setting of her patient in order to rehabilitate him fully to 'his world'. When working with a family with a young child it is imperative that the therapist is sensitive to the family background and its influences on child rearing. Therapists may quite inadvertently cause considerable difficulty and offence if they assume that their own child rearing experience is 'the norm' whether that is based on their experience of rearing their own children or the more distant memories of their own childhood. Many therapists work within multicultural societies and the breadth of their experience can be greatly enriched by taking time and using energy to discover more about their patients' family life. In some groups the expectations of boys are much greater than girls and considerably increase the families' anxieties if a boy is sick. In others the possibility of a good marriage is jeopardized if a girl has a visible physical impairment. It may be unacceptable for a woman to travel alone with a man who is unknown to the family, hence the breakdown of many well-planned transport arrangements. Maximum use of translators, link workers and racial awareness courses will lead to an enriched and harmonious working in many inner city areas.

Sadly not all family life is harmonious. Bringing up a family demands many personal and financial resources. The additional responsibility of a sick or disabled member of any household can tip balances that were previously frail. Stresses within family life can manifest themselves in many ways. Neglect of the children's fundamental needs of food, warmth and safety, an inability to provide adequate parenting and stimulation and possibly physical and sexual abuse are but a few of the manifestations of difficulties within a family.

Children growing up within a stressed household are particularly vulnerable. They are unable to run out of the home. They may have considerable ambivalence about the risk of disclosing their distress because, however unhappy they are, home is the place they know best. The child will have established an important bond with his parents even if at times he finds it difficult to make sense of his parents' behaviour towards him. Parents rarely consciously wish to harm their child. Therapists working with families must be vigilant. The physiotherapist in particular may have a regular need to undress a child to perform her treatment. This inevitably gives opportunity to assess how the parent and child respond to this request. A parent who is reluctant to undress a child may or may not be concerned that he or she has something to hide. The therapist should not immediately make assumptions of abuse. The parent may be well aware that the child is at a stage where he will be frightened at parting with his clothes in a strange place at an inappropriate time of day. The parent may know that the child will willingly *part* with his clothes but anticipate an embarrassing tantrum when he comes to getting dressed again. All of this is stage-appropriate behaviour. However, *the therapist should be concerned if* the child has bruises which cannot be explained by ordinary day-to-day bumps especially if they are to the face or trunk or if they demonstrate a characteristic row of fingerprints; if the child has unexplained burns especially small round cigarette-shape burns; or if the child is excessively preoccupied by, or defensive of, the genital areas. *The therapist should not act on her own if she has any cause for anxiety about the well-being of the child.* She should alert a senior member of her team or of the relevant social service team as soon as possible. She should be careful to report facts and not opinions. Sensitive exploration of these anxieties should then follow which frequently results in an innocent explanation. In the situation where abuse is taking place it is important that the therapist is supportive to the child, his family and any other agencies involved. Social services have a statutory responsibility to act in the best interest of the child. On rare occasions this may result in the removal of the child from the parental home for a period and seem to be to the detriment of the parents. Therapists who have worked with a family before such an incident may find this conflict of needs very difficult to come to terms with and should seek help from their teams in working through this.

Provisions for children and parents

Under various statutes the health authority, social services and education department have a duty to provide certain resources. Within these boundaries it is at the discretion of the local bodies of these authorities to interpret how they will make their provision. There are local and regional variations and the therapist will need to be conversant with her local arrangements.

Health Care　The development of neonatal intensive care support units is a priority area. Hospital in- and outpatient facilities are provided for children and should be in separate areas and at different times from adult wards and clinics.

Child health clinics and/or GP practices provide the basis of developmental screening and immunization programmes.

Health visitors have particular expertise in infant and child care, and a responsibility for visiting all under-fives at home.

There is a school health service.

Education　It is the duty of every local educational authority (LEA) to provide a place for children at a suitable school, or otherwise, for all children aged 5–16 living in their area.

It is the duty of all parents of school-age children to ensure that they receive efficient full-time education suitable to their age, ability and aptitude by regular attendance at school or otherwise.

Children with special education needs have a detailed statement prepared describing their strengths, weaknesses and needs. Parents and professionals contribute to this statement. The local panel then decides how and where these needs may be met and a place is offered to the child. The provision should be in mainstream school unless the child's needs require facilities or resources that cannot be achieved within a mainstream school, e.g. single-level access.

Nursery classes are provided in some schools for children aged three to five. Most of these are for half-days only.

Occasionally a home teacher may be provided for several hours a week for a child who is unable to leave his own home.

Social Services Under the Local Authority Social Services Act 1970 there are a wide range of services for children and families. Among these are responsibilities to:
- supervise children placed in private day-nurseries, playgroups and childminding services.
- consider the provision of day-nurseries, playgroups and child-minding services by the local authority.
- to take action to prevent the need for children to be received into care.
- to receive children into care whose parents under clearly defined circumstances are unable to care for them (Children and Young Persons Act 1969).
- to supervise children placed for adoption.
- to supervise children who live apart from their parents in private foster homes.

Optional Provisions for Children and Parents Many mothers-to-be meet on a regular basis and form mutual support groups. Sometimes these are informal and others come under the guidance of organizations such as the National Childbirth Trust. These groups provide social contact and practical advice and support for families preparing for the new experience of parenthood. Many continue to meet after the baby is born and well on into his pre-school life.

Local health clinics may offer the facility of mother and toddler clubs for mothers and their infants and toddlers to meet and the children to have their first opportunity to play and experience social contact outside the home.

Pre-school playgroups offer valuable play experience for children from about three to five. They are run on a local basis, usually on a sessional basis with children usually attending upwards of two half-days a week. Parents may be asked to help supervise some sessions on a rota basis. While a charge is made to cover the running of the group, this is variable and help can usually be found for families experiencing difficulties in meeting this cost.

Private nursery schools offer pre-school education for young children. They may be more formal in their approach than play-groups. There is a termly or yearly fee.

Opportunity groups are active in many areas and offer play facilities for disabled and/or disadvantaged children and their able-bodied siblings. Many offer considerable support to parents and may have professional input from various therapies.

Many voluntary groups exist to help families with a disabled child: the National Children's Bureau publishes a booklet entitled *Help Starts Here* which describes a large number of these groups. Your local library should have a list of local groups. National organizations, e.g. Contact a Family, Mencap and the Spastics Society provide newsletters, visitors and activities for families with special needs.

THE DEVELOPMENT OF THE CHILD

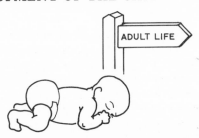

So far consideration has been given to the background and environment in which a child grows up. Now let us consider the processes that are taking place within the child.

As physiotherapists the most obvious area of interest is in the development of movement – motor development. But the child is a whole and integrated being and it is not possible to think about motor development in isolation from other parameters. Physiotherapists treating children must have a working knowledge of the cognitive, language and social skills that the child acquires. She cannot fail to become fascinated by the interrelationship of these skills and their dependence each upon the other.

The development from the total dependency of the infant to the independence of the mature adult is like a journey. As with any journey it is important to know when we are 'on-course'; so with child development. For convenience, those who are concerned with monitoring development have identified significant milestones which act as measures along the course. These include smiling, sitting, crawling, standing, walking, stair climbing and riding a tricycle.

Milestones are useful, identifiable measures. They may not represent the most useful and significant skills. Movement is a dynamic process and to be functional requires an interlinking of subskills such as rolling, balance and gradation of effort. Controlled, efficient and effective movement requires a harmonious sequencing and interplay of many isolated, individual motor skills. There is no absolute normal for a child's development. Children will proceed along various courses at a variety of paces. It is helpful to look at a range of activities that develop within certain average age bands. It should be remembered that any norm is arrived at from an average which spans wide extremes: for example, the norm for independent walking is 14 months, but some babies achieve this before nine months and others not until after 18 months. All fall within the normal range.

At birth

The new-born infant may, at first glance, appear to be totally dependent and lack any intrinsic motor abilities. Careful observation reveals more. Some activity occurs in predetermined and predictable patterns often described as *primitive reflex patterns*. Many of these behaviours are essential for the maintenance of life. Other activity is less stereotyped and there is clearly a voluntary element within it.

Typically the infant is happiest cradled within a parent's arms, often wrapped in a shawl. The baby becomes less settled if placed supine on a flat surface and may exhibit frequent, small *startle reactions*. The baby remains flexed into a fetal posture and has inadequate extension to enable him to 'balance' using the support of a flat surface. He will tend to 'roll' off his back and towards one side. His head will turn predominantly to one side although he has the ability to turn his head to either side. This is referred to as a *preferred head turn*. He will rarely lie with his head in mid-line. Placed on his tummy he will remain flexed, resting on his knees with his elbows tucked under his chest. He will automatically turn his face to one side or the other.

The need to suckle to sustain life is innate, although the processes of establishing efficient breast or bottle feeding may take a little while for mother and baby to achieve. Fundamental reflex activity underpins this behaviour in the infant, e.g. the *rooting reflex* whereby, if the infant's cheek is gently stroked, he will turn his head in search of the stimulus and attempt to suckle. Periods of wakefulness are erratic and not clearly defined in the neonate, but during such a period the careful observer may see the infant fix his gaze on his mother's face and watch intently as she talks to him. He is as yet unable to co-ordinate the visual tracking needed to follow her moving face. The hands are held predominantly fisted with the thumb adducted across the palm. The *grasp reflex* is present, i.e. if an adult places his finger within the hand of the infant and applies very gentle traction to the finger the infant will respond by firmly grasping the adult finger. The strength of this grasp is frequently adequate to raise the infant from the supporting surface.

0–3 Months

During this period the infant is establishing postural stability in supine and prone. This postural security is exhibited in an increasing ease of handling. He requires less support as he is lifted and carried. The postural flexion is gradually diminishing and his pelvis lies flatter on the supporting surface in both prone and supine. On his tummy, once he is able to lie flat and fix his pelvis, he has the stability to start raising his head. On his back he increases his ability to use the flat surface for support, and movements of all four limbs become more fluent and controlled. He gradually keeps his head in mid-line for longer periods. Early visual attention is focused on faces as they move very close to the baby's face. By two months most infants will follow a bright object, dangled at nine inches from their face, through a horizontal arc of 90°. In prone he will raise his head briefly to about 45°. By three months he will raise his head from prone to 60° for minutes at a time, watching with great curiosity. In supine he will follow freely through full range (160°–180°), both horizontally and vertically. Kicking has developed through a stage of symmetrical kicking where both legs move in unison, to the possibility of both symmetrical or reciprocal kicking. Head control is developing from simply balancing the head for a few seconds, through some stability of shoulder girdle to control of the upper trunk, shoulder girdle and head. The baby needs to be firmly supported around the chest when held in sitting. The hands are now open most of the time. Grasp is still partially reflex wherein the baby will firmly grasp an object placed in contact with his palm. This is a remnant of the *grasp reflex*. Grasp will fade out after a moment or two and the object falls. True release of an object is a complex motor behaviour and is not established for many months yet. The three-month baby is physically active most of his waking time.

3–6 Months

During this period the baby discovers and explores the mid-line of his body and starts to acquire the skill to change his position by rolling, pivoting and squirming. An immense variety of movements and combinations of movements start to emerge. Placed in supine his head is mostly in mid-line. He is able to take both hands to his mouth, engage his hands in mid-line and manipulate small light rattles with increasing dexterity. Early in this period his grasp is a *clutch grasp* involving mainly the ulnar aspect of the hand. He plucks at his clothes and blanket. He will attempt to reach out to an attractive toy. Once grasped, toys are held for minutes at a time and frequently taken to the mouth for exploration. At the latter end of this age period he will reach and grasp a toy with ease. Grasp now involves the three fingers on the ulnar side of the hand, as yet the thumb and index finger are rarely involved in manipulation. He now enjoys banging and waving toys.

He gradually acquires new skills in prone. First, he learns to raise his head to 90°; he sustains this posture for longer and longer periods. He then starts to take weight through his arms, initially through flexed elbows, then through extended arms and by the end of this stage he is learning to transfer weight from one arm to the other in preparation for creeping and crawling. The ability to take weight through his arms is also developing when he is placed and supported in the sitting position. His balance control is extending down from his head and upper trunk and the supporting hands of an adult may be moved down to his pelvis. By the end of this period he will be starting to prop his weight a little on his arms. At six months he can reliably prop his weight forwards, between his legs.

He may be starting to roll from prone to supine and on to either side. Some babies will be able to roll from supine to prone and/or move around in circles on the spot in prone, i.e. pivoting. Six-month-old babies are active, inquisitive and gaining a high degree of control of their bodies and some control of their immediate environment.

6–12 Months

It is within this period that most babies become mobile. At the beginning of this period they may be rolling and pivoting. Some will

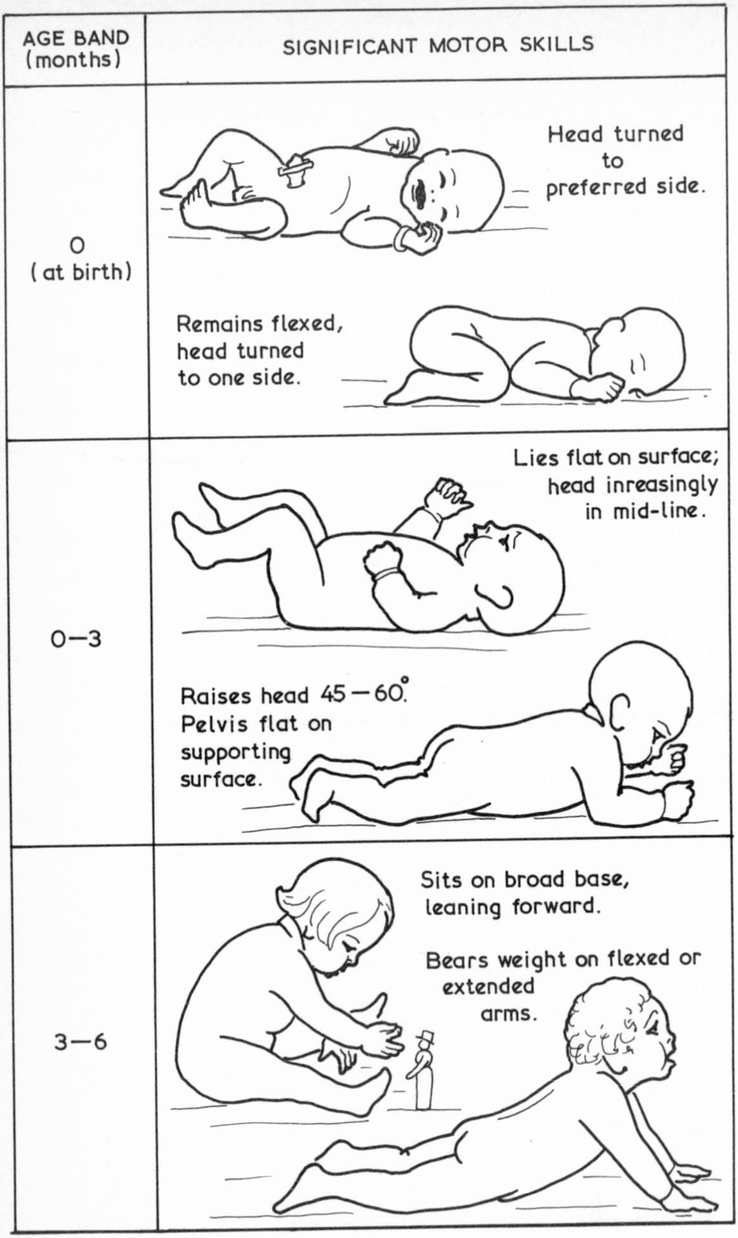

AGE BAND (months)	SIGNIFICANT MOTOR SKILLS
0 (at birth)	Head turned to preferred side. Remains flexed, head turned to one side.
0—3	Lies flat on surface; head inreasingly in mid-line. Raises head 45—60°. Pelvis flat on supporting surface.
3—6	Sits on broad base, leaning forward. Bears weight on flexed or extended arms.

Fig. 20.4 Milestones of motor skills development

AGE BAND (months)	SIGNIFICANT MOTOR SKILLS
6—12	Stands, holding on to furniture. Becomes mobile — crawling or shuffling.
12—24	Walks, using a wide base — arms raised to aid balance. Drops from and rises to standing in a variety of ways — eg 'bear position'. Uses variety of positions for play including semi-squatting. Runs, kicks ball; changes direction fluently.

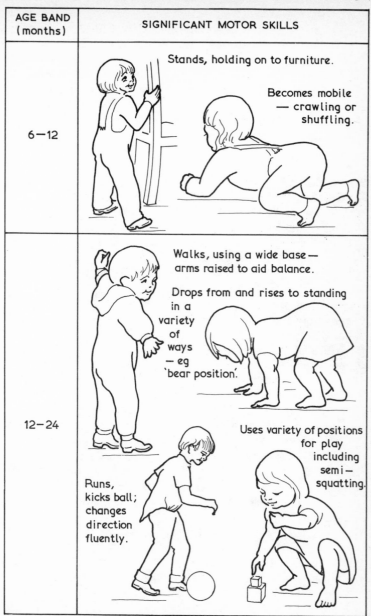

progress through commando creeping to crawling to pulling up to standing through kneeling. Others will develop through sitting, to pivoting in sitting to hitching to bottom shuffling to standing. Generally speaking children who take the bottom shuffling route will stand somewhat later than those who crawl. Once standing is achieved the baby will learn to transfer weight from one leg to the other, then cruise sideways around furniture and subsequently walk independently. Some children learn to push a toy on wheels to aid their stability, others learn to cruise across wider and wider gaps between furniture. Others yet may not take their first independent steps until they can safely rise to standing in free space (without the support of people or furniture). Many children use a combination of several of the above routes.

While this drive towards walking continues other skills are developing. The precarious sitting of the six-month-old evolves into a versatile dynamic skill through which the year-old child can get into and out of the sitting position from prone, supine kneeling and standing. Saving reactions become brisker, more varied and reliable. By around nine months the baby can reliably save himself sideways and at about a year he will be able to place his hands out backwards to save himself from toppling over. Many twisting, turning and rotational behaviours emerge, enabling the baby to link his move-ment skills of sitting and standing. Grasp and manipulation are developing fast. At the start of the period his grasp is crude and mainly palmar. He obtains objects by scooping them up using the ulnar side of his hand rather like a small shovel. He will handle objects of a variety of shapes, sizes, textures and weights, and transfer objects hand to hand and hand to mouth. He can vary his grasp and manipulation between banging toys and flicking them with his fingers to explore. There develops more involvement of the radial side of the hand, starting with the base of the thumb until by one year the baby has developed a pincer grasp in which he opposes the tip of his index finger and thumb and can approach small objects with increasing precision. His grasp is becoming more economical and he uses only enough movement for the task in hand. He is able to grade his motor activity alongside an increasing ability to estimate the size, weight and consistency of objects. Release of objects is emerging but remains crude, often relying on the added momentum of tossing the toy, knocking it against the side of a container or placing it into the accommodation hand of an adult. During this period baby is learning more about himself, his environment and the relationship between the two. He uses his freedom of movement to explore and discover. He is also becoming physically independent of his caring adults in respect of moving, doing and changing his own situation.

1–2 Years

By now the infant is rapidly becoming an active toddler. He can move freely by his chosen method and has an increasing control over the world around him. He will initially walk on a wide stable base using a somewhat rigid waddle. He will learn to drop from standing to crawling or sitting and rise up again in a variety of ways. He will need the ability to get into and out of standing without the aid of something to pull up on in order to become a truly independent walker. He is learning to climb stairs in a semi-crawling position. He may get stranded at the top for a while before he learns to descend safely on his tummy (feet first) or hitch down on his bottom. Now that balance is well developed his hands may be freed to acquire new and more refined dexterity.

He places objects into simple containers, rings on to posts and builds a tower of two cubes. Release of objects is now deliberate and precise. He often enjoys looking at books, turning the pages or walking around with one tucked under his arm. By the second half of this second year of life he will acquire the ability to climb up stairs placing two feet on each step. He will gradually use a narrower base for walking as his balance improves. He will run and change direction, push, pull and manoeuvre a variety of large objects, e.g. trucks, boxes and furniture. He adopts a range of positions in which he can play, including floor sitting, sitting on a chair, side sitting, standing, squatting and kneeling. He will start to paddle along on a ride-astride toy. He is starting to jump, lifting two feet together. By two years he will be almost independent (if a little messy) when feeding himself with a spoon. He will manipulate objects within his hand and start to construct in-set jigsaws and large Lego-type bricks.

The two-year-old child is emerging from toddlerhood to his pre-school years. He is equipped with a range of gross and fine motor skills which will form the foundation of his further movement development. Handwriting demands the ability to modify grasp and manipulate objects within the hand; football demands the ability to stand on one leg and to transfer from one position to another with speed and precision; riding a bicycle demands an integration of powerful leg movement and rapidly and efficiently adaptable balance. The first two years are crucial to the motor development of the child.

BIBLIOGRAPHY

Gassier, J. (1985). *A Guide to the Psycho-motor Development of the Child*. Churchill Livingstone, Edinburgh.

Gesell, A. (1971). *The First Five Years of Life: A Guide to the Study of the Pre-school Child*. Methuen, London.

Leach, P. (1980). *Baby and Child*. Penguin Books, Harmondsworth.

Matterson, E. M. (1970). *Play with a Purpose for Under Sevens*. Penguin Books, Harmondsworth.

Sheridan, M. (1975). *Children's Developmental Progress from Birth to Five Years: The Stycar Sequences*, 2nd edition. NFER Publishing Company, Windsor.

Sheridan, M. (1977). *Spontaneous Play in Early Childhood – Birth to Six Years*. NFER Publishing Company, Windsor.

Chapter 21

Paediatric Illness and Disability

by C. BUNGAY MCSP

Illness can be defined as 'a state of body or mind which interrupts the functioning of normal life'. In this chapter injury will be included with illness; a distinction between illness and disability will be made on the basis of duration. *Illness* will be regarded as a circumscribed event that is transient and reversible; *disability* as a state of body or mind which jeopardizes full functioning throughout a significant formative stage or the remainder of that person's life. Clearly it is not always possible to make firm distinctions between these two areas.

ILLNESS

If the imposition of illness is related to the developing child it becomes apparent that one is dealing with two parallel processes; the illness itself and the interruption of the child's innate development. The stage at which illness occurs has a greater or lesser impact, e.g. the toddler who is sick enough to require a stay in hospital is far more vulnerable to the change of environment and care-givers than the articulate seven-year-old; the one-year-old who is taken off his feet because of a fractured femur will miss out on many more stage appropriate experiences than the 10-year-old confined to bed for a similar period. Particular problems may arise if an infant or neonate requires in-patient medical support because this can inhibit the close relationship that should be forming between mother and child.

All health workers should foster a sensitive awareness of the needs of parents and children at each stage of a child's maturation and be prepared to modify and adapt their approach to treatments so as to minimize any frightening or damaging effects that they may have on the whole child. Parents will be worried if their child appears to regress in behaviour or skill level and may need reassurance that this is quite usual, and that with confident consistent handling their child will gradually return to his former self and continue to make progress. This fear is frequently more exaggerated in the parents of a child who has an intercurrent illness superimposed on an underlying development disability. Many of the child's attainments will have been hard earned and slowly gained. It is not surprising that the parents react strongly to any regression. Such parents will need consistent reassurance from all members of the medical team.

The family and the child's treatment

Any parent who is distressed or anxious will seek ways of expressing his/her fears and frustrations. Sometimes this will take the form of anger with the medical team caring for the child, appearing to be constantly criticizing hospital staff and 'getting in the way of proper treatment'.

Occasionally, parents may withdraw and become passive. Before criticizing them, just stop for a moment and think how their role as parents changes when the child is ill. Normally they are in control of the family; they make the decisions, decide what, when and how things are to be done. Suddenly, along with their anxiety about their sick child, they are no longer in the 'driving seat' – doctors, nurses, therapists and others are taking over and they are in danger of being excluded. We all react when we are in danger – some of us fight, some of us flee. Parents under threat are no different. The role of the parents should not be undermined, for they do know their child in a way that none of the medical team can. Parents can and should be partners in their child's treatment.

Visiting or residence should be encouraged and parents should be included and involved with any physiotherapy treatment given. Parents should not be asked to leave the room just because unpleasant processes such as suction are being used with their child. That is the moment when the child needs the support and comfort of his most trusted family and the parents need to be enabled to help him. They should, however, be given clear, reasoned and accurate explanations about treatment and they should understand how they can help and what is expected of them. Parents should be told what will be done to their child, what he will feel, how long it will last and how this will help him. If a parent is not able to participate in the treatment session, or the older more mature child elects that parents should be excluded, time should be allowed within the treatment session to explain to the parents what has been done and how they can assist. This is not an optional extra but an integral part of any good treatment.

Communication with parents

Thoughtful planning may considerably influence the effectiveness of conveying information to the parents. Research related to patients attending doctors' clinics, shows that only a small proportion of what is said is retained immediately after a patient leaves the consulting room. Even allowing for the fact that physiotherapy sessions are longer and less formal it is reasonable to assume that the spoken word needs reinforcement. There are a number of strategies for doing this. The therapist can *model* the activity by showing the parents how to perform it. She can give the parents the opportunity to experience the *feel* of a movement that she is trying to encourage by enabling them to have hands on during the treatment. The therapist can make it a priority that the parents themselves *practice* within the treatment session by carrying out the exercises with their child. She can provide *written* instructions or individual pro-grammes. Care should be taken not to lapse into technical shorthand and to use clear concise language and pictures and diagrams to convey meaning. When a technique is frequently repeated it may be

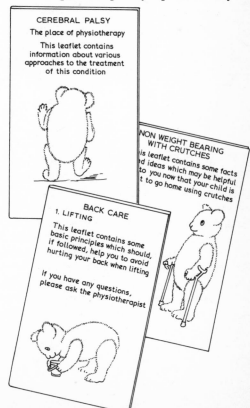

CEREBRAL PALSY

The place of physiotherapy

This leaflet contains information about various approaches to the treatment of this condition

NON WEIGHT BEARING WITH CRUTCHES

is leaflet contains some facts d ideas which may be helpful to you now that your child is t to go home using crutches

BACK CARE
1. LIFTING

This leaflet contains some basic principles which should, if followed, help you to avoid hurting your back when lifting

If you have any questions, please ask the physiotherapist

Fig. 21.1 Written
information for parents

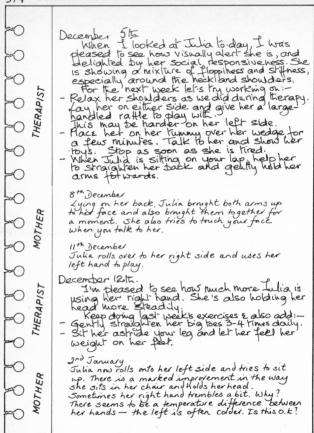

THERAPIST

December 5th
When I looked at Julia to-day, I was
pleased to see how visually alert she is, and
delighted by her social responsiveness. She
is showing a mixture of floppiness and stiffness,
especially around the neck and shoulders.
For the next week let's try working on:-
- Relax her shoulders as we did during therapy.
Lay her on either side and give her a large-
handled rattle to play with.
This may be harder on her left side.
- Place her on her tummy over her wedge for
a few minutes. Talk to her and show her
toys. Stop as soon as she is tired.
- When Julia is sitting on your lap, help her
to straighten her back and gently hold her
arms forwards.

MOTHER

8th December
Lying on her back, Julia brought both arms up
to her face and also brought them together for
a moment. She also tries to touch your face
when you talk to her.

11th December
Julia rolls over to her right side and uses her
left hand to play.

THERAPIST

December 12th.
I'm pleased to see how much more Julia is
using her right hand. She's also holding her
head more steadily.
Keep doing last week's exercises & also add:-
- Gently straighten her big toes 3-4 times daily.
- Sit her astride your leg and let her feel her
weight on her feet.

MOTHER

2nd January
Julia now rolls onto her left side and tries to sit
up. There is a marked improvement in the way
she sits in her chair and holds her head.
Sometimes her right hand trembles a bit. Why?
There seems to be a temperature difference between
her hands — the left is often colder. Is this o.k?

Fig. 21.2 An extract from a family's therapy diary

worth considering producing a hand-out or leaflet that can become
the basis of communication (Fig. 21/1). Material should be
presented in an attractive way, if possible on coloured paper so that
it makes a greater impact. Where there are language problems help
should be sought in getting translations of written material and, if
possible, a translator should assist in some treatment sessions.
Working with and through a translator requires care, and the therapist must ensure the accuracy of what is being translated and keep
her communication free of ambiguities which may become magnified
across the language barrier. By definition, communication is a two-
way process.

Parents should be allowed the opportunity to communicate with
the therapist. Thought should be given as to whether the child

should be exposed to all of this communication. There may be instances where the parent wishes to express fears or anxieties that it would not be appropriate for the child to hear. The therapist may need to be resourceful and create a situation where the child can continue to play safely for a few moments while she takes the parents discreetly aside to give them the freedom to talk. If the child is too young or insecure to be left playing alone it may be necessary to use another person to distract the child. If neither of these work it could be useful to encourage the parent to telephone at a pre-arranged time to discuss the child's treatment and progress. A *home treatment diary* (Fig. 21/2) can be an effective way of encouraging parents to feed-back information and to store-up questions. If this is used, time must be allowed within the treatment to read and discuss the contents of such a diary. Its importance should not be reduced to a few moments just as the next patient is hammering on the door.

Who is the therapist treating?

Treating a child, even for a similar condition, e.g. a knee injury, is not quite like treating an adult. It is reasonable to suppose that the adult patient can be expected to take responsibility for his own therapy, getting himself to the department, actively participating in treatment and making a commitment to continuing it at home. A child is not independent of his parents. Legally he cannot consent to his own treatment until the age of 16 years. His parents are bound to make decisions for him and see that his needs are met. Indeed if they fail to do this then they may be accused of neglect and have their parental rights removed. It follows therefore that physiotherapists have a responsibility to equip them to meet these needs; thus, there is a dual treatment obligation to the child and his parents. It is not adequate just to teach the child how to walk with his crutches, it is essential to give guidance to the parents about how to supervise him and to establish a line of communication should they feel that they are in difficulty. The wise therapist will remain vigilant as to how she is working with the parents and keep adequate informative records of instructions given to them as well as to the child.

THE TREATMENT ENVIRONMENT

It is important that patients feel comfortable and reassured by their surroundings during treatment. For children this is of enormous importance. The treatment environment starts as the child enters the waiting area; where children are seen in the same area as adults it is important that provision is made for their specific needs. Many very young children will have little experience outside their own homes. For the pre-school child the size and furnishing of rooms should be as home-like as possible. Children become anxious about large pieces of mysterious equipment which they don't understand. They are distressed by large bare rooms. The natural play environment of young children is on the floor and the treatment environment should have suitable floor coverings of washable carpet, mats or safe rugs. Toys and games for children of varying ages should be available both for reward or distraction as well as to facilitate treatment.

Much treatment will take place on the floor. Parents should be invited to join the therapist or given low chairs to sit on and not left isolated on high seats inappropriately removed from the site of activity. Frequently, siblings will accompany the patient and may need to play in the room while treatment takes place. It is important that they are made welcome and encouraged to join in the treatment where this is appropriate. They may need to take a turn at trying out what their brother or sister is doing and the therapist must use her discretion as to when this is helpful to the child or his sibling.

The wearing of formal uniform in paediatric practice is a subject of much debate to which there is no single right or wrong response. Perhaps individual units might like to ask themselves such questions as:

Why do we wear uniform?
Is it possible to maintain a professional presence without it?
Is it necessary for reasons of cleanliness or hygiene?
What effect does a uniform have on the child?
What effect does a uniform have on the parents?
What effect does a uniform have on co-workers who do not wear a
    uniform?
Does the task require a uniform or do I as a person need it?
How should I maintain my professional integrity without it?

Honest answers may help the decision-making process.

Dealing with the crying child

Just like laughter so tears are a natural part of childhood. They signal a number of emotions including anxiety, insecurity, hunger, pain, discomfort, distress and anger. They are an important mode of communication for the young child and it is not always possible or appropriate to avoid them. It is more beneficial to help a child work through his distress or anger than to suppress it for now only to return to the same frustration next session. It may be quite appropriate to continue the activity and offer support, reassurance and understanding. However, a child crying during the treatment can be as distressing and distracting to the people around as to the child itself. A calm accepting attitude can settle much anxiety. The therapist may need to remove the family discreetly to a quieter room or plan to have them at a time when they do not cause too much disturbance to the department as a whole. Causes should always be sought for the crying child, and it should never be assumed that a child will cry during treatment just because . . . . Changes of technique, time of treatment, environment or even of therapist may be necessary.

Where might treatment take place?

Treatment could take place in a number of areas, e.g. hospital ward, department or home, and for children there is an increased possibility of venues. They may include health centre, nursery group, school or recreational group if this is where the appropriate work needs to be done. A two-hour visit to work with a child's gym teacher and enlist her help, may be a better investment than half an hour twice weekly for an indefinite period in an isolated treatment environment. Many skills may be safely shared with other workers; the physiotherapist's expertise lies in identifying the child's problems, selecting and initiating suitable techniques and activities and monitoring his response to this. There are situations where other people may just as appropriately carry out the day-to-day work with the child provided they have good communication with the responsible therapist.

It is not possible to say that any one place is the best place for treatment. The basis of any decision may be made after considering questions such as:
- what techniques are needed?
- what equipment is needed?
- how much space is needed?
- are the family mobile?
- where will the child benefit most from treatment?
- what back-up services are needed?

CHILDHOOD DISABILITY

When considering childhood disability it is important to remember that one is dealing with *a child and family with a disability*. That is to say that one is working first and foremost with a child within a family who happens to have a disability or defect that may potentially become a handicap. All that is known about family life, normal development and childhood needs applies to this area of work just as it does to any other.

Disability has already been defined as a state of body or mind which jeopardizes full functioning throughout a significant developmental stage or the remainder of that person's life. This distinguishes disability from illness which runs a circumscribed course. Not all conditions fall neatly into one or the other category.

It is perhaps important to consider some of the terms that are used in relationship to the child with a disability. Unfortunately any terminology is open to abuse and for many families particular words carry with them the stigma of preconceived and often erroneous assumptions. Care should be taken in discussion with families to ascertain that they are comfortable with the terminology that is used about their child and that the medical/educational team have explained the precise meanings of the words that they are using:

- defect: a structural or physiological abnormality.
- disability: a lack or impairment of a particular capability or skill.
- handicap: a condition or set of conditions that hinder or prevent the pursuit or achievement of desired goals.

The degree of handicap that results from any defect or disability will depend on the individual child or family, their expectations, resources and ability to use appropriate adaptation and compensation. Paradoxically, a child with significant defects and major disabilities may function with the minimum of handicap, whereas a child with what appears to be minimal disability may struggle with major handicap. It is the aim of all workers in the field of childhood disability to nurture and develop the child and the family's strengths and abilities and to reduce to a minimum the effects of his defects and disabilities.

Disabling conditions may present at birth, gradually evolve over the first few years of life or occur as a result of illness or trauma at any stage throughout childhood. They may involve the impaired or inadequate development or integration of movement, language, sensory or intellectual skills. They may involve the inadequate or impaired development or functioning of any of the body's major systems, e.g. cardiovascular, respiratory, musculoskeletal, endocrine, etc. A significant number of children present with a mixture of disabilities – sensory, motor, intellectual and cardiovascular and thus will live with multiple handicaps. While the physiotherapist's main involvement is in areas of movement and respiratory disability, she may be called upon to help assess any child with any disability and assist the family with the practicalities of day-to-day life.

Congenital conditions: These are conditions that *are present* at birth. It would, however, be misleading to imply that all congenital conditions *present themselves* at birth. Some are clearly apparent, e.g. Down's syndrome, talipes and major cardiac defects. Others do not reveal themselves immediately but only become apparent as the infant or child matures, e.g. muscular dystrophy, neurofibromatosis, most cerebral palsy and many hearing and sight defects. This group includes intra-uterine infections the outcome of which may or may not be apparent at birth, e.g. cytomegalovirus, rubella and toxoplasma. Some conditions are genetically linked, e.g. muscular dystrophy, and may occur in several children within the family.

Acquired conditions: These are conditions that are acquired as a result of, for example:
illness: encephalitis, meningitis, juvenile chronic arthritis, dermatomyositis, neoplasms, malnutrition, poliomyelitis, etc.
trauma: head injury, child abuse, road traffic or playground accidents.

Diagnosis of disability

For no family is the diagnosis of disability welcome news. At whatever age the presence of a developmentally threatening condition is recognized the news will cause much pain for the parents. Their hopes and expectations for their young child will suddenly be undermined. They may even feel that they have lost the infant they thought they were nurturing and be left holding a new baby, almost a stranger whom they have yet to get to know. As with any news that shocks, this produces responses and reactions in the people that hear it. Shock may lead to fright, flight and anger before adaptation and reorientation occur. The degree of trauma that this news-breaking brings can be considerably reduced by teams developing good practices in how they work with the parents.

It is essential that information should be shared with parents at the earliest opportunity, usually by the paediatrician with another team member, e.g. social worker or therapist. The information should be concise and factual; it should, whenever possible, be given to both parents simultaneously and in a private, unhurried and friendly environment. The baby should be present at the time. Many parents are greatly reassured if the person breaking the news handles the baby, demonstrating that he or she finds the baby an 'acceptable and lovable' person. Opportunity should be given for the family to be seen very soon after the initial news-breaking and then at regular intervals so that they can start to seek answers to the many questions that will inevitably emerge as the shock subsides. Four stages of the psychic crisis which follow traumatic news have been described (Cunningham, 1982):

Phase of crisis	Presentation	Needs of the family
1. Shock	Emotional behaviour Disorganization Disbelief	Sympathy Support
2. Reaction	Expression of anger, grief, aggression, guilt and denial Search for cause or blame	Listening Honesty Facts Acceptance
3. Adaptation	Realistic appraisal	Information
4. Orientation	Search for help Planning for future	Regular advice and guidance

Adapted from Cunningham's Model of Psychic Crisis (1982)

Therapists working with the family of a recently diagnosed child will soon recognize these stages of response and become aware that their approach to treatment will need to be adapted to the stage at which the family is. Many families do not move precisely through the stages and from time to time will move back and forth among them. To be effective in her communication with the family the therapist must be adaptable in her approach and be prepared to move with the family at their pace.

After the diagnosis has been shared, the family may remain in a state of numbed shock for some time. At this stage it is important for the therapist to keep treatment simple and, if necessary, to repeat and reinforce information given to the parents. While in a state of shock people's ability to absorb and retain new information is reduced. The therapist should be sensitively directive and encouraging, generating an atmosphere of acceptance of the child as he is with realistic hopes for his future.

After the phase of shock the parents may enter one of extreme reaction. During this stage they may fluctuate between aggressive searching for the cause of their child's problem, either within the family, the pregnancy or the attendant medical care, and total denial of the child's disability and a fervent assurance to the therapist that given a little time all will be well. This can be a bewildering time for anyone working with the family, never knowing what the mood of the day will be or what will be demanded of the therapist. She must accept this as a normal phase of the necessary adaptation, listen diligently, answer honestly, and hold firmly to the facts that she knows about the child's condition. She should aim to establish an accepting rapport with the family so that they feel able to express their feelings of anger, guilt and aggression. She should not collude with the family's unrealistic suggestions but calmly interpret her own understanding of the problems.

In due course the family will be able to adapt to the new circumstances. They will be ready to make a realistic appraisal of their child, his special needs and the effect that this is going to have on family life. They will require information not only about their child, but also about other children with similar conditions; the services that are available to them now and possibly into the future; the provision of education, recreation and, perhaps, even the ultimate employment and marriage for the child. Other team members may be called upon to assist in establishing an accurate assessment of the child's abilities and difficulties; voluntary and national groups may provide information about specific conditions, social workers about local services. An introduction to an educational psychologist may be indicated so that he can explain about educational provision. The physiotherapist should be able to explain the principles by which she treats the child and acknowledge that there are several approaches to the treatment of disabled children. She should know the strengths, weaknesses and limitations of her own approach and be able to indicate to parents how and where they might explore other approaches for themselves. At this stage, parents may be susceptible to the emotive claims made by some media presentations, and this will need to be handled with considerable tact.

Not until the family has moved through the stages of shock, reaction and adaptation can they truly make any judgement or plan for the future of their family. This process takes a very variable course, often with frequent regressions and leaps forward. It is rare for a family to reach a stage of orientation in less than two years from the time of diagnosis, and not uncommon for the process to remain insecure for five or more years. At this stage the therapist is able to enter an effective working partnership with the parents. They will be able to continue a programme of treatment at home. Short-term goals should be established that are attainable. The parents may be encouraged by recording their activities and observations in a diary (see p. 374). This can be shared with the therapist during treatment sessions. The therapist may use this to make suggestions about treatment and activities to encourage. Longer-term aims and objectives should be discussed with parents, and the therapist needs to encourage parents to voice their objectives also. If the parents' expectations are clearly unrealistic, once you know what they are, you are in a stronger position to modify and re-model them. You may be able to negotiate short-term goals that lead towards the parents' desired goal thus helping the parents to learn to appreciate the sub-stages along the route.

Significant events in the child or family's life may make a family more vulnerable and cause intermittent crises. These include birthdays where progress is measured against a peer group; times when the child's development seems to plateau; the stage where the child enters a life outside the family circle, e.g. playgroup; and again as the child approaches school. Later the family may once again become less secure when there is a change of school; the onset of puberty; the approach of school leaving and when there are changes in the provision established for the adult disabled person. At these times the family will need informed communication and access to people in whom they can put their trust.

Assessment of disability

Before any treatment can be contemplated the therapist must be conversant with the child, his strengths, his weaknesses and his needs. This must be based on a firm knowledge of child development, a detailed knowledge of motor development and its relationship with other parameters of development, a knowledge of the underlying pathology if it is identifiable and an estimate of the child's present level of functioning. She must evaluate any areas of deficit or disability. She must be aware of the prognostic possibilities: Will any deficits remain the same, become more marked or go on to some degree of recovery? What is known from past experience about the condition? What are the likely parameters for the outcome acknowledging the variation of each individual? What are the family's personal resources? Are there environmental factors that may influence the child's eventual level of disability? In all of these areas:

- What will change with time and maturation?
- What can be changed by intervention?
- What is unlikely to change?
- What will need augmentation in order to give the child the optimum quality of life?

An assessment of this level may need a number of sessions to establish. It may be necessary to supplement one's 'head knowledge' with background reading and discussion with colleagues. It may be necessary to watch the evolution of a problem in a very young child before any reasonable assessment may be made. It is important to share with the parents what you are hoping to derive from these early sessions. Some therapists find it helpful to explain to the parents that she is unable to advise fully until she has a firm understanding of their child. Parents can be useful partners in the assessment process and thus their understanding of their child can be harnessed and developed. It is useful to ask the parents to help your assessment by carrying out one or two specific observations between sessions, e.g. how much of the time does he lie with his head turned to the right? Care must be taken that the task given to the parents is specific and that it is fully explained, and, more importantly, is understood, so that the resultant feedback is reliable.

Planning of treatment

The basis of any treatment plan relies on objectives, both short and long term. The establishment of long-term objectives is not always easy. In the young developing child there are additional factors such as latent intelligence, emergent personality, and level of motivation which would require nothing less than a 'crystal ball' to narrow down the extended future. It may be necessary to introduce middle-term goals. The definition of short and middle term will change with the age of the child. Middle term for an infant of two weeks may be six months, for a toddler of two years it may be one year and for a child of six it may be two or three years:

Baby Sam aged two months has Down's syndrome.

Long-term goal   – Sam will achieve maximum independence in mobility.

Middle-term goal – By 12 months Sam will have one means of independent mobility by creeping, rolling, crawling or bottom hitching.

Short-term goal   – By three months Sam will roll from his side to his back.

Josie aged six years has spina bifida.

Long-term goal   – Josie will be able to live in a warden-assisted flatlet.

Middle-term goal – By secondary school (aged 11) Josie will be independent in her dressing needs.

Short-term goal – By primary school (aged 8) Josie will be able to deal with all her outdoor clothing and able to go out to play and return to the classroom without assistance.

Having established objectives the necessary sub-stages will become apparent. The physiotherapist now needs to decide which techniques are the most useful to develop these skills. She will make an individual or institutional decision as to whether she will adhere closely to one particular approach to treatment, or whether she will use a blend of approaches deriving from an evaluation of what she finds works best in her own practice or is shown to be the most applicable to the situation by research studies. If she is confronted with a very complex problem she must know where the extent of her own knowledge and skills ends and where it may be appropriate to seek advice from a more specialist centre, refer on, or ask for help from a colleague within another discipline.

The physiotherapist will need to decide on the frequency, duration and venue of treatment. Rarely is it possible or desirable for the physiotherapist to deliver all the necessary treatment to the child. It is her function to identify the child's needs, the particular techniques and activities that will help that child and to communicate and teach these skills to the child's care-givers who will be with him for the major part of his day. The therapist should continue to monitor, revise, update, and modify the child's treatment.

Communication

To be effective communication must be two-way, a blend of listening, looking, processing and only then talking. When working with children the need for effective communication is increased because of the child's dependence on the people around him. At the very least it may be necessary to communicate with the child and his principal care-giver, usually a parent. If the child is seen by several members of a multidisciplinary team or a number of different agencies it is imperative that communication is adequate to avoid duplication, confusion and waste of resources. The most effective teams are those where a key worker evolves as the main supporter to the family. Other team members meet regularly and discuss difficulties,

Fig. 21.3 The multidisciplinary team

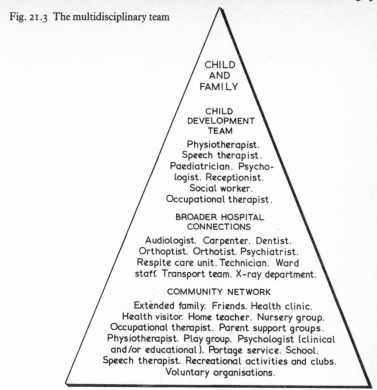

CHILD
AND
FAMILY

CHILD
DEVELOPMENT
TEAM
Physiotherapist.
Speech therapist.
Paediatrician. Psycho-
logist. Receptionist.
Social worker.
Occupational therapist.

BROADER HOSPITAL
CONNECTIONS
Audiologist. Carpenter. Dentist.
Orthoptist. Orthotist. Psychiatrist.
Respite care unit. Technician. Ward
staff. Transport team. X-ray department.

COMMUNITY NETWORK
Extended family. Friends. Health clinic.
Health visitor. Home teacher. Nursery group.
Occupational therapist. Parent support groups.
Physiotherapist. Play group. Psychologist (clinical
and/or educational). Portage service. School.
Speech therapist. Recreational activities and clubs.
Voluntary organisations.

share ideas and deliver the necessary services to the family. The number and nature of team members directly involved with the family will vary from stage to stage but should be limited to those needed by the child and family. Through the key worker the family will have access to the entire team (Fig. 21/3).

PHYSIOTHERAPY TECHNIQUES

The infant and young child

The importance of play to the child cannot be overstated. Play is the vehicle through which the child encounters, discovers, experiments and learns. It is the vessel through which he regains skills lost as a result of illness or injury, practises existing skills and learns new ones. Play is an integral part of his daily life and is an essential part of parent–child interaction. It is a valuable tool for the physiotherapist. Very few children under the age of five will work directly on an exercise programme although many can be harnessed to work gain-fully by combining treatment with play (Fig. 21/4).

Arm exercises may be combined with ball work or drawing pictures on a large sheet of paper on the wall.

Leg exercises may be combined touching well-placed objects with the toes. Any exercise may be reinforced by using an action song.

Standing may be encouraged by placing an attractive activity on a suitable height surface.

Movement may be encouraged by fetching and carrying games, e.g. shopping. Obstacle courses provide endless possibilities for the therapist and fun for the child.

The child should not be allowed to become bored. His attention span will vary with his age, stage and personality. The therapist should try to keep her activities simple and have a selection to choose from if the first one fails or fades out quickly. Most children enjoy a balance of repetition of activities which increases their security and new ones to stimulate their interest. It is advisable to have at least a consistent starting and finishing activity. Children's perceptions of time are not as established as adults' – the child needs a signal and a little time to adjust, e.g. 'This is going to be our last game today' or 'It is nearly time to finish. We shall put your shoes on when these toys are in the box.' Try to finish the treatment while the child is happy and before he is too tired; if not, all sessions will end up with a tantrum and the next session is likely to start where the last one ended. It is important to explain to parents that sometimes it may be possible to treat for only a short period within the child's tolerance. Sometimes the remainder of the session can be used to talk to the parents about what has been done and how they can continue at home.

The older child

From about the age of seven children's awareness of their own bodies has matured enough to enable them to co-operate more actively in their treatment. They have sufficient body and spatial awareness to be able to carry out simply explained exercises and activities. The therapist must remain aware that the use of complicated adult language will be confusing to the immature child. If one observes a class in a primary school one becomes aware of how frequently the child in this age-group changes position and activity. Treatment should be adapted to this pattern of behaviour; the therapist should plan a number of short activities lasting five to ten minutes. She could allow time for play as a reward between or after

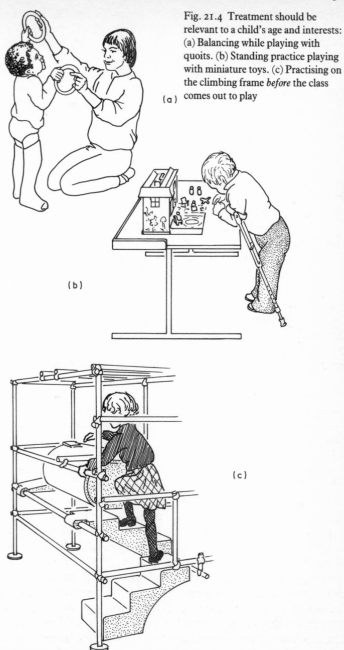

Fig. 21.4 Treatment should be relevant to a child's age and interests: (a) Balancing while playing with quoits. (b) Standing practice playing with miniature toys. (c) Practising on the climbing frame *before* the class comes out to play

therapeutic activities. She should always explain to the child what is expected of him. At this age it may be more appropriate to treat the child without the parents being present. It may take a while for him to establish confidence in the treatment setting and it is important to assure him that no invasive treatment will occur. This is especially important with children who have been referred via an accident and emergency department. Parents who are not present during treatment need to be kept informed about their child's treatment, his progress and any treatment that should be continued at home.

The adolescent

This is a group which is neither child nor adult, often fluctuating daily between the two extremes. These youngsters require special resources in those who treat them; the therapist must be prepared to respond to the fluctuations of maturation and expectation. Most adolescents will want to feel in control of their lives and the necessity to receive physiotherapy may be seen as an invasion of this independence. Where possible involve young people in the planning of treatment; invite them to set their goals under your guidance. Remember they need understandable measures of success, e.g. being able to return to disco dancing. Some adolescents may be unable to cope with their new-found independence and may attempt to establish highly dependent relationships with their therapist and resist the termination of treatment. An awareness of this risk and the setting of realistic and attainable treatment goals can help to avoid this situation.

THE USE OF EQUIPMENT

All children use some form of equipment as a part of daily life, e.g. they may use a pushchair, feeding chair or baby walker. All children have toys of some description. There is a very thin line between ordinary baby gear and therapeutic equipment.

Judicious choice of well-designed chairs, pushchairs and toys can reinforce the work of the therapist throughout the child's early life. It may be necessary to make small adaptations by the addition of cushions or larger play surfaces. As the child becomes older and larger it may become necessary to explore more specialized chairs, standing aids and toys to enable him to participate in play activities while continuing his treatment.

During the early months many babies will use a fully supporting chair or bouncing cradle seat. Some of these are designed for use as a car seat and indoor chair and are recommended from birth. They give total support at a reclined angle in order to protect the infant's spine from damage. These seats are particularly useful for the floppy infant and can in many instances contain the young baby with strong extensor spasms. A baby placed in one of these seats for planned periods each day will have an increased opportunity to watch his surroundings and they may assist the development of a mid-line awareness and early reaching and grasping.

A little later a less supporting seat may be introduced at a more upright angle. If plastic baby chairs do not offer enough support consider using a car seat with added foam cushions. It is sometimes easier to provide support from the upholstered surface of a car seat than using vinyl or plastic which tends to be slippery.

High chairs and feeder chairs enable the child that is establishing sitting balance to be safely seated for meal-times and play. Many high street models of high chair are designed to allow for growing. It is essential that the child with a musculoskeletal or developmental problem has adequate support and the seat size reduced to his dimensions. This can be achieved by adding towelling-covered foam cushions. As the child's sitting ability increases the support given can be reduced by the gradual removal of the cushions. There is an ever-increasing range of purpose-built chairs for the child with special needs, and if good functional seating cannot be achieved by modifying an 'off-the-peg chair' advice should be sought from the nearest seating clinic or specialist manufacturer.

Early mobility is likely to be in a sling attached to the parent, a pram or a pushchair. Models of all these flood the market continuously with claims for excellence, durability and prestige; the most expensive is not always the best. Therapists working with young children should help the parents (and often grandparents) not only to identify their child's needs, but also, their own needs in respect of height, weight and function, and enable them to go out and choose a pushchair to meet them. Where a child has substantial seating needs in excess of his peers the Disablement Services Authority (DSA) may help with this provision. The therapist working with the child is expected to evaluate the child's difficulties and indicate his needs, e.g. total support, modular seating system, etc.

Later, independent mobility may be aided in a number of ways. Some babies enjoy using a bouncing sling suspended from a frame or doorway. These must be placed at the correct height and used for planned periods only. For some children the use of this type of baby bouncer is ill-advised:

Very floppy children may be in danger of obstructing their airway.

Stiff children may increase the use of their extensor spasm and disrupt the development of sitting skills.

Children with learning difficulties may reinforce a tendency to perseverate a limited number of movements and fail to broaden their repertoire of experience.

For other children baby bouncers may be a useful adjunct to treatment. For the upper limb deficient child who has difficulty in establishing standing balance they can aid him through that stage; for the child who is recovering from a chest infection they can encourage activity and stimulate coughing; and used with careful planning they can provide a new experience for the learning disabled child.

Baby walkers have similar pros and cons. The judicious use of a well-chosen baby walker can enhance the developing skills of a young child. Indiscriminate use of a badly fitting or inappropriately designed walker can undo the work of child, parents and therapist.

Specialist equipment is available for children with delayed or disordered motor development (Figs 21/5, 21/6). This ranges from

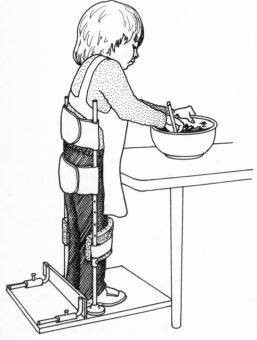

Fig. 21.5 The place of equipment in daily life: standing frame aids participation in cake making

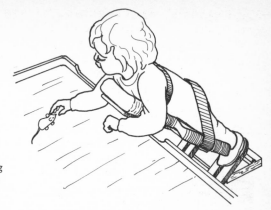

Fig. 21.6 The place of
equipment in daily life:
prone board enables
table play while working
on extension of the hips
and spine

simple foam wedges to assist prone development, to prone-standing boards, to standing frames, walking aids and a whole range of wheelchairs, manual and power operated.

For any piece of equipment the question What do we want this to do for the child? should be asked of both the parents and the therapist. Does it give him or us something that we can't get any other way? Does he lose anything by using it? Is the gain greater than the loss? Well-chosen and well-used equipment can help to carry treatment through into daily life. It can enable a child to participate in activities appropriate to his age while he continues to develop the motor skills needed to perform the task independently.

THE USE OF APPLIANCES

An appliance may be defined as a piece of body-worn equipment. The term includes splints, footwear, calipers and spinal braces. The use of appliances for children poses one special difficulty – the younger the child the faster he grows. To function effectively an appliance must be a good fit, lightweight and durable. It is not unknown for a child between two and three years to outgrow a pair of shoes in three months during a growth spurt. The elbow crutches of the paraplegic toddler may be worn out in a month.

If an appliance is functional it will be used; if it is used it will wear out. If it is going to wear out it will need replacing, and to replace appliances takes time. Careful planning and early ordering are needed so that the child is not to be left stranded without his essential support.

Splints that are required for a short period only may be made by the therapist from one of the many splinting materials available.

Each has different qualities and can be used for specific purposes, e.g. Hexcelite is a lightweight medium that has proved very versatile for making lightweight splints for infants and young children. Orthoplast may be useful when making splints that require greater strength and durability. Both these materials are malleable using hot water at a temperature that even young children can tolerate. Because they require little apparatus for their application this type of material is easy to use in the community and in conjunction with home treatment.

If splints are required for an extended period it is probably more cost-effective to use an orthotic company. Ideally the therapist should work with the orthotist and explain and interpret what is required for the child.

Appliances should be used to achieve a specific function such as supporting a weak limb or preventing deformity. Parents and children need to understand what the therapist hopes to achieve by using an appliance. Even cosmetic appliances are rarely pretty. Many families value advice on how to find suitable clothing for the child while using calipers or spinal supports. When boots are recommended for support, thought should be given to the choice of style and colour, and when new boots are being ordered child and parents can often be given a choice of colour. This can add new interest for the child and increase his motivation to wear and use his boots.

SPECIFIC THERAPEUTIC APPROACHES AND OTHER INTERVENTIONS

Physiotherapists and all who are in contact with sick/disabled children need to remind themselves continuously of the individuality of each family and the uniqueness of each child. Regardless of the medical condition each child and family present with their own particular blend of personality, expectation, life-pattern, strengths, weaknesses, resources and needs. It would be presumptuous to assume that any one approach to treatment was the only right, proper and effective method to use. The therapist working in this field will develop her own range of techniques, so that with an individual child and family she can draw upon them and supplement them as the situation requires.

Debate is continuous as to which term should be used in relationship to working with long-term disability; treatment/management/therapy/intervention/care? Words come into and out of fashion and subtly different meanings are endowed upon them with each cycle. However, all workers have the one common objective – to be as effective as possible in minimizing the handicapping effect of the condition thereby helping the child to enjoy the optimum quality of life. Within the conventional boundaries of physiotherapy much is owed to the work of Bobath and Peto. Other systems that offer help and direction to parents include the Portage Teaching Service, and increasing numbers of families are exploring the methods offered by the various 'Institutes for Human Potential' based on the work of Doman and Delacato.

Bobath

A neurodevelopmental approach to the treatment of cerebral palsy was established in England in the 1940s by Karel and Berta Bobath: the approach continues to evolve and is based on the principle of using techniques of handling and positioning in order to inhibit abnormal postures and movements and facilitate desirable normal motor patterns of movement. Parents are taught how to continue treatment into the child's daily life activities such as carrying, dressing and feeding. This approach is in use throughout many countries.

Peto

The system of Conductive Education was developed by Dr Andras Peto in Budapest in the 1960s. The inscription above the institute in Budapest bears the inscription: 'Not because of, but in order to'.

Work is based on the principle that cerebral palsied children consciously learn movement by constant practice and repetition. This learning is reinforced by the use of voice and rhythmical intention. Professional demarcations are abandoned and a single 'conductor' is trained in all aspects of therapeutic and educational work. Most activities take place within a group setting and are task-based and functionally related. At present (1989) this method is attracting much media interest and a number of families are prepared to journey to Budapest to explore the possibilities of this approach.

Portage

This early intervention teaching approach was developed in Wisconsin and used for work with socially deprived children. This system has been introduced to Great Britain and offered to families with learning disabled children. Most services work on a home visiting basis, the visitor aiming to teach the family how to break down learning tasks into small attainable steps. The parents are given a chart that describes the teaching activity and records their work with their child. This service is now in use in many areas, often being offered to children with motor disabilities. It works in parallel with other services and therapies and can be a useful reinforcer. To avoid overlap and confusion there must be good, effective liaison between the therapist and the portage worker.

Doman–Delacato

This approach derives from the work of Temple Fay. In the 1960s Glen Doman and Delacato extended the premise that children must develop through the evolutionary stages of reptilian squirming, amphibian creeping, mammalian crawling to attain the primate upright gait. To this they added elements of vestibular stimulation and techniques of re-breathing. Working through the institutes for human potential, assessments are offered and home programmes devised and monitored. Programmes are arduous for the child and his family, frequently occupying 12–14 hours a day. The child is patterned by up to five workers at a time and exposed to interludes of selected stimulation re-breathing and vestibular stimulatory activities. The aim is to bombard and exploit the areas of the brain that are presumed to be undamaged.

Summary

No one approach to therapy will ever meet all children's needs. Each system has its strengths and its limitations. Each system has something to teach one in establishing one's own way of working and repertoire of skills.

For the ill or injured child the aim of the physiotherapist is to restore him to full function in the shortest possible time with the minimum interference to his normal life. She may use many resources to assist her, including the parents, the extended family, caregivers, teachers and recreational leaders.

For the child with a disability the physiotherapist will have a long-term commitment not only to him but also to the family in helping to mitigate the effects of whatever the disability. She too will be part of the many sources of help available to disabled children.

A good paediatric service should be able to respond flexibly to the child's and the family's needs, offering the most effective treatment, in the most appropriate place at a time that causes minimal disturbance not only to education but also to family life.

REFERENCE

Cunningham, C. (1982). *Down's Syndrome: An Introduction for Parents*. Souvenir Press, London.

BIBLIOGRAPHY

Cunningham, C. and Sloper, P. (1978). *Helping Your Handicapped Baby*. (Human Horizons Series.) Souvenir Press, London.
Education Act (1981). HMSO, London.
Education Act – DES Circular 8/81 (1981). HMSO, London.
Finnie, N. (1974). *Handling the Young Cerebral Palsied Child at Home*, 2nd edition. William Heinemann Medical Books Limited, London.
Hall, D. M. B. (1984). *The Child with a Handicap*. Blackwell Scientific Publications Limited, Oxford.
Lansdown, R. (1980). *More than Sympathy*. Tavistock Publications, London.
McCarthy, G. T. (ed.) (1984). *The Physically Handicapped Child: An Interdisciplinary Approach to Management*. Faber and Faber, London.
Mitchell, R. (1973). *Defining Medical Terms*. (*Developmental Medicine and Child Neurology*, vol. 15.) Blackwell Scientific Publications Limited, Oxford.

Chapter 22

Some Paediatric Conditions

by C. BUNGAY MCSP

NEONATAL RESPIRATORY PROBLEMS

Premature, low birth-weight and other very sick infants may be cared for in special units in regional centres or large hospitals. Many of these babies have respiratory problems which will at some stage require physiotherapy. Work in such a unit is highly specialized, and it is necessary to be acquainted with local procedures and to work closely with the medical and nursing staff.

It is possible for infants to survive from the age of about 24 weeks' gestation and with birth weights below 1000 grams. Their special requirements are:

1. *Minimum handling*: Small, premature and very sick infants respond badly to handling, and will show signs of apnoea, bradycardia and cyanosis.
2. *Warmth*: Babies lose heat very rapidly because of their relatively large surface area.
3. *Oxygen*: Immature or damaged lungs may require an increased supply of oxygen. It is important that this should be adequate but *not* in excess of requirements. High levels of oxygen for long periods can damage the baby's eyes.
4. *Ventilation*: The premature baby may be physiologically unable to maintain respiration without mechanical assistance. Low birth-weight and other sick babies may also need to be ventilated.
5. *Feeding*: By intravenous catheter or by nasojejunal or nasogastric tube. In the latter case physiotherapy should be given before feeds; continuous tube feeds should be discontinued and the stomach aspirated before treatment, with the contents being returned to the stomach afterwards.
6. *Constant observation and monitoring*: It is essential that any change in condition is noted so that deterioration or improvement may be acted upon immediately.

Equipment

There is a large amount of equipment which must be confusing for anyone entering the unit for the first time.

1. *Incubators* enable infants to be nursed and observed in a constant warm and humid atmosphere with minimum disturbance.
2. *Ventilators* are required by many of the babies. Intermittent positive pressure ventilation (IPPV) may be used initially progressing to continuous positive airways pressure (CPAP) as the infant begins to initiate his own respirations.
3. *Oxygen* may be administered via the incubator, sometimes into a headbox if it is necessary to maintain a high concentration. Oxygen can also be given directly into the endotracheal tube through the ventilator or via nasal prongs when using CPAP.
4. *Suction apparatus and catheters* must always be ready for use. The size of catheters used in these infants is usually number 6, 8, or 10.
5. *Monitors* come in many shapes and sizes and are used to record ECG, heart rate, blood pressure, respiratory rate, temperature, oxygen concentration in the incubator and levels of oxygen in the blood. When the machinery is available the latter is measured using a transcutaneous electrode which gives a continuous reading of $tPCO_2$.

Apnoea alarms may be in use either in the form of a highly sensitive pad on which baby lies or a disc electrode attached to his chest. In either case the alarm sounds if the baby ceases to breathe for more than the pre-set number of seconds.

It is important to note the readings on monitors before, during and after treatment. For this age-group normal heart rate ranges from 120 to 140 beats per minute. Normal respiratory rate is 35–40 per minute, but may rise to over 80.

Physiotherapy (Fig. 22/1)

In spite of the difficulties it is possible for physiotherapy to make an effective contribution in suitable cases. The most common of these are:

1. Chest infection with increased secretions.
2. Increased secretions following prolonged intubation.
3. Collapse of lung due to mucus plug or aspiration of feed.
4. Meconium aspiration.

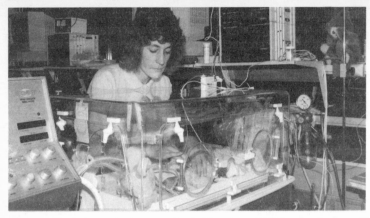

Fig. 22.1 Physiotherapy in the neonatal unit. Note the multiplicity of technology aids

Before commencing treatment it is important to check that all necessary equipment, e.g. gloves, catheters, suction apparatus, is to hand and in working order.

Techniques must be adapted to each baby's condition. *Postural drainage* may not be tolerated if the baby is very sick. In any case it is rarely possible to treat more than two areas at any one treatment. *Tipping* can be accomplished by winding the tray of the incubator up or down. *Percussion* is possible using three fingers of one hand and supporting the chest with the other. As an alternative a small Bennett mask may be used for percussion, which must be given firmly enough to influence underlying tissues. *Vibrations* using two or three fingers with pressure on expiration can be effective in clearing secretions. It is quite easy to do this in time with the ventilator. If not ventilated the baby's respiratory rate may be high – the vibrations can then be given on every second or third expiration. In some units the padded head of an electric toothbrush may be used to give vibrations by nursing or physiotherapy staff.

Suction　The removal of secretions is an important part of treatment and may be required before, during and after physiotherapy, as well as at other times. It is most important to acquire a good technique in order to minimize the almost inevitable damage caused by introducing a catheter into the delicately lined airways. There is need to be aware of the dangers of both inadequate and over-enthusiastic use.

Secretions may be removed from the nasopharynx via the nostril, or from the oropharynx via the mouth. Before suction 0.1–0.3ml of normal saline may be instilled into the endotracheal tube. Suction should only be applied during withdrawal of the catheter, which should be the largest size that can be introduced with ease. When suctioning through the endotracheal tube it must be borne in mind that the catheter will, in effect, fill the airway, and speed is essential so that the child can breathe. Suction pressure should be no higher than 50cm H_2O(5kPa).

Instructions for positioning and turning babies between physiotherapy sessions should be worked out with the nursing staff, together with the times of treatment.

RESPIRATORY PROBLEMS IN BABIES AND YOUNG CHILDREN

Babies and young children present with a number of respiratory conditions that are 'peculiar' to childhood due to the relative size and maturity of their respiratory system, e.g. bronchiolitis.

The principles of physiotherapy and postural drainage need some adaptation from the adult model. Small children often feel more secure by being treated on a person's lap or on the floor rather than on a bed. Many children associate bed with sleep and are disturbed and puzzled at the idea of going to bed during the day and in a strange place. A child's tolerance of lying down is considerably less than that of an adult. Treatment sessions will need a careful balance of postural drainage and active games and exercises. This is especially important if the child has a long-term condition, e.g. cystic fibrosis. He needs to enjoy his treatments and see them as fun, not as an imposition on his life. Therapists and parents will need to be resourceful and inventive in order to introduce new variations to alleviate boredom.

Suggestions for chest physiotherapy for babies and young children

Postural Drainage (Fig. 22/2) This is most easily done with the baby lying on a pillow on the physiotherapist's lap (A, B). The baby feels comfortable and secure and can lie in the prone, supine, side- or half side-lying positions with additional support provided by the physiotherapist's hands on his chest. The physiotherapist should sit on a low chair so that she can regulate the degree of tip by moving her knees. In (D) she achieves this by having her right foot on a low platform; in (C) she produces the same effect by extending her left knee.

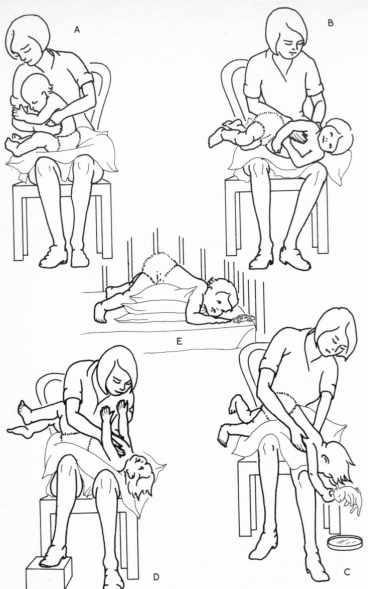

Fig. 22.2 Postural drainage positions for babies and small children. A. Apical segments of the upper lobes. B. Right middle lobe. C. Posterior segment of the lower lobes. D. Anterior segments of the lower lobes. E. Draining the posterior segments of the lower lobes by lying over pillows in the cot

Thus, all areas of the lung can be drained with minimum disturbance. If possible, the baby should be positioned so that his face can be seen, so that his colour can be checked frequently. A toy unbreakable mirror can be useful if arranged so that the physiotherapist, and the baby, can see his reflection, particularly when draining the posterior segments of lower lobes. Other toys, mobiles, or musical boxes may also be arranged to hold the attention of toddlers who are often happier treated on the lap, but still tend to get restless. They can also be tipped over pillows and are often found afterwards administering the treatment they have received to their favourite doll or teddy.

Details of the correct drainage positions for each area of the lungs are shown in the diagrams.

'Exercises' It is quite easy to give vibrations and shaking in time with the baby's natural expiration. Toddlers will often imitate sounds and may 'sing' Ah-Ah-Ah while their chests are clapped or vibrated. Laughing is good exercise and, if not too ill, most babies enjoy being tickled and encouraged to use their arms, by grasping the physiotherapist's thumbs while she performs 'circles' or 'hugging and stretching'. They quickly learn to participate; and so help to maintain mobility of chest and shoulder girdle, which can become quite stiff even in very young children.

All children love bubbles and blowing them is often a good introduction to the very young as well as helping to overcome the fears of many slightly older children, who may be away from home for the first time and view any new face or treatment with apprehension. Bubble-blowing requires little effort and therefore does not cause tension in the muscles of the throat or chest – even if the child does not blow them he enjoys watching and will reach out to catch them and a great deal of activity can be stimulated in this way.

Fat, lethargic babies are sometimes 'chesty' and may benefit from a spell in the baby bouncer. The activity improves their general musculature as well as increasing the rate and depth of respiration.

Simple direct breathing exercises should be commenced as soon as it is possible to get the child's co-operation. This varies from about the age of two years to four or even five years. The easiest starting positions are side lying or supine with knees bent. The child's hands rest over his diaphragm and he feels his 'tummy get smaller as the air goes away' and larger as he fills up again with air. This can then be repeated with hands on the lower ribs.

Older children will benefit from activities such as swimming and trampolining. Whistles and wind instruments may help some children provided they do not require excessive effort.

CONGENITAL TALIPES EQUINOVARUS (Fig. 22/3)

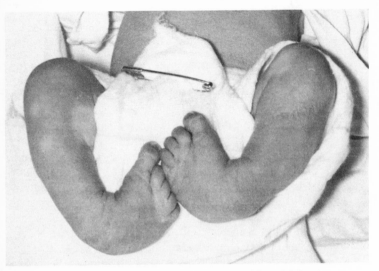

Fig. 22.3 Congenital talipes equinovarus showing severe bilateral deformity

The foot is twisted downwards and inwards. The head of the talus is prominent on the dorsum of the foot, the medial border of which is concave. In severe cases the sole of the foot may face upwards and, if untreated, the child will walk on the dorsum of the foot. The majority of cases are bilateral.

Aetiology

The cause is uncertain, but there is often a genetic element and other congenital abnormalities may also be present. One explanation is that the development of the foot is arrested before birth as a result of an unidentified intra-uterine infection. The initial abnormality may be in the bones with secondary soft tissue changes. Alternative theories suggest that moulding of the foot occurs when the fetus lies awkwardly in the uterus, and that the primary change is in soft tissues – the bones only become misshapen later if the deformity is not corrected. A congenital neuromuscular abnormality may be the precipitant.

There are three components of the deformity:

1. Plantar flexion of the ankle (equinus). The talus may lie almost vertically instead of in the horizontal position.
2. Inversion of the sub-taloid and mid-tarsal joints. The calcaneus faces inwards (varus).
3. Adduction of the forefoot at the tarsometatarsal joint. Some cases also present internal rotation of the tibia.

There is shortening of tibialis anterior and posterior, and the long and short flexors of the toes. The calf muscles are wasted and the tendo calcaneus is drawn over to the medial side of the heel. Similarly, the ligaments and joint capsule on the medial side of the ankle and foot are tight and the plantar fascia forms a tight thickened band on the medial side of the sole. On the lateral side of the leg, the peronei and lateral ligaments and capsule are over-stretched and weak.

Treatment

It is very important that treatment is commenced early, if possible on the first day of life. It must be continued until the child walks. Treatment consists of gradual, steady over-correction of the deformity by manipulation, and maintenance by splinting and the encouragement of the development of active use of all the leg muscles, particularly the peronei. Some cases will require surgical intervention. Aggressive stretching should never be contemplated and the physiotherapist should work in close co-operation with the orthopaedic surgeon. Soft tissue operations may be performed within the early months of life. Bone surgery is rarely indicated before the age of one year. The timing and nature of any surgery will vary with the individual surgeon. For good conservative results it should be possible to obtain, if not hold, full over-correction of the deformity within the first three to four weeks. When full correction is obtained splinting and stretching *must* be sustained until active movement can maintain the position. This may necessitate intermittent strapping for a period of several months in order to avoid the danger of deformity recurring. This can occur in less than two weeks and diligent supervision is essential when the change is made from continuous to intermittent strapping.

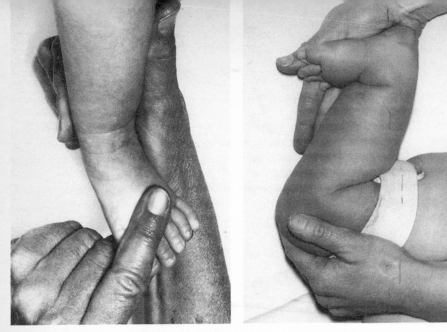

Fig. 22.4 (*left*) Manipulation to abduct forefoot
Fig. 22.5 (*right*) Manipulation to gain combined eversion and dorsiflexion

Manipulation (Figs 22/4, 22/5) Manipulation to obtain over-correction may be performed on young babies by either the doctor or physiotherapist without anaesthesia. In mild cases where no splinting is necessary the parents are taught to manipulate the foot regularly, e.g. at each nappy change or feed time.

During the manipulation the baby's knee is flexed and the lower leg held firmly to prevent any strain on the knee. Each part of the deformity is stretched separately. The manipulations are:

1. *To correct the heel*: The heel is grasped and pulled down and out, stretching the tendo calcaneous and structures on the medial side. For a good result the heel must be fully correctible in the first three to four weeks of life. After this time an inverted heel is unlikely to respond to manipulative measures.

2. *To abduct the forefoot*: The baby's left heel rests in the palm of the physiotherapist's right hand so that her thumb supports the outer side of his leg, and her index and middle fingers hold his heel. The physiotherapist uses her left thumb and index finger to grasp the base of the toes. The ball of her right thumb acts as the fulcrum as she stretches the inner border (Fig. 22/4).

3. *To combine eversion and dorsiflexion*: The fully correctible foot can be pushed up and out so that the dorsum touches the outer side of the leg. Care must be taken to ensure that the dorsiflexion takes

place in the ankle joints and not within the sole of the foot. Tightness of the tendo calcaneus will inhibit this and may indicate a need for surgery.

Strapping (Figs 22/6, 22/7) Strapping is the most effective way to hold the infant foot in a corrected position; it may be applied by the doctor or the physiotherapist. Cast materials, e.g. plaster of Paris or Delta-Cast, may be used. Many splints and bootees are becoming available – although they rarely help to obtain correction they may sometimes help to maintain the corrected foot.

Keeping the infant's skin in good condition is imperative if the programme of strapping is to proceed uninterrupted. The following suggestions will help to promote this:

1. Prepare the skin by painting with compound benzoin tincture (Friar's balsam) or Opsite before applying the strapping. If in spite of this the skin becomes sweaty or soggy, a drying agent may be liberally applied and the strapping continued. (Gentian violet may no longer be used – the hospital pharmacist should be consulted about a suitable agent.)

   Once initial correction has been obtained it may be possible for the parents to remove the strapping 24 hours before re-applying thus allowing a bath and exposure of the skin. Very rarely a baby may be allergic to zinc oxide tape but tolerate one of the non-allergic plaster tapes, e.g. Dermicel.
2. Reinforcement of the corrective straps to prevent them from dragging on the skin.
3. Careful padding of pressure points with adhesive felt. Remember that the exact distribution of these will alter as the foot changes shape with correction.

The method of strapping to be described has been used for many years and still proves satisfactory. Minor adaptations can be made to suit the individual case. The lateral malleolus is protected by a small piece of adhesive felt. Another piece of felt 1.25–2.5cm (½–1in) wide, depending on the size of the foot, is wrapped around the medial side of the great toe and under the base of the other toes. Care should be taken to place the foot on to the pad and not to drag it across the underside of the foot.

Three strips of 2.5cm (1in) wide zinc oxide strapping tape are used to correct the three elements of the deformity. In very tiny infants and pre-term babies the strapping will need to be reduced in width.

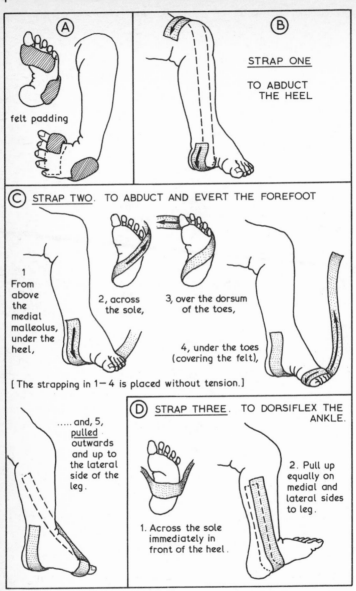

(A) felt padding

(B) STRAP ONE

TO ABDUCT
THE HEEL

(C) STRAP TWO. TO ABDUCT AND EVERT THE FOREFOOT

1
From
above
the
medial
malleolus,
under the
heel,

2, across
the sole,

3, over the dorsum
of the toes,

4, under the toes
(covering the felt),

[The strapping in 1−4 is placed without tension.]

..... and, 5,
pulled
outwards
and up to
the lateral
side of the
leg.

(D) STRAP THREE. TO DORSIFLEX THE
ANKLE.

2. Pull up
equally on
medial and
lateral sides
to leg.

1. Across the sole
immediately in
front of the heel.

Fig. 22.6 Strapping for talipes equinovarus

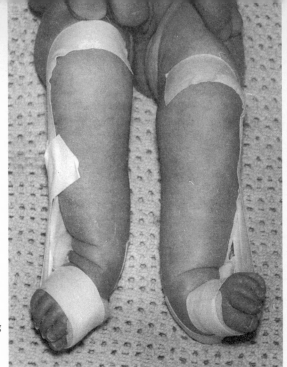

Fig. 22.7 Strapping
for bilateral talipes
equinovarus

1. *Strap 1* starts below the medial malleolus and passes under the heel, up the outer side of the leg and over the flexed knee (Fig. 22/6 A, B).
2. *Strap 2* starts above the medial malleolus and passes diagonally across the sole of the foot, and is placed around the forefoot (covering the felt). NB: It is important that no tension is applied up to this point. The strap is then applied upwards and outwards to the lateral side of the leg (Fig. 22/6 C).
3. *Strap 3* maintains dorsiflexion. It passes stirrup-like under the sole of the foot, immediately in front of the heel and is drawn up equally on both sides of the lower leg (Fig. 22/6 D).

Reinforcement by short strips of zinc oxide tape placed diagonally across the corrective straps helps to prevent dragging on the skin. Care should be taken not to allow these straps to run right around the calf as this could impede circulation.

A simple cotton weave bandage, applied over the strapping and secured with zinc oxide tape, protects the strapping and can be replaced in the event of soiling.

Initially, strapping is inspected, renewed or reinforced daily progressing to twice weekly until full over-correction can be maintained without undue circulatory disturbance. If treatment is started early this is usually within the first three weeks. It is then re-applied weekly to fortnightly. Some form of splinting must be maintained until the child is standing when his own body-weight will act as a corrective force. There is a strong tendency for this condition to relapse. Splints or bootees may be useful at this stage. They must be well fitting and reviewed frequently during this period of rapid growth. Parents need to understand the function of their child's splints and be competent and conscientious in their application and use.

Exercise   Even while strapping and splinting are being used the baby should be encouraged to kick. He may do this against his mother's hands, the end of his cot or pram and, when he is old enough, against the floor. This strengthens his muscles and reinforces the correction of the deformity. Each time the strapping is removed the peronei should be stimulated by stroking or brushing over the muscles or along the outer border of the foot. When intermittent splinting is introduced the baby should be encouraged to exercise without his splints. Parents should be taught how to manipulate the foot through a full range of movement, how to stimulate the peronei and to stand the child frequently.

Advice to parents   Parents must understand:

1. The importance of continuous treatment.
2. The danger of relapsing if treatment is stopped too soon.
3. The necessity of keeping the strapping or splinting dry.
4. The importance of inspecting the toes to check the circulation. They should be told to return to hospital urgently if the toes become blue or swollen.
5. As soon as possible, parents should be encouraged to remove their child's strapping one day before it is due for replacement. This will enable them to enjoy the important experience of bathing their baby.

TORTICOLLIS

Torticollis (wry neck) is occasionally seen by the physiotherapist. The child's head is held tilted to one side so that the ear is drawn towards the shoulder on the tight side. At the same time the face is turned towards the opposite side.

Aetiology

Structural torticollis: Anomalies of the cervical vertebrae may be the cause of the neck posture. These occasionally present as a feature of a more extensive syndrome, e.g. Klippel-Feil. Physiotherapy is not indicated.

Ocular torticollis: Occasionally older children present with their head held to one side. There is a full range of passive movement and the posture becomes more exaggerated when concentrating on visual tasks. This is due to imbalance of the eye muscles and requires the attention of the ophthalmologist not the physiotherapist.

Infantile torticollis (Fig. 22/8): This is the type most commonly seen. It is often associated with a palpable small hard lump of fibrous tissue in the muscle belly of the sternomastoid muscle. This is described as a sternomastoid tumour – a term which can cause undue anxiety to parents who may be fearful of malignant disease. If this term is used the therapist should be careful that the parents understand its meaning and allay any fears. The fibrous tumour may present before birth or a haematoma may result from a traction injury during birth. Facial asymmetry and moulding of the head is often a factor. If the muscle is stretched and head mobility improves this asymmetry will slowly improve over the first year of life. In untreated cases facial asymmetry may persist and after some years become irreversible and disfiguring.

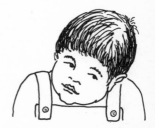

Fig. 22.8 Infantile torticollis
showing 'tilted' head posture

Treatment Physiotherapy consisting of stretching, active exercises and general handling and management should be started early, usually at about four to six weeks. Treatment started after six months is generally less effective. After this time the muscle is more difficult to stretch and the baby more resistant. A tenotomy of the sternomastoid may have to be considered at a later date.

Stretching   The movements in stretching the sternomastoid are:

1. Side flexion of the head away from the tight side.
2. Rotation of the head so that the face is turned towards the tight side.
3. Both movements combined, side flexion followed by rotation.

If the infant is small the stretching is best performed while he lies on the therapist's or parent's lap (Fig. 22/9). She will need to sit on a chair that is low enough to rest both feet firmly on the floor. The baby will feel secure and relaxed on a lap. In the case of a right-sided torticollis he lies across his mother's lap with his head on her right knee. She places her left arm across him and firmly grasps the point of his right shoulder to steady it; her forearm keeps his arms and trunk tucked securely to her own body. She places her right hand on the right side of baby's head, avoiding his ear and slowly brings his chin to mid-line before performing side flexion (bringing the head towards her) and rotation (turning the face away from her). If the baby is too big, the stretching may be performed on a firm flat surface, and a second person will be needed to help. The assistant holds the baby's shoulders, while the mother performs the movements as before.

Each movement should be through the fullest range possible, performed five or six times at each session and repeated two or three times daily. Because it is so important that the mother performs these stretches the physiotherapist must realize that the mother needs reassurance that she will not harm her baby. She will be frightened, especially if he cries, and will need opportunity to practise

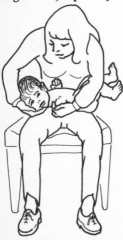

Fig. 22.9 Mother
practising manipulation
and stretching

and gain confidence. She may need one or two weeks of close supervision before she feels confident to stretch the baby at home. All treatments should end with a pleasurable reward for mother and baby, e.g. a cuddle or a feed.

Active Exercise From about 10 weeks the baby is mature enough to play an active part in his treatment. He can be encouraged to turn his head through the full range of rotation by attracting his attention with a coloured rattle or toy. At first this is done in supine, later in prone and later still in sitting. It is important to move the rattle slowly, giving the infant time to fix his vision on to it and then accommodate the movement. By changing his position, and gently holding down one shoulder, the movements of flexion, extension and side flexion can be isolated and encouraged.

General Handling and Management The baby should be encouraged to lie on alternate sides. Frequently one side is easier than the other and parents may need guidance in supporting him comfortably, e.g. with a rolled towel behind his back.

The cot or reclined chair should be placed so that the baby is encouraged to look towards the tight side; toys may be hung along the side to attract his attention.

The baby should not be sat upright too early or for too long; his head will drop to the tight side if the opposing muscles are still weak or fatigued.

The following pages offer a summary of a number of conditions which may be encountered by the physiotherapist working with children. It is only a resumé and full details may be found in specific textbooks.

Condition	Brief description	Physiotherapy indicated
Arthrogryposis	A congenital condition in which there are multiple joint abnormalities	Early treatment consists of stretching and passive movement Later treatment involves splinting and mobilization within the residual deformity
Asthma	Respiratory condition that may present at any age. May be exacerbated by infection, anxiety or allergy	During acute episodes physiotherapy is rarely effective. Between acute episodes the therapist may teach relaxation, postural drainage and the use of nebulizers, etc

Condition	Brief description	Physiotherapy indicated
Ataxia	A condition affecting the organization of balance and fine co-ordination. It may be congenital or of later onset May be associated with cerebral palsy or other diseases, e.g. ataxia telangiectasia or Friedreich's ataxia	Differential diagnosis has an important effect on prognosis A number of ataxias are progressive Treatment includes work on balance, functional seating and suitable recreational activities
Brachial palsies	Usually result from birth trauma. *Erb's palsy* – damage to 5th and 6th cervical nerve roots. Resulting paralysis of shoulder and whole arm *Klumpke's paralysis* – damage to 7th and 8th cervical nerve roots. Resulting paralysis of wrist and finger extensors and intrinsic hand muscles	Early treatment aims to reduce the risk of joint deformity by passive movement, positioning and splinting As movement recovers active movements can be encouraged through play When full recovery does not take place surgery may be required to give adequate joint stability
Brain damage	A non-specific term used to describe functional and movement difficulties due to malfunction, malformation or injury to the brain	Each child requires individual evaluation of his specific difficulties and a plan tailored to meet his needs
Bronchiectasis	Chronic dilatation of smaller bronchi. May follow repeated infection or inhalation of foreign body, e.g. small part of toy or peanut Child fails to thrive and may produce purulent sputum	Postural drainage If the condition is limited to a well-defined area surgery may produce good long-term results
Bronchiolitis	An acute viral infection occurring in small infants usually under one year. There is	The sick baby requires oxygen, humidity and diligent nursing observation

Condition	Brief description	Physiotherapy indicated
	cough, wheeze and marked dyspnoea The baby may become floppy and cyanosed	Physiotherapy is not indicated during the acute stage but may be required later if some consolidation remains
Bronchitis	Wheezy respiratory condition often associated with childhood asthma	See asthma
Cerebral palsy (CP)	A group of conditions in which there is impairment of movement due to a non-progressive lesion of the developing brain The lesion is static but the condition will appear to alter with growth and maturation Terms used in connection with the distribution of CP include hemiplegia, diplegia and quadriplegia. Terms used to describe the type of movement disorder include spastic, ataxic, athetoid and dystonic	There are many approaches to the treatment of CP: the most effective include elements of prevention of deformity, facilitation of movement, maximization of residual skills and full participation in educational and recreational activities
Chickenpox	Common childhood illness occasionally complicated by encephalitis	Physiotherapy may be needed to rehabilitate the child who has had encephalitis
Clumsy child	A child who has a specific difficulty in learning to perform, select and sequence motor tasks	The physiotherapist should make a full assessment of the child's movement skills, being careful to eliminate specific disease, e.g. cerebral palsy or muscular dystrophy. A remedial programme may be indicated

Condition	Brief description	Physiotherapy indicated
Congenital dislocation of the hip (CDH)	Displacement of the head of the femur in relationship to the acetabulum – usually superior and posterior. CDH is more common in girls than boys, and is usually unilateral Several tests are used to assist diagnosis including Barlow's	Orthopaedic management is initially with splinting, occasionally surgery is required Physiotherapists may apply the splints and advise the family on management of their child in splints or plaster
Cystic fibrosis (CF)	A disorder of the exocrine glands in which secretions are abnormally viscid. There is failure to thrive due to pancreatic deficit. Respiratory complications are common Digestive problems may be treated with Pancrease or Creon	Postural drainage should be carried out daily Parents learn to carry out chest care at home
Diplegia	Sub-group of cerebral palsy where the lower limbs are significantly more affected than the upper limbs	See cerebral palsy
Down's syndrome	Commonest of all syndromes associated with mental handicap, occurring in about 1 in 660 live births Infant may be floppy, and there is an increased incidence of cardiac, sight and hearing problems	The physiotherapist may advise the parents on how to assist their child's motor development
Encephalitis	Sudden and occasionally catastrophic illness which may be viral in origin. Can result in damage to sight, hearing, movement and learning	Assessment and rehabilitation

Condition	Brief description	Physiotherapy indicated
Epiglottitis	One cause of stridor, and croup. It is an acute obstruction of the upper airway in young children and is associated with a hoarse dry cough. Can result in rapid total collapse. Intubation and intensive care support may be required	Chest care may be indicated, particularly if a tracheostomy is necessary
Erb's palsy	See brachial plexus lesions	
Head injury	May occur in childhood, often as the result of a playground accident or road traffic accident	Rehabilitation and co-ordination with other team members
Hemiplegia	Movement disorder affecting one side of the body. It may be congenital, e.g. cerebral palsy, or acquired, e.g. post-trauma	See cerebral palsy
Hypertonia	Raised basic muscle tone due to upper motor neurone lesion. It is usually associated with cerebral palsy or head injury	
Hypotonia	Lowered basic muscle tone. It manifests itself in some types of cerebral palsy, Down's syndrome and dystrophies	
Intra-uterine infections	These may include, cytomegalovirus, rubella and toxoplasma, and they can result in damage to any of the developing systems, e.g. hearing, sight or motor	

Condition	Brief description	Physiotherapy indicated
Meningitis	Systemic infection, often bacterial, which may occur in the pre-term infant or at any stage in childhood Acute, life-threatening early illness may be followed by complete recovery or there may be residual damage to the central nervous system resulting in cognitive, motor and/or sensory deficit	During the acute phase the child may require respiratory support During the recovery phase physiotherapy may assist effective rehabilitation Residual deficit will require long-term support and management
Microcephaly	A pathologically small head usually well below the third centile. The affected child usually presents with mental retardation with or without visual, auditory and/or motor problems. Epilepsy may be an additional problem	The physiotherapist may advise on motor development and treat specific motor disorders
Mucopolysaccharidoses	This group includes the Hunter, Hurler and Morquio syndromes. They are lysosomal storage diseases and are characterized by growth disturbance, mental and motor deterioration and corneal clouding In Morquio syndrome the intellect remains intact	Kyphosis and other spinal problems often arise. There is an increased risk of atlanto-axial subluxation As the disease progresses many children will need chest care
Muscular dystrophy	A number of types may present with varying prognosis, *Duchenne* being the most common. It is X-linked therefore affects only boys. May be apparent between three and six years. Classically	The physiotherapist may have much to contribute in the management of this group of disorders. She can maintain mobility and joint range for as long as possible and adopt a positive view

Condition	Brief description	Physiotherapy indicated
	identified by Gower's sign. Ambulation is usually lost by the early teens. Most youngsters succumb to respiratory failure by their early twenties *Becker* form of muscular dystrophy similar but less severe and progress slower. Also X-linked *Limb girdle dystrophy* variable in severity. Autosomal recessive and may be seen in girls	when a wheelchair becomes necessary Diligent care should be taken with regard to sitting posture As the disease progresses chest care will be necessary
Paraplegia	Term reserved for paralysis of lower limbs usually as a result of a spinal lesion Most commonly associated with spina bifida or spinal injury Sensory loss and bladder dysfunction are common	Assessment of muscle power and sensation Passive movements to reduce secondary deformity Mobilization using splints, calipers, wheelchairs, etc
Pertussis (whooping cough)	Common infectious disease of childhood characterized by paroxysmal cough and vomiting. Runs a long and often debilitating course which may go on for months. Pneumonia and lung collapse may occur as complications	During the early stages this condition may be exacerbated by chest physiotherapy causing further distress Residual areas of lung collapse may respond to physiotherapy
Poliomyelitis	Viral infection which in a small percentage of cases travels from the alimentary tract via the circulatory system to the anterior horn cells of the spinal cord and brainstem. Results in	Rarely seen in an *acute* form. Children with residual paralysis may present for assessment prior to splinting or surgery. In the developing child therapists should be

Condition	Brief description	Physiotherapy indicated
	flaccid paralysis, joint instability and reduced growth of the affected limbs. Rarely seen in countries which have a vaccination programme but still occurs in epidemic form in underdeveloped areas	aware of the problems of inequality of growth
Psoriasis	Skin condition characterized by scaly lesions varying from small pink areas to large red patches Causes considerable distress to schoolchildren who are frequently teased by their class mates	Sometimes responds to UVL combined with lotions including tar preparations (see Chapter 13)
Quadriplegia	Sub-group of cerebral palsy in which all four limbs and trunk are affected. Head control, swallowing and speech may also be involved	See cerebral palsy
Scoliosis	Describes curvature of the spine in which there is a lateral curve in excess of 10°. May be postural or structural. Grouped as congenital, paralytic, idiopathic	The therapist may be involved in the management, monitoring and treatment of all types of scoliosis. Close co-operation with the orthopaedic and orthotic management is essential
Spina bifida	Congenital abnormality in which there is incomplete closure of the vertebral canal Effects of the cord lesion may vary from negligible to total flaccid paraplegia Hydrocephalus (ventricular	See paraplegia

Condition	Brief description	Physiotherapy indicated
	enlargement) is present in the majority of children with spina bifida	
Spinal muscular atrophy	Group of hereditary conditions in which there is progressive atrophy and weakness associated with degeneration of the anterior horn cells. Three types are usually described: *Severe* (Wernig-Hoffmann): Early onset. Poor feeding and respiration. Death usually in first year of life *Intermediate*: Significant and progressive weakness. Failure to develop standing or walking. Respiratory involvement. Death usually by early adult life *Mild* (Kugelberg-Welander): Some proximal weakness and occasional tremor. May be mistaken for early Duchenne but walking is sustained and condition remains static	Physiotherapy will include respiratory care, the maintenance of joint range and developing as much functional independence as possible. Attention must be paid to posture and seating

BIBLIOGRAPHY

Bleck, E. (1987). *Orthopaedic Management in Cerebral Palsy*. Blackwell Scientific Publications Limited, Oxford.

Gordon, N. and McKinlay, I. (eds.) (1980). *Helping Clumsy Children*. Churchill Livingstone, Edinburgh.

Griffiths, M. and Clegg, M. (1988). *Cerebral Palsy: Problems and Practice*. Souvenir Press, London.

Levitt, S. (1984). *Treatment of Cerebral Palsy and Motor Delay*, 2nd edition. Blackwell Scientific Publications Limited, Oxford.

Roberton, N.R.C. (1986). *A Manual of Neonatal Intensive Care*, 2nd edition. Edward Arnold, London.

Scrutton, D. and Gilbertson, M.P. (1975). *Physiotherapy in Paediatric Practice*. Butterworths, London. (Out of print. Available in libraries.)

Shepherd, R. (1980). *Physiotherapy in Paediatrics*, 2nd edition. William Heinemann Medical Books Limited, London.

ACKNOWLEDGEMENTS

The author extends her thanks to the following for their advice and help in the preparation of these three chapters:

Dr Richard West MD, MRCP, DCH, consultant paediatrician, St George's Hospital, London.

Members of the Departments of Child Psychology and Child Psychiatry, St George's Hospital, London.

Colleagues in the Health, Education and Social Services Departments in the Wandsworth, London, area.

The staff, parents and children of the Child Development Centre, St George's Hospital, London.

In particular, the author is grateful to Miss Barbara Kennedy MCSP for her unfailing encouragement during the writing and planning of the chapters and for her contribution on paediatric conditions in chapter 22.

Chapter 23

Psychiatric Illness

by H. LAWLER BA, MCSP

In the United Kingdom physiotherapy in psychiatry is an expanding field of work, and many physiotherapists have developed a high degree of expertise in the specialty. They have combined the skills which they acquired when working in the general field with their knowledge of psychiatry to develop an approach to dealing with the mentally ill patient. To be successful the physiotherapist must be flexible and adaptable, she must have the ability to listen carefully to what patients say and to observe their mood and reactions.

The help given to the patient with a mental illness by the caring professions lays great emphasis on the multidisciplinary approach to problem solving. Each member of the team is respected for their particular contribution towards the care of the patient. Depending on the patient's needs the amount of input given by each profession will vary. It is important that all members of the team meet regularly so that everyone concerned has the same aims and objectives.

The team, led by the consultant psychiatrist, comprises doctors, hospital and community nurses, physiotherapists, occupational therapists, psychologists, social workers, the chaplain, and the pharmacist.

The patients with whom the physiotherapist has main contact can be divided into the following categories:

- the acutely ill
- the long stay
- the elderly
- forensic.

THE ACUTELY ILL PATIENT

The acutely ill patient when admitted to a psychiatric ward may be just as ill as the patient admitted to an intensive care unit in a general hospital. The problems presented can be of a mental or physical nature; an improvement in one may well result in the improvement of the other. Admission may be on a voluntary basis or under a section of the Mental Health Act. If the patient is under section then he/she is not free to discharge him/herself until the period of the section is passed. A voluntary patient may discharge himself at any time just as a patient in a general hospital. The vast majority of patients are admitted voluntarily.

The acute ward will be a caring, informal environment within which the multidisciplinary team are able to assess and treat the patients. The patients are encouraged towards independence for their personal care activities. Therapeutic programmes are compiled for each patient to suit their individual needs. These activities may include social skills groups, relaxation classes, exercise therapy and health and fitness education. All of these are intended to help the patient to get back into the community and to resume his usual activities.

THE LONG-STAY PATIENT

Many of the patients who presently occupy long-stay wards in the large mental hospitals in this country have been there for many years. It was once the policy for them to reside permanently in these institutions and consequently they regard the hospital as their home. There is a great effort being made to rehabilitate many of them back into the community. The work of the multidisciplinary team here is to teach and encourage the patients to take responsibility for their personal care, develop their social skills and raise their general level of fitness.

THE ELDERLY SEVERELY MENTALLY ILL (ESMI)

These patients may be admitted to an acute ward for the elderly for assessment and treatment and then return home. However, it is sometimes necessary for them to remain in hospital permanently (see Chapter 27).

FORENSIC PATIENTS

These patients are assessed, diagnosed and treated in secure units. Their behaviour, as a result of mental disorders, has brought or is likely to bring, them into conflict with the law. They are usually referred from special hospitals, prisons, psychiatric hospitals, or the courts. The mental disorders from which they suffer are similar to those seen on any open psychiatric ward.

Commonly presenting disorders which the physiotherapist will see are as follows.

SCHIZOPHRENIA

The main clinical features observable in schizophrenia are:

(a) impaired thinking
(b) alteration in behaviour; it becomes indecisive and apathetic
(c) emotions become chaotic; the usual feelings one experiences become muddled and may quickly change
(d) hallucinations – most commonly these are auditory – may be voices telling the person what to do or commenting on what they are doing. Sometimes they are tactile and the person has the feeling that things are crawling over or in their body
(e) delusions – thinking that they are someone famous, often a member of the royal family
(f) the patient has no insight into the above features.

Treatment Usually chemotherapy, psychotherapy, social skills training, industrial therapy, recreational therapy, and preparation for return to living in the community.

Physiotherapy It has been found that regular physical activity for these patients can contribute to their easier management in the ward. Competitive activities should be avoided as the patients do not respond well to stressful situations.

Drug regimes for schizophrenic patients may possibly lead to tardive dyskinesia. This manifests itself as repetitive involuntary movements principally orofacial, but can include the neck, trunk and the extremities. The physiotherapist as an expert in movement disorders may be the first person to notice the onset. It should be reported to the medical team. The therapist must avoid reinforcing the delusions and hallucinations which the patient may be experiencing.

DEPRESSION

Depression may appear either without warning and for no obvious reason or following a crisis such as bereavement, the break-up of a relationship or the loss of a job. It may present with the following clinical features:

(a) significant weight loss continuing until the patient begins to recover
(b) sleep pattern is disturbed with patients showing initial insomnia and early morning wakening. Suicidal thoughts will often occur at this time
(c) there is a diurnal variation in mood. The patient will often feel better as the day progresses, but their mood tends to drop again towards the evening
(d) lack of energy and an inability to concentrate
(e) loss of interest in what is happening around the person; activities which used to give pleasure no longer even raise a smile
(f) unremitting lowness of spirits and the feeling of worthlessness
(g) deterioration of general appearance, the patient becoming unkempt
(h) in severe cases there is total motor retardation. This is characterized by a complete loss of motivation to the extent that there is no eye contact, mutism, and any movement performed is extremely slow.

Treatment   This condition is often successfully treated by the use of one or more of the following methods: antidepressant drugs, tranquillizers, sedatives, electro-convulsive therapy (ECT), or psychotherapy.

Physiotherapy   The physiotherapist has a very important role to play in the treatment of this condition. It has been shown that exercise, both aerobic and anaerobic, plays an important part in lifting the mood state (Doyne et al, 1987).

These patients have a tendency to self-harm. Careful observation of the patient is essential in order to detect any changes in their mental state. The physiotherapist should listen to the patient's speech content and monitor his approach to the exercise.

If the patient is depressed due to long-term physical disability such as a stroke, neuromuscular disease, or amputation it may be appropriate for the physiotherapist to give specific treatment to the person to gain/maintain functional independence.

MANIC DEPRESSIVE DISORDER

This major illness is characterized by severe mood swings which alternate between the state of mania as described below and an overwhelming feeling of misery and despair (see depression).

There are various signs that a person is manic, among them are the following:

(a) restlessness, overactivity and marked euphoria
(b) never showing fatigue and needing little sleep
(c) rapid speech, flight of ideas, and grandiose thoughts
(d) poor judgement resulting in inappropriate behaviour such as irresponsible spending of money and sexual promiscuity.

Treatment The condition is often successfully treated with lithium which is a drug which acts to stabilize the person's mood. Tranquillizers may also be used and in some cases ECT.

Physiotherapy In the manic phase physiotherapy may not be appropriate. However, if the patient is being seen as an outpatient, possibly in a depressive phase, the physiotherapist should be alert to any significant alteration in the patient's behaviour.

HYSTERICAL CONVERSION SYNDROME

A subconscious attempt by the person to get themselves out of a stressful situation. It may take the form of mutism, paralysis, deafness, sensory loss. Unlike malingering it is not deliberate or conscious and so the person has no fear of being found out because he genuinely experiences real symptoms.

Treatment To some extent the problem will resolve itself when the underlying conflict has been sorted out or in the process of being so. Chemotherapy and psychotherapy both have a place in the treatment.

Physiotherapy If the patient has been paralysed for a long time the physiotherapist will be an important member of the team as there is likely to be disuse atrophy of muscle groups affected. It will be vital to re-educate the limb and restore function.

Physiotherapy allows the patient to rationalize his improvement and may also be important in providing him with an acceptable reason for recovery.

PHOBIAS

These may be an excessive fear of situations or objects such as eating out, open spaces (agoraphobia), enclosed spaces (claustrophobia), animals, fire and many others. The phobic person realizes the fear is unrealistic but will still take steps to avoid the situation.

Treatment This usually takes the form of behaviour modification techniques by trained psychologists and nurses.

Physiotherapy The physiotherapist may be asked to help by teaching relaxation techniques to enable the patient to cope with the tension that they feel when presented with the cause of the phobia.

ILLNESS PHOBIAS

These patients present with a multiplicity of problems concerning their physical health. Extensive investigations have usually been carried out with no definitive diagnosis.

Physiotherapy Full use of the whole body is encouraged and general fitness is aimed for. Praise is given for improvement and illness behaviour is ignored. (Treatment is very much on the lines of the 'School for Bravery' as practised in Doncaster (Williams, 1989).)

ANXIETY STATES

Anxiety is a normal reaction experienced in everyday life in a mild form; however, when it becomes excessive and pervasive it is an illness. This may occur alone or as often happens in combination with other psychiatric illness.

Patients may complain of symptoms such as dizziness, palpitations, tremor, cold clammy palms, chest pains, inability to swallow and pins and needles.

Treatment This may be by the use of tranquillizers. They have their place, but patients can become dependent on them and withdrawal can have unpleasant effects. Psychotherapy and desensitization are methods of treatment often used.

Physiotherapy After a careful physical examination it is explained to the patient that the physiological feelings experienced are the body's normal reaction to anxiety. The patient should be reassured that he does not have a life-threatening illness. Relaxation techniques need to be taught, both to do at home when resting and at the time when the feelings of panic occur. Exercise may be taught to the patient as a means of dissipating their symptoms, for instance running up stairs, doing step-ups.

OBSESSIVE COMPULSIVE STATES

The person continually repeats certain ideas or actions. This takes such forms as continual washing of the hands, a special routine for getting dressed, counting objects, doubt about whether doors are locked, or gas turned off, etc. The obsessions become so troublesome that they interfere with normal everyday activity.

Treatment   Psychotherapy is the main treatment used, and in some cases chemotherapy and ECT may be appropriate.

Physiotherapy   This may take the form of relaxation techniques if there is an associated anxiety. Exercise therapy may be appropriate as a diversional activity avoiding any repetitive process which may encourage the obsessive behaviour.

PSYCHOSOMATIC DISORDERS

These are physical conditions which are also the result of psychological influences. Onset can often be seen to have taken place following major emotional events in life.

Some of the illnesses often associated in this way are: asthma, hay fever, eczema, tension headaches, migraine, low back pain, rheumatoid arthritis, psoriasis.

Physiotherapy   Where appropriate in these conditions physiotherapy takes the usual form. It is useful to bear in mind the probable psychological factors when planning the long-term management of the patient.

ANOREXIA NERVOSA

This is a body image disturbance. The patient shows a need to maintain a pathologically low body-weight. Onset is usually during adolescence and occurs more frequently in women than men.

Treatment   Anorexic patients are usually only admitted when their weight has become extremely low. They have a regime of bed rest and regulated food intake with careful observation following meals. As their weight increases they are gradually allowed to increase their activity.

Physiotherapy   In the early stages isometric exercises are gently introduced. This provides the physiotherapist with the opportunity to build up a rapport with the patient and to introduce the idea of a good body image at an early stage. As their weight increases active exercise can be introduced. The aim is to improve tone without allowing over-activity as this will tend to 'burn off' weight, therefore avoidance of aerobic exercise is essential. Weight-lifting exercise with a high weight/low repetition formula is ideal, the patient being reassured that this will not produce large muscle bulk.

SUBSTANCE ABUSE

Street drugs

These patients will be admitted to hospital for detoxification. They often present in a poor physical condition suffering from malnutrition, showing behaviour which may be aggressive, agitated, uncooperative or lethargic.

Treatment   A detoxification regime is used.

Physiotherapy   This must be given in a non-judgemental environment. Evidence of injections, tattoos, and abscess scars may be obvious but should be ignored. Concentration may be poor at first so short bursts of varied activities is most successful. In view of the patients' poor physical condition the exercise regime should be built up slowly. Development of a regular exercise regime will encourage the return to normal biological rhythms.

Prescribed drugs

After years of dependence many people are now trying to withdraw from minor tranquillizers, namely benzodiazepines. This is achieved by a gradual reduction in the dosage under medical supervision. Various withdrawal symptoms are often experienced by these patients and may include severe panic attacks, profuse sweating and musculoskeletal pains.

Physiotherapy   Support and encouragement are very important during the withdrawal phase. Patients are often helped by an exercise regime and relaxation to enable them to cope with the panic attacks. The patient needs to understand that the feelings experienced during the panic attack cannot harm him although at the time he may feel terrible. Musculoskeletal problems are assessed and treated in the usual way.

Alcohol

This is a chronic disorder represented by the repeated and excessive intake of alcohol which affects the drinker's health, social and economic functioning. Chronic alcoholism may result in various conditions including mental deterioration and personality changes.

Treatment Admission for detoxification by various methods.

Physiotherapy Co-ordination is usually poor so it is especially important to make sure that the exercises are performed correctly. Patients soon get tired so there is a need to build up stamina.

The physiotherapist has an important role in building up the self-esteem of the patient and should encourage a regular exercise regime. It has been shown that abstinence rates are higher for people who have undertaken regular exercise (Palmer et al, 1988).

PERSONALITY DISORDERS

These people have disorders of feelings and behaviour. They are inadequate and behave in an antisocial manner finding it difficult to get on with other members of society. Due to this behaviour they often become involved with the courts and may go to prison, special hospitals or forensic units. Physiotherapy for this kind of patient can be found in the forensic section (p. 432).

PHYSIOTHERAPY

The department

It is important that the department provides a friendly, relaxed atmosphere. The overall feeling conveyed should be one of positive good health. For some of the patients the nature of their illness is such that they have a feeling of worthlessness; they may think that people do not want to be bothered with them and such patients must know that time will always be made available for each and every one of them.

The department needs to be of a reasonable size so that vigorous activities can be carried out without endangering other people. It is also useful to have a separate room or cubicle where individual treatments can be given, and confidentiality maintained.

Equipment It is advantageous to have a multigym as it provides a number of 'stations' at which patients can perform their exercises. A static bicycle, bouncer and jogger are additional apparatus which can be well utilized. These items enable the patients to familiarize themselves with their use and encourage the progression to facilities in the community. If this equipment is not available a circuit can be set up from the usual type of apparatus that is found in a physiotherapy gym. It is an added benefit to have sports facilities and equipment available.

A good department will have the usual electrical equipment for the treatment of specific physical conditions. Mats and pillows are essential if relaxation classes are to be held and also a cassette player and tapes. Small apparatus such as beanbags, balls, quoits and balloons are useful on the wards when taking general exercise classes.

General aims of treatment for the acute psychiatric patient

(1) To promote health and fitness – exercise tolerance, co-ordination, strength, stamina and concentration.
(2) To help patients develop a knowledge and understanding of their own bodies – in particular to teach correct breathing patterns, and to help patients to understand the effects of the autonomic nervous system.
(3) To encourage alternative ways of controlling stress levels by exercise, relaxation and lifestyle adjustment.
(4) To provide a friendly, relaxed, and supportive atmosphere where problems can be comfortably discussed.
(5) To help patients regain their self-esteem, and to return to normal function.
(6) To help patients deal with the disturbing effects of their psychiatric symptoms.
(7) To assist patients in coping with the effects of drugs and give helpful feedback on performance to other team members.

Method

Referrals: These may be made by any member of the multidisciplinary team, however the doctor in charge of the case is always kept informed.

Assessment: It is useful to make an outpatient's first appointment during a quiet period in the department so that he is not overwhelmed. In-patients may be seen either on the ward first or in the department on an individual basis, whichever is appropriate.

Information about the patient is collected before the first visit including such things as social, medical and psychiatric history, and prescribed drugs.

At the first attendance an unstructured interview takes place during which time the physiotherapist elicits the following information:

(a) what the patient sees as the problem, and

(b) whether the patient really wants to do something about it.

The physiotherapist explains what the department can offer in the way of equipment, the atmosphere, advice and support. It is emphasized that it is the patient who will have to supply the effort if he wants to achieve results – he will not be attending to have something done for, or to, him! For some patients it is appropriate to do a simple fitness test. This would include peak flow, height, weight, step-up test for one minute followed by the pulse being taken immediately on finishing and then two and five minutes afterwards. The therapist also discusses any previous sporting activity undertaken.

Treatment

Physiotherapy forms part of the in-patient's programme which is individually designed to suit his needs. A session usually lasts about an hour and a patient attends as often as is appropriate for him. The ideal size for the group is 8 to 10 people. This allows the physiotherapists time to talk to anyone who feels down or concerned about something. Outpatients may also be attending other departments, such as occupational therapy, and the physiotherapist needs to liaise with them so that a balanced programme is devised. The use of the apparatus must also be carefully supervised so that it is used correctly as well as ensuring that patients are not being over-enthusiastic and doing too much. Social interaction between patients is encouraged and a supportive atmosphere fostered.

PHYSIOTHERAPY FOR LONG-STAY PATIENTS

The philosophy of care for the mentally ill has changed radically in recent years. It has moved from one of custodial care, with locked wards and high walls surrounding the hospital as a means of containing people who are mad, through literally the knocking down of the walls, to the present concept of care in the community for as many people as possible. Modern developments in the drugs' field have revolutionized the mangement of some conditions and thus enabled patients not to have to remain in hospital.

These patients may have been in hospital for many years and have become institutionalized. Their general level of fitness, and their social skills will have deteriorated. It has been found that this decline can be stemmed by group physical activity (McEwen, 1983). The nature of their illness often means that they have developed poor posture; the side-effects of some of the drugs will result in parkinsonism. Many will lack motivation and self-esteem.

Treatment

Regular exercise groups help not only to restore function and prevent further deterioration in posture and general mobility, but they also increase the patient's body awareness. All of which will help to improve the body image.

Most patients find it beneficial to use the multigym or exercise circuit as used by the other patients. Swimming, badminton, table tennis and other sports are also useful activities for both physical development and in helping to improve co-ordination. It is important that patients who are going to take on the more strenuous activities should be physically checked over by the doctor before embarking on them.

The physiotherapist as part of the multidisciplinary team will be helping some of the patients who have been in hospital for a long time to prepare for discharge into the community. Many of the patients have odd gait patterns. Usually the physiotherapist does not attempt to alter them unless they are causing pain or distress. Chest infections are common especially in the winter as a large proportion of the patients smoke.

The patients can also present with any of the usual problems which one might meet in the outpatient department. Careful assessment is required here, and care taken about apparatus used. Skin sensation may be unreliably reported and the patient may be tempted to interfere with electrical machines. Some patients may find these machines upsetting due to their psychological problems.

PHYSIOTHERAPY IN FORENSIC PSYCHIATRY

The physiotherapist works as a member of the multidisciplinary team. The development of their role within this group of professionals is still at a fairly early stage and so must be approached with an open mind. New techniques and strategies need to be developed alongside regular reappraisal of present practices so that a worthwhile contribution is made to the team approach of problem solving. It should be borne in mind that the role will probably vary from unit to unit depending on the particular skills and interests of the physiotherapists. It may not always lie totally within the traditional physiotherapy parameters. The approach to physiotherapy described here is that which has been developed at the Unit in Norwich.

General recreation

This is an area which has an established role. When dealing with patients whose activities are restricted it becomes increasingly important that they are provided with activities for relaxation/enjoyment. This combined with the obvious physical benefits provide the primary aims of these activities.

The less obvious secondary aims are:

(1) Competition within a group which can be used as a form of education for patients with obvious personality problems, especially when relating to others.
(2) Provision of a controlled, acceptable and positive area for the release of feelings of aggression/anxiety which some patients have difficulty in controlling.
(3) To develop a feeling of trust. Individual sessions to introduce an activity which a patient enjoys can often be used to initiate some interest/motivation which can then be channelled into other areas of activity.

Mental health

In this area the physiotherapist is able to form part of a purposeful, therapeutic individual care plan thus continuing the work carried out by other professionals.

In order to understand the philosophy behind the physiotherapist's approach it is worth while comparing a list of attributes, which to a greater or lesser degree are present in all keen sports people, with the problems exhibited by a large number of the patients seen at the forensic unit.

Sportsman	Patient
Motivation	Lack of motivation
Ability to communicate	Limited communication skills
Ability to assert themselves	Limited/inappropriate assertion skills
Ability to make decisions	Impaired decision-making ability
Ability to work as part of a team	Isolation
Awareness of surroundings	Unaware of surroundings

It can be seen that the basic attributes of a sports person are lacking in this patient group. In isolation this information is of little use; however, when combined with information on basic child development and the ability to learn through play and copying elders there is the foundation of a therapeutic activity. Games can be educational if organized correctly and even adults can learn by copying others.

The aim of the physiotherapy department is to provide:

1. A structured programme of games/physical activities designed to highlight the use of particular social skills, e.g. communication.
2. Provide patients with the opportunity to copy members of staff taking part in the same activity.

By fulfilling these two aims the patients are offered an arena for both fun and personal development, in a relaxed and natural environment which we all experience at some times in our lives.

Admission/treatment ward

Observation is vital during the assessment period. The physiotherapist will be looking both at the patient's physical abilities as well as his behaviour. The following are particular areas of interest which form the basis of the physiotherapist's assessment:

Level of participation/activity/motivation
   Does the patient require prompting to participate?
Communication
   Does the patient communicate spontaneously?
   Is the content appropriate?
Assertion
   Does the patient assert himself in any way?
   Is he inappropriately or over-assertive?
Group/individual relationships
   Does the patient respond to a particular individual?
Organization/leadership abilities
   Is the patient capable of performing basic organizational tasks?
   Does he shy away from responsibility?

Aggression
Has the patient shown any sign of verbal or physical aggression?
Mental state
Is the patient preoccupied?
Does the patient present with odd behaviour?

It can be seen from this that many very important observations can be made about a patient in a recreational setting.

Intermediate ward

Three specific areas can be identified for which groups can be organized. Their activities are arranged so that the patients can be helped to overcome their particular problem areas:
The aims of each group are as follows:

Communication
(a) Provide a structured but informal environment where patients can be encouraged to practise communication in a large group.
(b) Assess the appropriate use of communication skills.
(c) Provide advice on appropriate use of communication skills.

Assertion
(a) Provide an area in which patients may be taught appropriate assertion skills.
(b) Provide a structured environment in which patients may be encouraged to develop assertion skills.
(c) Provide an area where patients can be placed in a position of responsibility/authority.

Trust
(a) Provide activities which require trust in others.
(b) Provide activities which act as a starting point for discussion of factors affecting trust and general behaviour.
(c) Provide activities which present patients with a challenge, for example, overcoming fear or anxiety.

Pre-discharge patients

Much of these patients' time will be spent outside the unit as they adjust to life in the community again. It is appropriate for the physiotherapist to be involved in putting the patients in contact with sports clubs and facilities in the locality in which they will be living after discharge.

THE THERAPEUTIC EFFECTS OF EXERCISE

The physiological effects of exercise on cardiac output, venous return, respiration, and muscle development have been understood for many years. However, research – mainly in the USA – into the psychological effects have shown there to be many benefits, but it is difficult to ascertain the exact physiological processes behind them (Harber and Sutton, 1984).

Exercise promotes the release of endogenous opiates which have the following effects:

– reduces anxiety and tension
– raises the mood state
– increases pain tolerance.

Regular exercise promotes a feeling of well-being, improves the body image and thus raises the self-esteem. It develops strength, stamina and tolerance to fatigue. It has a role in helping to prevent heart disease, gastric ulcers (often the result of stress), obesity and postural problems.

People with psychological problems often find social situations difficult to handle. As most physical activity encourages social inter-action this must have a beneficial effect.

COUNSELLING

It is vitally important for physiotherapists in all spheres of work to develop their counselling skills. It is of particular importance that they learn to listen, not only to what is being said, but also what is not being said – topics which are being avoided, questions which are not fully answered, and, of course, body language. Such things as gaze avoidance, wringing of hands and restless movements can give clues about people's feelings and anxieties. The physiotherapist must not be frightened to ask straightforward questions, and to confront difficult situations. The atmosphere of the department must be such that the patient feels safe and therefore able to respond.

The physiotherapists must feel at ease with themselves and their attitudes towards various moral and ethical issues. The relationship between themselves and the patient has to be non-judgemental. The patients need empathy and genuine regard for themselves as people. Any sign of disapproval of the patient's feelings or lifestyle is likely to destroy any relationship which has been built up. The physio-therapist needs to get alongside the patient to try to understand his difficulties, and from there to help him to find a solution.

DRUGS

Some of the drugs used in psychiatry have side-effects which are of relevance to the physiotherapist:

Neuroleptics or anti-psychotics (major tranquillizers) In the short term they are used to calm disturbed patients, and in the long term to prevent a relapse when the patient has been psychotic. Relevant side-effects commonly include dizziness, drowsiness and extra-pyramidal symptoms (parkinsonism). Postural hypotension is possible and occasionally tardive dyskinesia (repetitive muscle movements) and agitation.

It should be noted that some anti-psychotic drugs may cause extreme sensitivity to ultraviolet light.

Lithium carbonate This is used in the treatment of mental illness to stabilize mood. In the long term it is used prophylactically in the treatment of manic depression.

Relevant side-effects of too high a dose of lithium are dizziness, drowsiness, fatigue, ataxia, tremor and hyper-reflexia, all of which require a reduction in dose.

Excess exercise and perspiration may alter the serum levels.

Anxiolytics (minor tranquillizers) The drugs, almost exclusively the benzodiazepines, can be used to treat short-term definite anxiety states as a first-aid measure. The main side-effects are drowsiness, poor co-ordination and impaired concentration. Longer-term treatment with benzodiazepines risks dependence in some patients and should be avoided.

Beta blockers can be used occasionally to treat the physical symptoms of anxiety such as tremor, sweating and tachycardia.

Hypnotics These can be used for the short-term treatment of insomnia. Continued use risks dependence, rebound insomnia and morning hangover.

Antidepressants There are various kinds which include tricyclics, monoamine oxidase inhibitors (MAOIs) and some other drugs used in the treatment of depression. Relevant side-effects here include postural hypotension, drowsiness, dizziness and often fatigue.

Anticonvulsants These are used to prevent seizures, and careful monitoring of the dosage is required until the fits are controlled or until there is a toxic effect.

The side-effects vary depending on the particular drugs. All commonly cause dizziness and drowsiness, some fatigue and ataxia and occasionally there may be parkinsonism/tremor, tardive dyskinesia, postural hypotension and hyper-reflexia. Some of the drugs are also likely to cause skin rashes.

Miscellaneous Anticholinergic drugs are used for treating the extra-pyramidal side-effects of the neuroleptics.

It is important that the physiotherapist is aware of the effects of these drugs as it may well be to her that the patient first reports any problems. The physiotherapist might observe in a patient a movement disorder or the fact that the patient seems to tire quickly when exercising.

Further information on the drugs used in psychiatry can be obtained either from the pharmacist in the hospital or from the *British National Formulary*.

THE MENTAL HEALTH ACT

One of the aims of this Act is to ensure that mentally ill and mentally handicapped patients have their rights regarding treatment, care and discharge observed.

There are various sections under which patients may be detained for assessment and treatment in hospital. The time varies from six hours to six months. Treatment in the context of this Act does not include physiotherapy, so therefore the patient has the right to refuse physiotherapy.

REFERENCES

Doyne, E. J. et al (1987). Running versus weight lifting in the treatment of depression. *Journal of Consulting and Clinical Psychology*, 55, 5, 748–54.

Harber, V. J. and Sutton, J. R. (1984). Endorphins and exercise. *Sports Medicine*, 1/2, 154–71.

McEwen, B. (1983). An evaluation of the need of the long-stay psychiatric patient for organized exercise. *Australian Journal of Physiotherapy*, 29, 6, 202–6.

Palmer, J., Vacc, N. and Epstein, J. (1988). Adult inpatient alcoholics: physical exercise as a treatment intervention. *Journal of Studies on Alcohol*, 49, 5, 418–21.

Williams, J. I. (1989). Illness behaviour to wellness behaviour. The 'School of Bravery' approach. *Physiotherapy*, 75, 1, 2–7.

BIBLIOGRAPHY

Atkinson, R. C., Atkinson, R. L. and Hilgard, E. R. (1981). *Introduction to Psychology*, 8th edition. Harcourt Brace Jovanovich, New York.

Berne, E. (1970). *Games People Play: Psychology of Human Relationships*. Penguin Books, Harmondsworth.

Dunkin, N. (1981). *Psychology for Physiotherapists*. The British Psychological Society and Macmillan Publishers Limited, London.

Hamilton, M. (rev.) (1984). *Fish's Outline of Psychiatry*, 4th edition. John Wright Limited, London.

Hare, M. (1986). *Physiotherapy in Psychiatry*. Heinemann Medical Books, London.

Hill, P. et al (eds.) (1986). *Essentials of Postgraduate Psychiatry*, 2nd edition. Grune and Stratton Limited, London.

Oldfield, S. (1983). *The Counselling Relationship*. Routledge, London.

Mechenbaum, D. (1987). *Coping with Stress*. Facts on File.

Stafford Clarke, D. and Smith, A. (1983). *Psychiatry for Students*, 6th edition. Unwin Hyman, London.

ACKNOWLEDGEMENTS

The author thanks the following for their advice and help in the preparation of this chapter:

Dr D. Rumball, Consultant Psychiatrist, Norwich Health Authority.

Mrs N. Hardy MCSP, Senior Physiotherapist, Hellesdon Hospital, Norwich.

Mr S. Bazire, Pharmacist, Mental Illness and Handicap Unit, Norwich Health Authority.

Mr A. Hadley MCSP, Senior Physiotherapist, Regional Forensic Unit, Norvic Clinic, St Andrew's Hospital, Norwich.

Chapter 24

Adult Mental Handicap

by M. E. JEFFERIES srp and J. M. MORGAN mcsp

Physiotherapy for mentally handicapped adults of all ages is an expanding field. Medical advances have increased the life-span of the profoundly handicapped, so a greater percentage of these people survive into adulthood.

The accent on community care means that people will be seen in many situations, home, adult training centres (ATCs), group homes, special care units, health centres or their equivalent. This policy also means that care for acute conditions will be given in general hospitals. A basic understanding of mental handicap, and the approach needed, is therefore necessary for physiotherapists working in other fields.

Ignorance leads to unnecessary fear. It is important to remember that however handicapped each patient is an individual and will respond to a caring approach.

HISTORICAL BACKGROUND

There has always been a distinction between those retarded from birth and those temporarily affected by madness. In England a statute of Edward I (1272–1307) distinguished between those 'born fools' and those 'temporarily mad'. The Victorians produced the Idiots Act 1886 for those handicapped from birth, and the Lunacy Act 1890 for the insane. These, with the 1913 Mental Deficiency Act, were mainly custodial and a more enlightened act was not passed until the Mental Health Act 1959. Recently, the Mental Health Act 1987 reflects the results obtained by a multidisciplinary approach resulting in most mentally handicapped persons being cared for in the community.

CRITERIA OF MENTAL HANDICAP

Social criteria have always been the principal boundary markers, but they are vague, being influenced by local conditions and support.

Factors to be considered include low intelligence, low standard of behaviour, and a poor achievement at peer group level.

Low intelligence

Although there are many drawbacks to intelligence quotient (IQ) testing, it has been found that of persons with an IQ below 50 and the most profound handicap, a very high proportion show demonstrable central nervous system (CNS) abnormality and are therefore capable of remarkable improvement with correct treatment.

Low social behaviour

It has been understood for years that deficiency of mind is not the same as intellectual deficiency although it includes it.

Poor achievement at peer level

There is difficulty in normal education and in finding work in an industrialized society.

The criteria of the American Association of Mental Deficiency
Mental retardation refers to sub-average general intellectual functioning which originates during the developmental period and is associated with impairment of one or more of the following:

1. Maturation – the rate of attaining self-help skills.
2. Learning – acquisition of achievements during school years.
3. Social adjustment – ability to maintain oneself in adult life, in community living, employment and conformity to accepted standards.

MENTAL HANDICAP

A person who is mentally handicapped does not develop in childhood as quickly as other children nor attain the full mental capacities of a normal adult. It can vary from the profound, associated with gross physical abnormalities, to the milder degree covering a wide spectrum ranging up to and merging into the normal.

Classification and terminology

The wording used varies from country to country as well as from time to time in the same country. In the US/Canada, the term *mentally retarded* is used. The World Health Organization (WHO) and the UK use the term *mentally handicapped*, but use different terminology for classification of the severity. The following table indicates the present (1988) terminology:

WHO Term 1986	IQ	Old term	Other term	UK Mental Health Acts 1959	1987
Profound	0–20	Idiot	Low grade	Severely subnormal	Severe mental impairment
Severe	20–35	Imbecile	Medium grade		
Moderate	35–50	Imbecile	Medium grade	Severely subnormal	Severe mental impairment
Mild	50–75	Feeble-minded	High grade	Subnormal and/or psychopathic	Mental impairment psychopathic disorder

MENTAL HEALTH ACT 1987

The new classification, while similar to the 1959 categories, has a new restrictive definition which gives it an important difference.

Severe mental impairment means a state of arrested or incomplete development of the mind, which includes severe impairment of intelligence and social functioning and is associated with abnormally aggressive or seriously irresponsible conduct on the part of the person concerned and severely mentally impaired shall be construed accordingly.

Mental impairment means a state of arrested or incomplete development of the mind not amounting to severe mental impairment, which includes significant impairment of intelligence and social functioning and is associated with abnormally aggressive or seriously irresponsible conduct on the part of the person concerned and mentally impaired shall be construed accordingly.

Psychopathic disorder means a persistent disorder or disability of mind, whether or not including significant impairment of intelligence, which results in abnormally aggressive or irresponsible conduct on the part of the person concerned.

All types of mental handicap can be aggravated by added physical and psychological problems, the most common ones being epilepsy, deafness, anxiety states and behavioural problems such as self-mutilation and pica.

The mentally handicapped person is also liable to contract any of the diseases found in the general public. Accidents are more common, due to lack of awareness and poor physique.

CAUSES OF MENTAL HANDICAP

Chromosomal abnormalities
Primary genetic disorders
Acquired conditions – pre-natal
                  – perinatal
                  – postnatal

Chromosomal abnormalities

Accurate identification of chromosomes became possible in 1956 and early descriptions allocated chromosomes in order of size. 1–23 similar pairs plus the X and Y sex chromosomes.

A number of chromosomal abnormalities have been demonstrated in syndromes associated with mental dementia abnormalities. They are an important group because, if the diagnosis is made by amniocentesis early enough in pregnancy, the mother can be offered an abortion. Should diagnosis be made postnatally it is accurate and gives a prognosis; it also determines the need for genetic counselling.

Down's syndrome (trisomy-21) is the commonest autosomal abnormality. There may be a completely extra chromosome at the 21 position, or part or the whole of another chromosome may be attached to one of the 21 pair giving a similar clinical picture. The frequency is 1:600 of all births equally male to female. The frequency increases with maternal age. Down's syndrome accounts for approximately one-third of all cases with an IQ of less than 50. Some of these people may develop sufficient intelligence to read and write, but the majority require supervision for life.

Trisomy involving the sex hormones produces a number of clinical entities, the commonest being:
XXY Klinefelter's syndrome: Male feminization.

XO Turner's syndrome: Female genital malformation and webbing of the neck.

Primary genetic disorders

Genetic disorders are of major importance in many forms of mental retardation; although the specific mechanism is not known, it is possible to show that their pattern of transmission follows Mendelian laws. It is of interest that some of these conditions have a unique biochemical abnormality, almost certainly in the primary structure of a specific protein coded by a specific portion of the genetic material. Antenatal diagnosis and counselling are important to prevent the birth of some conditions, while others need correct treatment from birth to prevent some abnormal clinical patterns developing.

At present, Duchenne type muscular dystrophy, Huntington's chorea and Friedreich's ataxia are untreatable, but phenylketonuria and congenital hypothyroidism (cretinism) are treatable.

Acquired conditions

Prenatal: The myth that the baby was safe within the uterus (womb) protected by the placental barrier has been destroyed, by the linking of cataract, deaf mutism and congenital hip dislocation (CHD) with rubella, or physical abnormality following the ingestion of thalido-mide by the mother.

It is also recognized that factors including the mother's health, the ingestion of drugs, including alcohol, smoking and x-ray exposure, can affect the fetus.

Perinatal: Anoxia from any cause during birth, including heavy sedation of the mother, or trauma due to a difficult or precipitate delivery causing intracranial bleeding are potent causes of handicap. Neonatal hypoglycaemia or ineffectively treated jaundice due to Rhesus (Rh) factor or any other reason can lead to mental handicap.

Postnatal: In early childhood infections, especially encephalitis and meningitis, can be followed by mental handicap. Bacterial meningitis may also lead to hydrocephalus.

Poisons such as lead ingested from old paint, or breathed in beside a busy road, can be associated with reduced levels of intellect. Non-accidental injuries can cause permanent physical and mental handicap.

Finally, the lack of early stimulation is more adverse where the IQ is near the 50 level. A normal child will produce its own stimulus.

PHYSICAL AND NEUROLOGICAL ASSESSMENT

Today, treatment is multidisciplinary. Besides specific physio-therapeutic techniques, it is the role of the physiotherapist to educate other disciplines, giving practical, sensible guidance and support to the parents and key workers. Accurate reassessment monitors the efficiency of, or need to amend, the regime. (It is assumed that the reader understands the motor development of children from birth to five years (see Chapter 20) and the development of neurological reactions.)

Before beginning the assessment, the patient should be with some-one he knows and trusts. Use a quiet warm room, free from noise or distraction; mat roll, wedge, tape-measure and goniometer should be at hand. The patient should be wearing the minimum of clothing, trunks for men, bra and pants for women.

The first assessment may not be a true guide to the condition and it may take several sessions to obtain a true picture. Some form of record must be kept (Fig. 24/1). This is meant to be of use to all carers, not just the physiotherapist.

Use of the chart

General appearance: Consider the look of the patient. Does he look happy? Sad? Contented? Miserable? How does the parent or carer relate to him? Fussily or quietly supportive? It is as well here to spend a few moments settling both patient and parent/carer into a quiet frame of mind; as well as allowing a chance to make an evaluation of how the parent or carer will respond to advice about treatment in the future.

Head: Look at head control, remembering that it is the key to good posture.

Spine: Note curvatures. Time will increase abnormalities unless specific treatment is given.

Upper and lower limbs: These are examined for joint movements, type of muscle tone present or any deformity.

Reflexes: In mental handicap, besides the normal spinal reflexes, the primitive and pathological tonic reflexes are also assessed.
 The primitive reflexes are:

- Primary standing
- Automatic walking
- Sucking and rooting
- Placing reaction
- Moro or startle reflex.

PHYSIOTHERAPY ASSESSMENT

Date of Assessment: *Consultant:*
Name: *Date of Birth:*
Ward: *Home Address:*

History and Diagnosis   E.P. Yes/No   I.Q.

General Appearance

Head Control
Spine
Rib Cage
Upper Limbs
  Right Arm
  Shoulder
  Elbow
  Forearm
  Wrist & Hand
  Left Arm
  Shoulder
  Elbow
  Forearm
  Wrist & Hand

Lower Limbs
  Right Leg
  Hip
  Knee
  Ankle
  Foot
  Left Leg
  Hip
  Knee
  Ankle
  Foot
Prone Lying
Sight & Hearing
Reflexes   Moro Reflex
         Asymmetrical Neck Reflex
         Symmetrical Neck Reflex
         Parachute Reflex
         Patella Reflex Rt.   Left
         Babinski   Rt.   Left
Sensation

Postural and Locomotor Development

Basic Activities

Ambulant Gait

Balance and Co-ordination

Volition and Response to Command

Functional Activities

Walking Aids/Wheelchairs

General Conclusions

Assessor

Fig. 24/1   Assessment form

Modification of these plays an important part in some treatment regimes.

The pathological tonic neck reflexes are:

1. *Labyrinthine tonic reflex*: In supine there is increased extensor activity in all groups. In prone there is increased flexor activity.
2. *Asymmetrical tonic neck reflex*: If the head is turned to the side, the arm on the same side extends while the opposite arm flexes. Therefore there will be feeding difficulties. The patient is unable to bring the hands together in the mid-line, is unable to get the hands to the mouth, and is in danger of developing scoliosis.
3. *The symmetrical neck reflex*: This produces changes of distribution of tonus in the arms and legs. In the prone position, if the head is raised, the arms extend and the legs flex. If the head is flexed, the arms collapse and the legs extend. This is very similar to a cat drinking. The patient has difficulty in taking up an all-fours position and will be unable to crawl properly. This may cause him to sit back on his heels with contractures developing as a result.

A mention here of the *parachute* or protective extension of the arms reaction. This is a saving reaction which has to be developed in the sideways, forward and backward directions.

Functional assessment shows what the patient can or cannot do and the way in which it is done. The section on aids and wheelchairs is a reminder to consider the patient's present and future needs.

To sum up, the data should reflect an accurate assessment of the patient's present position and enable a plan for treatment to be drawn up for the physiotherapist and key workers. This should aid and sustain maximum development of the individual.

Sensory deprivation

The profoundly handicapped frequently have additional sensory loss. The type and degree of deprivation can only be assessed by observation over a long period, and the correlation of information from all sources.

Sight: The loss of sight ranges from myopia to total blindness. Lesser defects may be suspected by observing:

– The distance at which objects are held.
– Are they held to one side as in hemiopia?
– Is the head held in a position to allow a forward field of vision?
– Is attention held only in a limited central field of vision, as in tunnel vision?

Developmental defects of the eye obviously lead to blindness; where the eyes and optic nerves are physiologically intact but the information cannot be processed, there is central blindness. Eye poking is often seen in this condition.

Hearing: Partial or total hearing loss may be suspected in severely handicapped individuals. However, lack of response to name may be due to lack of comprehension or central deafness. If there is no response to sound, the help of a speech therapist should be sought in the first place.

Poor speech can be allied to hearing loss. Comprehension but no speech due to motor aphasia can be helped in several ways. If signing is used the speech therapist can help with teaching the signs to those involved with the person. A communication board may be used; in co-operation with the speech therapist, the physiotherapist should help in attaining the optimum position for the arm or arms. This is important in the use of the board, and so head control is vital where eye pointing is the best method of communication.

Matching games help discrimination, short-term memory, attention span, hand–eye co-ordination, colour and even counting.

Body image: Particularly in hemiplegia, the body image is of one side only. Where the physical signs are slight the reluctance to walk through doors or other narrow spaces, learned by striking door posts, may be put down to behaviour problems. Careful questioning of the carers is required to discover the real cause. Many mentally handicapped people cannot tell left from right or mirror copy. This can be due to lack of body image or the development stage reached.

It is only by acute and prolonged observation that sensory defects or combination of defects can be established. Treatment for other conditions must be decided in the light of any sensory loss present.

PHYSIOTHERAPY

Many forms of physiotherapy may be required to treat general diseases that affect the mentally handicapped, although traditional treatments may need modification, and to encourage the maturation of the incompletely developed brain a number of specialist regimes have been devised.

Treatment aims

1. To suppress abnormal patterns which prevent progress towards a more normal state, remembering that development unfolds in a sequential pattern.
2. To facilitate alternative pathways of movement.
3. To control gross motor function, thus encouraging normal movements.
4. To improve hand–eye co-ordination needed for manipulative skill.
5. To maintain as normal a posture as possible, preventing contractures.
6. To produce therapy that is interesting and so improve both physical and mental well-being.
7. To give advice to key workers and relatives that will help maintain and progress the patient's achievements.

Acute Conditions   The ills of the population at large are also the ills of those who are mentally handicapped. The aims of treatment are the same as those for anyone else, except the approach has to be varied according to the degree of handicap.

History-taking from the moderately handicapped can have pitfalls. In an effort to please, a positive answer may be given to every question. There may be echolalia (parroting). Indication of pain may also be unreliable, moving rapidly around the body. The cause of this may, in part, be due to lack of comprehension, lack of body image or inability to name the parts of the body correctly.

Where the handicap is severe, with no comprehension or speech, the history must be elicited from the carers. They may know the reason for distress, tears. Is it pain, rage, frustration or attention-seeking? Note the reaction to handling, increase in tone, flinching, etc.

Treatments

With those who are moderately handicapped, the goodwill of the patient must be gained. In some cases, the physiotherapist will be well known by the patient. If not, time will be needed to achieve rapport. Where possible, have a relative, friend or carer present for the first few sessions. Explain what is being done and why.

The volition to co-operate fully may be absent, and treatment needs to be continued longer than normal. The patient may have short-term memory loss and be unable to remember the regime. There may be no time sense but meal times can be used as reference points for performing exercise regimes. Where available, those caring for the individual must be carefully instructed in the regime to be followed.

The multihandicapped person with a chest infection presents a challenge, especially where there are gross spinal and rib cage deformities, with rigidity. The patient is unable to co-operate, so the active principle must be applied to the patient. Careful positioning with the use of wedges, pillows, allied with active shaking, may start the cough reflex. A mechanical vibrator is of great assistance in these cases. Where sputum is produced, if the developmental age is less than five years, it will lie at the back of the mouth, and may need removal by suction.

Following epileptic seizures, trauma can occur. In the non-ambulant patient there is poor calcification and fragility of the bones, especially the femur when the fracture site is usually at the junction of the lower and middle-third of the shaft. Where the individual is normally ambulant mobilization may be difficult following a lower limb fracture or a period of non-weight-bearing. Firmness, patience and perseverance are needed, while suitable rewards for attempting to stand and walk may be the answer.

Splinting This form of treatment is useful for the prevention and correction of deformity and also in the distressing condition of self-mutilation, the causes of which are many and not fully understood.

The physiotherapist may be approached to help with splinting and the material used should be effective but not in itself damaging. The heat-formed foam-type materials with carefully placed reinforcement appear best.

An example of splinting being of use is where the individual repeatedly strikes the eyes, ears or face. At best, repeated cuts around the eyes result, at worst detached retinas. The ears suffer repeated haematomas (the boxer's cauliflower ear) and hearing loss can follow. By splinting the elbows in an extended position, the hands can still be used, but the eyes cannot be struck with the fists, the ears and face are protected by the soft material, and the force which can be exerted reduced. In some cases, the behaviour will reduce or disappear. The psychologist has an important role to play in behaviour change, and the physiotherapist should be aware of, and continue, any regime.

Hyperactivity When the mentally handicapped person is also hyperactive treatment for other conditions presents difficulties. Postural drainage will need help to maintain the position. The distractability and very short attention span indicates short treatment sessions, with interspersed rest periods.

Firmness during sessions is important, so that each small step towards the final target is achieved. This may take a long period. When a new target is set, the previous attainments must be maintained.

Special Forms of Treatment Most special forms of treatment rely on progressive patterning movements with inhibition of primitive and abnormal tonic reflexes. Some treatments may cause discomfort and apparent distress to the patient, therefore it is important that the physiotherapist fully understands the reasoning behind the treatment so that she is able to explain the method, and the advantage gained, to parents and other carers. Failure to do so might lead to misunderstanding and suggestion of cruelty. It is advisable for the physiotherapist to have postgraduate experience of the method she intends using. Some of these methods are:

- *Temple-Fay*: Progressive movement patterning.
- *Kabat*: Mass movement patterning with a diagonal direction and the use of sensory afferent stimuli to initiate movement.
- *Bobath*: Reflex inhibition and muscular facilitation (see p.393).
- *Rood*: Developmental sequences of respiration, sucking, swallowing and speech. Brushing techniques and ice therapy are also used.

- *Vojta*: Reflex creeping patterns.
- *Doman-Delacato*: Homo-lateral patterning.
- *Peto*: Conductive education (see p.393).

Hydrotherapy The importance of this treatment in mental handicap is now widely recognized. These patients enjoy the same advantages of warmth and alleviation of body weight as anyone else. There is a reduction of spasticity and the ability to perform active exercises that would be impossible on dry land.

In some cases a hyperactive individual is helped by pool sessions. Adequate staff must be available to ensure the safety of both the individual and the staff. A high level of activity in warm water leads to relaxation later.

In the authors' opinion, hydrotherapy gives confidence, enjoyment and fellowship. It aids individual movements and allows mass patterns of movement to be initiated.

Riding for the Disabled (see Chapter 25) This is a valid form of treatment. There is an improvement in balance aided by the interaction between horse and rider. The increased muscular development of the pelvic region and thigh muscles aids incontinence. The self-image is improved; it is often the first time that wheelchair users find themselves looking down on others. The unusual environment produces an exciting stimulus.

Additional treatments

Drama, art and play therapy are all part of the recognized treatments available to those who are mentally handicapped. They should lead into the next level of developmental activity and increased movements, and be happy experiences. The physiotherapist can obtain specialized catalogues to help in the selection of suitable apparatus and aids.

MUSIC

The initiation of active treatment is made difficult by the lack of understanding, communication difficulties and the reduced power of concentration inherent in some mentally handicapped patients. In this situation, movement associated with music is found very rewarding. The constant repetition of a movement to popular music, usually a song or nursery rhyme, becomes accepted and remembered by the patients, producing both pleasure and treatment. Meanwhile, they are not aware that a fully structured treatment is being carried out.

In the profoundly handicapped, music may be applied to individual treatments or group therapy. When used individually, it often involves the use of percussion instruments, drums, tambourines, etc. on a one-to-one basis, the hands of the therapist guiding the patient's hands to produce the range of movement required. In group therapy, the music sets the mood and pace of the exercises to be performed. Music increases motivation, co-ordination and sense of well-being. It stimulates social development, concentration span and learning capacity.

Group treatment

Moderate Handicap The aims of the groups must be tailored to fit the needs and abilities of the individuals in the group. The staffing levels should reflect this. Music is essential to most groups. Close co-operation with a music therapist, where one is in post, is ideal. Generally, taped music has to be used. The choice should be carefully made, relating to the reaction times of the group, the activity and the mood being set. The tapes should be pre-set to the start point, and be in correct order. The cassette player should be simple to operate, robust and suit the room being used. Ideally, one person should operate the player while the leader prepares the group for the next activity. Equipment, like the cassette, should be robust. Balls, where used, should be the soft foam type, in various sizes and bounce. Colourful parachutes are expensive, but sheets firmly stitched together make a good substitute. Skipping ropes, hula hoops, bean bags, skittles, floor games are all useful and ingenuity will find other equipment or substitutes.

The group should be held in a suitable area, free from distraction at an agreed time and day. Where possible involve the carers in the group.

The Overactive A small group is most suitable. The aim should be to achieve stillness and relaxation. The first goal should be to gain attention. At the commencement of the course, the members may wander aimlessly, leave the room or interfere with the equipment. Use quiet music, encourage the members to stay in the room and be still. Movement can then be introduced, using physical guidance at first, and gradually withdrawing the prompt as the movements are learnt. End the session with lying still on the floor. One-to-one staffing may be needed; very disruptive members may need to be excluded from time to time. The mood of the group will vary; don't despair that you have failed – next time may be totally different. The progress of the group and the individuals should be monitored and recorded at regular intervals.

Moderate to Mild Handicap   Many of this group have poor musculature and posture. Their self-image is poor and their reaction times slower than normal. The overall aim of the group should be physical improvement, enhanced self-image, confidence and co-operation. The group should enjoy the activities.

As with the hyperactive group, the music should be carefully chosen to suit the reaction time of the members and the mood the leader wishes to set. A fast rhythm cannot be achieved by many of this group. Favourite tunes will emerge and can be used as incentives. Sequences of movement have to be taught step by step; achieve step one before teaching step two. Add on and then progress onwards. Speed and difficulty can be increased over a period of time.

One of the group may perform an exercise well – encourage him/her to lead the group in this exercise to increase self-esteem. Be careful to involve as many of the group in this activity as possible.

To foster co-operation, ball and passing games are excellent. Parachute activities involve the whole group. Monitor and record progress.

SEATING AND POSTURE

Posture and seating for the multi-handicapped are vital from the earliest days. Monitoring and adjustment must be continued throughout life. A wide and up-to-date knowledge of the types and sizes of chairs available is essential. Some occupational therapists specialize in this type of seating, and their help should be sought.

The following remarks apply to all chairs, furnishing or wheelchair. The size of the chair should fit the person using it. A matching set of chairs in a room may look superb, but fit none of the residents, leading to poor posture and increasing deformity.

Criteria for fitting a chair

Seat depth:	Back of knee to back minus 5cm
Seat width:	Hip width plus 7.5cm
Height. Floor or footrest:	Heel to back of knee minus 5cm
Back height:	To crown of head
Armrest:	Elbow supported at right angle

All measurements are taken in the sitting position.

Problems arising

With the non-ambulant patient, the hips and legs are often small in relation to the torso (hindquarter disproportion). In such cases, the width of the chair should be reduced by using firm cushions which must be attached to the chair so they do not slip. If the seat is too long, again a firm cushion can be used, reaching from the seat to the top of the chair.

Too wide a seat encourages side sitting, leading to windswept hips and scoliosis. Where the seat is too long, the legs may be drawn up, to relieve the pressure on the calves. Alternatively, the buttocks may be slid forward, resulting in kyphosis and head poking.

The hips may also be slid forward by spasm or as a behaviour pattern. A lap strap at hip level prevents this and is more comfortable than groin straps.

Where trunk control is poor, backward tilting of the whole chair may help. Side flexion is aided by the use of supportive pads at the back of the chair.

Where there is gross spinal and hip deformity, a moulded seat is required. In the UK these are now supplied by the Disablement Services Authority and are fitted to issued wheelchairs. As with any equipment the moulds must be carefully monitored for fit and wear.

However carefully a chair or mould is selected and fitted, unless the user is correctly placed in it, the posture will be wrong. All those caring for the user must be carefully instructed in the correct positioning of supports and user.

Lifting and Moving   The general principles of lifting and moving should be used by all those handling the multi-handicapped, but where the deformity is severe, the physiotherapist may be asked for help. Thought and skill must be applied to solving the problem on an individual basis.

In addition, the physiotherapist should teach the carers how to handle the individual so that lifting or moving is achieved in the safest manner.

The treatment of the multi-handicapped by physiotherapy is interesting, demanding and often intuitive. One may be treating an adult with the understanding and reactions of a child. Treatments often have to be presented in an enjoyable form but must not be allowed to sink into meaningless exercises. Tact, understanding and compassion are important in helping the patients, carers and key workers.

BIBLIOGRAPHY

Carr, J. (1979). *Early Care of the Stroke Patient*. William Heinemann Medical Books Limited, London.

DHSS. *Better Services for the Mentally Handicapped*. HMSO, London.

DHSS. *Wheelchair Handbook*. HMSO, London.

Hari, M. and Akos, K. (1989). *Conductive Education*. Routledge, London.

Heaton-Ward, W. (1975). *Mentally Subnormal*, 4th edition. Wright Books, London.

Mental Health Act 1987. HMSO, London.

Illingworth, R.S. (1987). *The Development of the Infant and Young Child*, 9th edition. Churchill Livingstone, Edinburgh.

Morgan, J.M. (1985). Musical route to laughter and increased self-confidence. *Therapy Weekly*, October 17, 7.

Tredgold's Mental Retardation, 12th edition. (1979). Baillière Tindall, London.

Wood, M. (1982). *Music for Living*. British Institute of Mental Handicap, Kidderminster.

ACKNOWLEDGEMENT

The authors thank Dr J.H. Morgan for his help with the sections relating to the Mental Health Acts, historical background and the causes of mental handicap.

Chapter 25

Riding for the Disabled

by S. SAYWELL MA, FCSP

Riding for disabled persons whether with physical, mental or mixed disabilities, emerged in the later years of the anterior poliomyelitis epidemic which swept through Great Britain and Scandinavia during the 1940–50 period. Much dedication from physiotherapists, working with the medical profession, was required to maintain clear airways and lung function for those victims of respiratory paralysis. These life-saving efforts demanded and received day and night attention seven days a week. This total involvement of physiotherapists in the field of intensive care left little opportunity for the treatment of sub-clinical and ambulant clinical patients who required advice, supervised exercises and a programme of progressive rehabilitation. It was this group of poliomyelitis victims whose plight alerted certain married physiotherapists, who were not free to offer their professional services to hospitals, but whose young children had ponies, to consider riding as an effective treatment programme. Physiotherapists owning suitable ponies, or with riding experience, also used their animals and skills to provide greater mobility for partially paralysed children. The determination and resourcefulness of those early workers created another limb of programmed progressive exercises, mobility and motivation from which have developed international organizations for riding for the disabled in many countries.

This chapter sets out to introduce physiotherapists to this useful form of exercise and recreation for disabled persons. It will show how accepted methods of treatments such as Bobath, Petö and others can be adapted and used with the patient mounted. It will also discuss the need for pony suitability. The application of such techniques in certain conditions is fully described.

PHILOSOPHY

The declared aim of the Riding for the Disabled Association (RDA) is to give an opportunity for any disabled person, who wishes to do so, to ride, as a means of benefiting his general well-being. The range

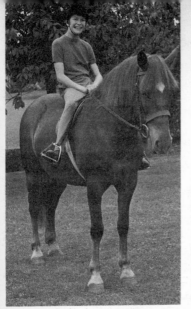
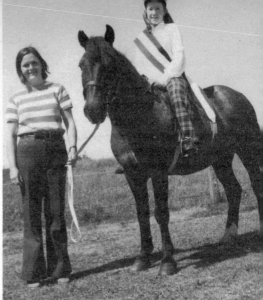

Fig. 25.1 An athetoid girl. Note the use of a safety stirrup

Fig. 25.2 The rider is a spina bifida who is wearing below-knee calipers. This is a perfect example of the right size of pony for its rider

of disabilities among those who are now enjoying this opportunity is remarkable (Figs 25/1 and 25/2).

The age-range falls mainly between the school-age child and those in the late fifties and above, for whom the benefits are as great as for children. Many of the adults have ridden in all types of equestrian events before becoming victims of accidents or disease. Such riders may require a period in which to assess their riding ability and find, for themselves, local RDA groups who may provide an opportunity to take up the reins again. These groups provide the ideal atmosphere for them to make their decisions and, where necessary, the adaptations and alterations which allow for years of enjoyable riding. Other chronically disabled adults and young people, especially school leavers, join riding for the disabled sessions to gain mobility, exercise and a leisure activity in which friendships may be formed among a wide group of both able-bodied and disabled contemporaries.

The structure of RDA groups includes both professional and knowledgeable lay helpers. A *riding instructor*, who may hold professional qualifications, or be a very experienced instructor in the Pony Club, is the acknowledged leader at the riding session. The main element in all groups is the *voluntary helper* who works with the instructor and chartered physiotherapist. The voluntary helper will (1) translate instruction to the rider, allowing each individual to gain as much independence as possible during the riding session; (2) help the rider achieve maximum correct range of movement when special exercises are selected; and (3) report any particular problem arising either from the rider, the saddlery or unexpected reactions of the pony.

The general turnout and appearance is important for all members of the group; suitable clothing and sturdy shoes are as essential for helpers as the regulation hard hat is for the rider.

All RDA affiliated groups are covered by adequate insurance policies and chartered physiotherapists in full work are protected by their membership. Chartered physiotherapists who offer help and who are not working can enrol with the Chartered Society of Physiotherapy's clinical interest section, Riding for the Disabled, when insurance cover at low cost becomes available.

For the physiotherapist to give the maximum benefit of her professional training to riders in RDA groups an ability to ride, or, at least, to experience the movements of the horse, is essential. Group instruction will help in providing basic riding lessons for this purpose, but all physiotherapists working with disabled riders should check, by observation, the instruction and progress of a *normal* rider. Attendance at ordinary classes of beginners and novice riders, under a good riding instructor, will provide an excellent introduction. The method of suiting rider to the pony/horse can be studied; the placing of each rider and pony in the ride to give maximum benefit to the whole class; the safety procedures; the management of classes of mixed riding skills; and methods of dealing with a variety of temperaments within the class can be observed and understood: all of which is to be recommended strongly.

Parents of disabled children are usually most concerned with sitting balance, standing, and taking some steps; riding can provide the motivation to acquire these skills – although more slowly, as normal chronological progressions are not applicable. Home exercises, an example of which is shown in Fig. 25/3, can be taught to parents to enhance the riding positions; they should be revised continuously. An excellent range of mounted exercises is to be found in the RDA Handbook, pages 78–85. Those most suitable and helpful to the individual rider can be selected and adapted in order to maintain and improve at home those skills which have been achieved in the saddle. It is sometimes necessary to restrain the over-enthusiastic parent from a too vigorous approach to home exercises. The acquisition of sitting balance frees the use of hands and arms for more functional activities, and appears to be more readily obtained by riding than any other activity.

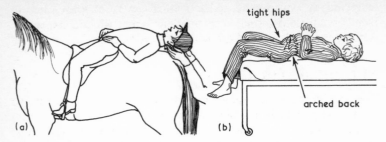

Fig. 25.3 (a) Stretching exercise (only to be used when the pony is accustomed to this type of activity); (b) home exercise showing the postural difficulties which require attention

Physical activity leads to mental activity even in those who are most severely intellectually impaired. The results of introducing riding to this group of disabled persons are exciting with much encouraging feedback coming spontaneously from parents, teachers and attendants who notice the changes in the individual rider. This may be simply a recognition of the riding day by putting on a hard hat, but it may result in greater independence of movement, improved social behaviour and general health. The physiotherapist will note the build-up of muscle tone (often low in the mentally handicapped person) and improved co-ordination of limbs and body movement. The clumsy child will show the same improvement. Those riders with previous problems of mobility, especially spina bifida or similar conditions, are provided with exercises and incentives to achieve mobility from the pony in stages: beginning with a simple walk forward, steering and stopping, to advanced and increasing balancing movements at varied paces with changes of direction within those paces. Class work gives ample opportunity to achieve goals, however simple, by creating a happy encouraging atmosphere, as well as experiencing the enjoyment of working together. This latter is often denied the disabled person who more usually is an individual within a group and rarely is a team member.

One aspect of handling disabled riders that is often overlooked, is the *natural* ability that many possess and which *can* be developed to give such riders opportunities to compete with able-bodied peers; or, alas, stifled by over-protectiveness. The physiotherapist can instil into group members professional views, give encouragement, create confidence and promote the principle of *keep trying*. The opposite is also true: when a rider who has a progressive disease is no longer able to benefit, the physiotherapist with her professional knowledge can recommend other activities. Such advice expressed with authority tempered by sympathetic understanding can be of great value to members of groups when such problems arise, who otherwise can become confused, worried and feel they have failed.

THE PHYSIOTHERAPIST

The link between the pony/horse and disabled rider presents an exciting challenge for the physiotherapist who is able to select from accepted methods of teaching patterns of movement those most suited to each rider, and adapt them to the individual rider's ability and potential. The opportunities for studying the principles of dynamic balance, co-ordination and acquisition of general agility offer the physiotherapist a series of projects (not as yet fully researched), which may lead to a change of conventional thought and traditional teaching, useful in the management of a variety of disabilities and in the appreciation of basic riding instruction for both able-bodied and disabled persons.

The Physiological Impact of Riding is Almost Immeasurable

The physiotherapist is well adapted to motivating patients, their families or guardians towards achieving seemingly impossible goals. She can therefore develop and encourage these skills through riding, by coaxing the timid to attempt a mobility for which they may lack the necessary mental or physical equipment; dampen the exhausting and unwelcome energies of the hyperactive; give opportunities for character training; enjoy socializing; and assist in the emergence of memory and retained instruction, all of which overflows into the activities of daily living.

Riding Offers a Lifetime of Opportunity to Acquire that Perfect Partnership with a Horse

This is enriching, not only in the satisfaction of achieving many skills, but also in the friendship formed by mutual affection and respect for horses. Once the basic skills of starting, stopping, steering at walk, trot and, often, canter, are acquired, the pony/horse then becomes the therapist.

Points of observation

Aims

1. To enable relevant advice to be given to the rider to improve posture and position (when he is able to appreciate this) by the instructor through lay helpers (through the instructor or by

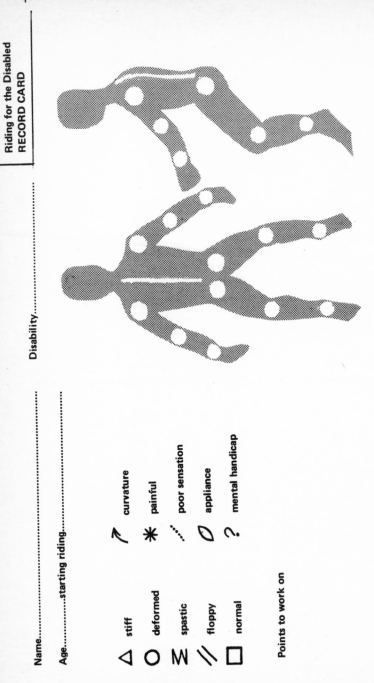

Fig. 25.4 Record card showing both sides. Produced by the CSP special interest group

RIDING ABILITY (continued)

DATE					
Mounting – unaided					
from block, ramp, pit					
from ground with help					
Walk – led					
free					
no. of helpers					
Trot – led					
free					
sitting					
rising					
no. of helpers					
Canter – led					
free					
no. of helpers					
Jumping – free					
no. of helpers					
Independent – school					
Control – field					

OTHER REMARKS

ADDITIONAL DATA — x, , number

DATE					
Cannot walk					
Walks with – calipers					
crutches					
sticks					
unaided					
Climbs steps					
Wheelchair					
Speech					
Sight					
Hearing					
Social					

RIDING ABILITY

Wheelchair transfer					
Aided – no. of helpers					
Lifting – one					
two					
three					

TYPE OF PONY

SPECIAL TACK

TESTS PASSED

Fig. 25·4 Record card showing both sides. Produced by the CSP special interest group

Printed by City Printing Works Ltd., Chester-le-Street

arrangement with the instructor).
2. To select possible corrections from application of physiotherapy techniques.
3. To encourage physical and mental targets towards a progressive improvement in riding skills. (Note: All those engaged in the active riding session should appreciate these progressive targets.)
4. Recording progress (Fig. 25/4).

Points	Aim	Suggested action
Head	Desired control	Steadiness (reflex action through trot work)
Arms	Independent action damping unwanted movement	Bobath/proprioceptive neuromuscular facilitation (PNF) techniques (Fig. 25/5)
Hands	Control of spasticity	Teach helpers correct grasps to hold fingers and wrist. Where to place hand slightly behind saddle and in what position
Seat	Central position and upright. Observe from in front, from the side and most importantly from behind the pony (Fig. 25/6). (Describe and illustrate normal result of sitting to one side)	Accept flexion of hip and shorter stirrup-leather length to gain upright position. Then reduce hip flexion and gain leg length
	Avoid pressure areas	Rising trot helps; or allow push-ups from saddle at appropriate intervals. Pressure changes occur naturally when instructor orders seat corrections
Hips	Relaxed, and angle with body as open as possible. Note: Leg length should come from hip	Exercises to reduce hip flexion contracture
Leg	↓ Extensor spasm	Reduce by appropriate physiotherapy
	↓ Adductor spasm	Riding without stirrups. Choice of pony/saddle by instructor. Note: Warmth of pony is also beneficial

Knees	Away from saddle	No gripping Helper to steady position
Lower leg	Hang from knee lightly against pony's side	Helper involvement. Teach correct holds (RDA Handbook, p. 40).
Heels	Lower than toe when condition will allow	Teach helpers correct physiological holds
Lumbar spine	Loose and supple	Corrections by appropriate exercises in all movement planes (RDA Handbook, pp. 78/86). Avoid stiffness and hollowing (Fig. 25/7)
Feet	Pointing forward	Correction from hips and directed by helper
	Avoid clonus	Discuss with instructor position of foot in stirrup iron. Riding for periods without stirrups
Note: Breathing	Asthma and allied conditions	Alert organizer. Rider should bring appropriate medication to the lesson. Remove rider from dusty conditions to recover/ remount

Remember: Hidden value of exercises, particularly in non-elimination games, in achieving success with rider's position. Freedom of movement. Avoid clinical assessments. Make exercises enjoyable. **The object is fun!**

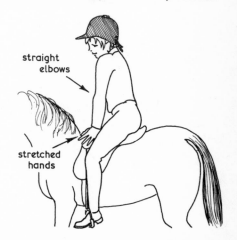

straight
elbows

stretched
hands

Fig. 25.5 A corrective position; taking weight through the hemiplegic arm

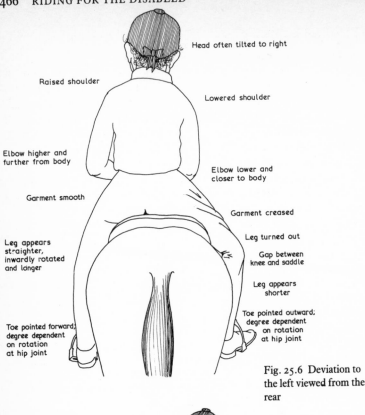

Head often tilted to right

Raised shoulder

Lowered shoulder

Elbow higher and
further from body

Elbow lower and
closer to body

Garment smooth

Garment creased

Leg appears
straighter,
inwardly rotated
and longer

Leg turned out

Gap between
knee and saddle

Leg appears
shorter

Toe pointed forward;
degree dependent
on rotation
at hip joint

Toe pointed outward;
degree dependent
on rotation
at hip joint

Fig. 25.6 Deviation to
the left viewed from the
rear

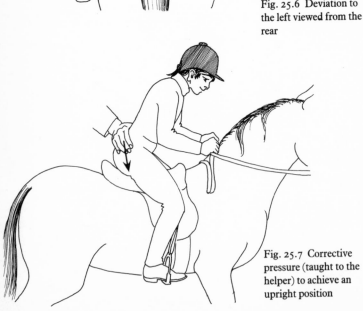

Fig. 25.7 Corrective
pressure (taught to the
helper) to achieve an
upright position

CEREBRAL PALSY

The result of a lesion or mal-development of the brain, i.e. non-progressive in character and existing from early childhood, is one of the most difficult groups of disability. The motor deficit in abnormal patterns of movement and posture is enormously varied, emphasizing to professional and lay helpers alike the danger of classifying disabilities under standard headings (Fig. 25/8). Medical research requires classification of disabilities for easy reference. However, for sport and competitive events, riders will know their own level, and train and enter for events of their choice. Instructors, trainers and therapists working together can advise on how the appropriate standard could be achieved; also which event is most suited to the rider's current skill and ability. Disabled riders demand

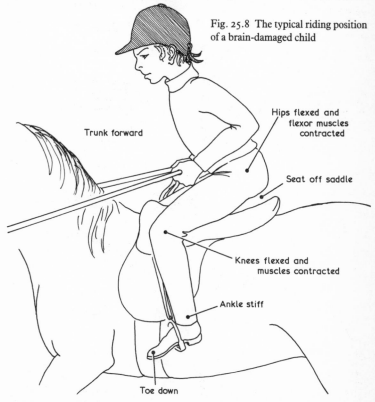

Fig. 25.8 The typical riding position of a brain-damaged child

Trunk forward

Hips flexed and flexor muscles contracted

Seat off saddle

Knees flexed and muscles contracted

Ankle stiff

Toe down

competition, which allows opportunities to be successful in their chosen activity, particularly when this leads to open competition with able-bodied horsemen and women, where the difference is often indistinguishable.

A good knowledge of normal child development and posture is required. An alert eye and constant observation will then show the therapist what is wrong in the movement and posture of riding pupils.

Each rider must be assessed as an individual. The focus of attention is the movement of the pelvis. Only if the pelvis can move freely will the rider be able to follow the movement of the horse – which is the basis of all horsemanship (Podhajsky, 1967; Watjen, 1979).

The work of the Bobaths first drew attention to the manner in which parents and friends could give the child the best opportunities for developing his capabilities, however limited they might be. The advent of the roller, large bouncing ball and the equilibrium board in producing three-dimensional movement in balance, provided an excellent stimulus to both patient and physiotherapist, offering greater input of reflex action by more intensive, continuous and faster repetitions than could formerly be maintained by the physiotherapist or accepted by the patient (Finnie, 1974).

These changing positions provided by roll, ball and board formed an appropriate basis for horse riding and allayed the fears of those solely engaged in Bobath techniques who quite naturally objected in the early years to sports or activities which might negate the desirable movement patterns. Two decades ago this was a real objection, often expressed, which led in some cases to rejection of riding by professionals and parents. Fortunately, by inviting those genuine objectors to riding sessions and demonstrating the incorporation of Bobath techniques into the exercise and riding programme, their fears were proved unfounded.

Problems arising when riding

Unsteady head position, particularly at the trot: Although this can be a matter of concern to spectators and riding instructors, the physiotherapist can give positive reassurance that only normal postural reflexes are involved and no restriction in the form of collars or splintage should be considered.

Sitting balance: For the young child, sitting astride the parent's lap is an essential position for acquiring sitting balance, damping out the tendency to straighten the hips and turn legs in. If the base is too

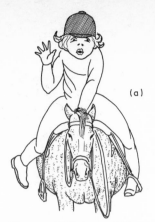
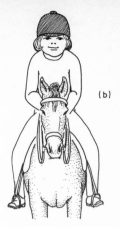

Fig. 25.9 (a) Unhappy child on too broad a base; (b) the same rider correctly mounted

broad, however, the position becomes exaggerated, a point to be discussed with the riding instructor who may have the opportunity to acquire a pony of the most suitable size for the rider (Fig. 25/9). This is not always a simple matter – best use has to be made of the availability of ponies which, in most British groups, are supplied voluntarily by their owners. Adjustment to saddlery – or the use of the vaulting pad – may be the answers for the beginner rider.

Observation by the therapist, and discussion with the instructor will be valuable when such problems arise. From this astride position, the correct riding seat can be encouraged and acquired, the arms and head controlled and a good functional position obtained for progress into achieving forward movement with the pony. The co-operation of parents and friends will be readily obtained once this riding position is explained, and exercises for use at home taught to reinforce and enhance this basic broad base from which balance can be obtained (see Fig. 25/3b).

VALUE OF VAULTING OR VOLTIGIEREN

Despite the daunting title introductory vaulting can be used in ordinary RDA sessions. It provides:

– Development of spring
– Strengthening of arms and shoulders
– Control of lower part of body
– Increase in suppleness and flexibility of the body
– General fitness
– Team spirit.

This activity can be carried out all the year round and is also useful if only one pony is available, provided the animal is strong, has a wide back, powerful hocks, a calm temperament and experience with vaulters. The local Pony Club members may provide such a mount. RDA has provided guidelines (RDA Ring Binder (Green Binder) Sec. D., Subsection 10) for groups intending to start vaulting sessions and recommends before selecting physically handicapped riders the group physiotherapist should be consulted.

It is important to understand the difference between *therapeutic vaulting* using the vaulting girth and *hippotherapy* as practised in Germany and Switzerland and becoming increasingly used in Great Britain by chartered physiotherapists. Therapeutic vaulting is entirely under the control and supervision of medically qualified personnel using the horse as a piece of mobile equipment.

Introductory vaulting builds up self-esteem, concentration, can diminish aggression and is of great value in the management of the autistic child or young person, the maladjusted child, Down's syndrome and those with behavioural problems.

Vaulting Pad The vaulting roller or girth has two handles set at an angle – one on either side. The handles stand away from the horse because of the padding underneath the roller. A *thick* piece of foam, approximately 30cm (12in) wide and 1.2m (4ft) long underneath the roller absorbs the pressure. In the centre of the roller is a long strap to help balance beginners. The girth buckles can be covered by a soft leather protector or a short girth used to prevent interference to the vaulter's legs. The vaulting roller can be used during the normal RDA riding session in place of a saddle when the saddle provided is too small or too large for the rider, if the rider is timid and needs to hold on, and to develop 'feel' of the pony's movement.

CONDUCTIVE EDUCATION AND ITS RELATIONSHIP TO RIDING

Riding instruction for disabled children, particularly the young child, is well adapted to the concept of conductive education which Professor Andras Peto of Budapest originated for children affected with cerebral palsy. This concept was designed primarily to produce an acceptable gait, since the Hungarian educational authority requires children to be able to walk before entering the school system. Conductive education is not a medical treatment and provides no cure of the underlying condition, but aims to achieve the ability to function in society without requiring special apparatus such as wheelchairs, ramps and other artificial aids. Conductive education is not a therapy but an education.

The principal aim is to achieve a high degree of *functional* independence for the handicapped person including proper sitting, balance, head control and to understand concepts of position in space, particularly in relation to the person's own body. In Hungary, a child *must* be able to walk to be admitted to school, even in the country's two special schools for the motor disabled (Sutton and Cottam, 1986).

Conductive education, as practised in Great Britain in special schools, makes full use of all staff working as a team – teachers, therapists, all assistants and parents – rather than specially trained conductors. Schools such as Ingfield Manor and Claremont (Bristol) have, over the past 20 years, adapted the Peto method; but this concept has not been accepted by those whose interests are to promote pure Peto-type institutions in Great Britain, although the principles have long been practised within existing educational and health systems and are spreading in an adapted form. It is also used successfully in the treatment of adults with neurological dysfunction (Kinsman et al, 1988).

It is emphasized that conductive education is a method of *education*, not a neurophysiological treatment approach such as Bobath, Kabat, Vojta, Temple-Fay, Rood, etc. All problems are treated as problems of learning. Teaching and medical treatment are inseparable.

Conductive education should be continuous throughout the day and involve all those concerned with the training, upbringing and development of brain damaged children. Therefore the riding session, with its complement of therapist(s), instructor(s) and helpers, offers an exciting challenge to activate and support *symmetrical balanced movements* which increase riding ability and skills. These achievements, in turn, feed back into activities of daily living through the attainment of sitting balance, head control, arm and hand steadiness and independent action; freedom of hip movement, correct position of the legs in sitting and independent action of the lower leg, feet supported in stirrups. School work, feeding and dressing then become easier; independence is achieved and the capacity for increased performance established.

The physiotherapist(s), instructor(s) and helpers should note each little progression, however small, which is important to the individual rider and also the whole group; one child's (rider's) progress assists the performance of others. This constitutes a normal situation in any riding class of able-bodied riders from the beginner to those with considerable riding skill. The physiotherapist must explain to the instructor – and her colleagues – the aim of Rhythmical Intention (that is, the use of speech to express intention). Movement is aimed at a goal and carries a certain motor task.

The sequence of movement must be explained, together with the aims of each progression.

1. The ability to sit in the saddle. This may occur on the pony before sitting balance is achieved in a chair without arms (Fig. 25/10).
2. Ability to keep feet in the stirrups – to give security of position – aided by a helper standing at each side.
3. Ability to move the head independently from body.
4. Ability to keep forearms and hands down – holding the reins (not attached to the bit) or a small stick.
5. Ability to move hands independently from one another – steering the pony through bending poles.
6. Ability to understand the position of the body – up, down, side, middle, left, right, out, in, apart, together, above, below, in front, behind.
7. Ability to understand where the hips are – in relation to the rest of the body – in order to achieve a good sitting position.

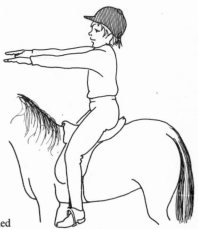

Fig. 25.10 Rider with arms outstretched

Exercises designed to achieve these positions and movements must be accompanied by a stated intention by the rider. As an example:

I pick up the reins.
I sit up tall.
My feet (legs) are hanging down.
I bend forward (Fig. 25/11).
I put my head on the pony's neck.
I touch my feet.
I press my elbows to my side.
I turn to the left (Fig. 25/12).
I turn to the right.
I turn to the left and touch my pony's tail.
I turn to the right and touch my pony's tail.

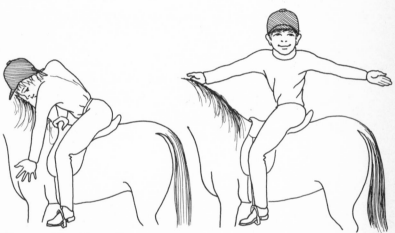

Fig. 25.11 'I bend forward'
Fig. 25.12 'I turn to the left'

With the whole class using speech and action, the individual rider's attention is drawn to the task. The helpers are also fully involved, interested in the achievements of the rider and therefore will concentrate on the instructor, repeating commands and aiding the intention when necessary.

The physiotherapist must explain that:

(a) These functional movements may take months to acquire, the progress made being scarcely discernible over a period of weeks.

(b) Constant repetition is essential, and therefore the exercise of great patience by the helpers is vital.
(c) Much praise for each small success is important, but praise must not be given if the target is not achieved. The rider will be aware of failure, understand and accept the situation and be ready to make another attempt.

SCOLIOSIS

Since the introduction of screening the school-age child, and the improved philosophy of the management of adolescent scoliosis, there is now an increased demand for riding as an acceptable activity during the developing years. Acceptable, that is, for the orthopaedic surgeon, paediatrician, the parents and family, and, most importantly, the young teenage girl who quite often flatly refuses to wear even the low-profile or Boston brace. *Note*: Young girls with idiopathic scoliosis and no other disabilities may own a pony and ride in ordinary classes or in Pony Club events. These youngsters may need only reassurance, adjustments to the brace (if cut too low), ride with longer stirrups and a little help in mounting.

The carrot of riding is often successful in overcoming this quite understandable resentment at a time of life when ordinary problems of growing up can make the developing years so difficult. The congenitally disabled child has further problems in the same period of development when spinal curvatures may progress rapidly, and bracing becomes a formidable task for surgeon, orthotist, physiotherapist and the wearer.

Exercises can maintain and enhance body tone, and are of value to the patient and family in bringing a positive attitude to the problems of management. The psychological benefits are considerable when riding is introduced, and the activity can be continued with care following surgical stabilization, including Harrington rod fixation, when the desire to do so is expressed by the child and agreed by the surgeon.

The problems requiring advice from the physiotherapist range from the normal attention to pressure areas (discussion with the orthotist and surgeon being necessary when adjustments are required to the brace itself), to a briefing session with the riding instructor and helpers on the management of brace-wearing riders. The modern materials used in low-profile and Boston braces are *slippery*, and outer garments therefore cannot be grasped securely for balancing support when necessary. It is this situation which demands the use of a firm belt, preferably with hand-holds, used in assisting mounting to steady the rider at moments of imbalance, when riding a circle or turn, or when the pony puts in a surprising sudden stop or turn. Other points to discuss are the restrictions of exercises; the difficulties of turning in the saddle, and therefore awareness of other riders coming from behind; or, if lead file, judging distance from those following.

For the severely scoliotic rider, balancing is achieved through constant small corrective movements especially on circles when centrifugal forces add further difficulties. In the top heavy spina bifida teenage rider (over-weight from limited activity) the percentage of body-weight displaced to one side can be 60 per cent (Fig. 25/13). Such a rider will restrict her type of riding experiences to circumstances which allow instinctive safety with maximum enjoyment. Hacking out, pony trekking and RDA dressage events leading to

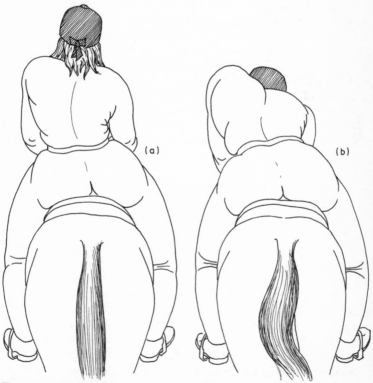

Fig. 25.13 (a) Showing the typical seat position when the body-weight is displaced due to spinal curvature; (b) showing the grossly distorted position when the rider leans forward

BHS Riding Club Preliminary and Novice competitions can be within the scope of some of the non-ambulant brace wearers when the curve is a simple one, not exceeding 20 degrees. Cantering is also possible. The adolescent with normal limb function will enjoy these activities and the spirit of competition with her peers.

BALANCE

The related sequence of balance features, from development of head control and sitting balance obtained normally in the seven/eight-month-old infant to the perfection of an athlete, ballet dancer or accomplished educated rider, is well understood. Laboratory investigations of vestibular influence by the brain, eyes, muscle pressure, skin pressure, stretch reflexes, and the effects of drugs on these mechanisms are responsible for our understanding of static and dynamic balance. For the serious student there are textbooks and journals such as *Physiology and Perception* from which to cull further information. In addition, readers may like to study a paper given at the 1987 WCPT Conference by Roberta Shepherd which discusses postural adjustments (Shepherd, 1987). Cotton (1987) believes the key may lie in the modern interpretation of the motor task.

What *is* open to further study is the acquisition of balance despite brain damage and allied disorders on a moving animal, horse or pony with ideas of its own! This is far more challenging for the student to consider than work already undertaken on the balance board, tilting table, roller or large 'bouncing' ball. The horse or pony provides a wide range of progressive balancing skills which should be acquired to give a good position in the saddle for the rider, and an ability to follow the movement of the horse. Apart from work done by the Bobaths, Finnie, Edinburgh Medical School and at Cambridge, an attempt was made in the gymnasium at Winford Orthopaedic Hospital to simulate the movement of a horse by using a wobble board on a section of the Westminster plinth system. This early experiment showed the effort required by two patients, one recovering from Guillain-Barré disease and one severely scoliotic heavy weight 14-year-old girl. Muscle activity flowed through the spine, accompanied with balancing movements from arms and legs, and, for the rider, gave some indication of the initial instability felt from an early riding lesson. This mock-up could be used with advantage in any group, particularly with the timid wheelchair bound prospective pupil. The experiment does not simulate the horse's influence to which the rider must adjust, and needs to be repeated possibly using a system of pulleys, weights and springs;

however, the pony gives the most complete three-dimensional movement therapy with the greatest number of possible variations.

Mechanical kinaesthesis

Apparatus: Tilt board, mirror, plumb line, flat plinth or broad stool (Fig. 25/14).

Activation: Pressure from seat bones, body sway.

Observer: Take photographs. Using a plumb line, note and record:
1. Muscle work
2. Curvatures
3. Joint and limb positions
4. Spasm

Use of record card: See Figure 25/4.

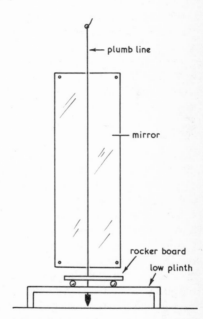

Fig. 25.14 Tilt board

The boards: Made of 19mm (¾in) wood, covered by a 6mm (¼in) layer of rubber with a non-slip surface. The essential feature of these boards is the shape of an attachment screwed to the undersurface. In one type of board (Type I) this consisted of two sections of a cylinder placed across the centre of the board so that the board was free to tip in one plane, like a see-saw. In Type II the attachment was shaped as a section of a sphere so that the board was free to tip in all planes.

In Type I boards the cylinder sections rose to a height of 5cm (2in) and were 20cm (8in) in length. In Type II boards the spherical attachment was of the same height and had a circumference of 20cm. The radii of curvature of these two attachments were therefore the same.

Type II boards were made in two overall sizes: 55×55cm (22×22in) and 55×100cm (22×40in). The larger board rocked about an axis parallel with its short side and it therefore gathered more momentum than did the square board. For this reason it was more difficult to control. Type II boards were circular with a diameter of 55cm.

Perception of movement, changes of direction, changes in the riders' posture, proprioception and vestibular inflow all contribute to achieving balance, but key questions about perception, movement, memory, mood, and body image remain unanswered. The pony, by offering such an enormous variety of alteration of pace (from walk, trot or canter, and with variations of speed within those paces), provides the most useful method of acquiring balance; together with constant enjoyment in the struggle for both brain-damaged riders and the clumsy child. Artificial aids could be used as pre-riding exercises, the tilting table or wobble board and the larger roller being especially useful and readily available to groups.

Each rider relies heavily on visual kinaesthesis, and is dependent on vision to sense how he is moving in relation to the static or active environment. The blind rider can lose track of how he is moving and requires additional mechanical information (i.e. sound assisted) such as bleepers out of doors, voices, sounding boards indoors (i.e. kicking boards) and a lowered general noise level while acquiring such help.

Apart from the physical aspects of acquiring balance, the visual cortex, perception and behavioural factors all have great influence in normal subjects. The pioneer work of Autrum Jung et al (1978) into the behavioural after-effects of brain injury provided a foundation for contemporary neuropsychology studies in young people, and in the congenitally brain-damaged patient. There are, however, important gaps in understanding and explanation of everyday perception of motion. At RDA sessions there are many objects, ponies and people all moving in different directions and at different speeds. The brain-damaged rider is receiving many complex stimuli, and may need a moment or two of freedom from too much input to adjust mentally to the task in hand.

The physiotherapist should explain in simple terms to the instructor and helpers the problems that riders suffering from impaired vision have in achieving balance, especially in the confusion of a free-riding session rather than a correctly planned and executed school ride (PC Instructor's Manual). The problem of directional letters, when the standard size cannot be appreciated by some riders with visual disabilities, can be overcome by the addition of a lower case letter, or picture. Pictures must be very clear, and not too artistic with a confusing if visually delightful background. Recognition of colour may be difficult – a point perhaps to be emphasized for those riders with mental handicaps (intellectually disabled).

Physiotherapists can benefit from taking a riding session wearing spectacles designed for a variety of visual handicaps. A selection of spectacles simulating partial vision through its many variations to complete blindness can be obtained from selected county council libraries. The Diamond Riding Centre, Carshalton, produced such spectacles for physiotherapists on special interest group courses. The experience was salutary, not only in directional finding but in the confidence in the instructor and with helpers. The bond with these needed to be strong!

Recording balance (balance coding)

Gabell and Simons (1982) described a system of balance coding. It is a simple method of recording functional assessment of ability to cope with different basic types of balance and could be applied to riding. As an example such recording can test the recovery point of leaning forward or sideways from the halt and on the moving pony at different paces and speeds.

Reasons for Recording It is essential to learn what the rider can or cannot achieve at any given position and pace: for example:

Numerical Coding 0 = No sitting balance
Therefore support from side helper required
I = Safe when sitting in saddle and being led forward
II = Safe when sitting and being led on 20m circle
III = Safe when sitting and being led on 10m circle
IV = Safe when sitting, being led, on sharp turn.

Variations are equally applicable with the introduction of head, arm and trunk exercises; progressions to independent riding free from the leading rein; more advanced movements at other paces, walk, trot, canter, jumping small spreads at low heights and at varied speeds.

Coding (1) can indicate how the rider should be managed; (2) is a swift compact method of recording, easily translated by helper; (3) indicates progress; and (4) helps in planning individual programmes.

MENTAL HANDICAP

Riding sessions provide opportunities to improve physical skills; assist mental development; adjust behavioural problems; and improve general health in children, young people and, perhaps most dramatically, in adults, especially those remaining in institutions and those now living in the community. Stimulation, motivation and learning is achieved through the visual, auditory, tactile, olfactory and gustatory experiences which the special school teacher develops and is continued at the riding session. Preparation for riding, putting on riding hats, seeing the ponies being groomed, tacked up, led from their boxes and the people working with the ponies, add fresh experiences (visual, tactile, auditory, olfactory) – feel of the pony, saddle, leathers, stirrups – hearing shod feet at different paces, the smells of pony, stables, hay and grass. But most of all, the kin-aesthetic sense, with the appropriate language, is greatly developed. Progressive exercises in groups or for individuals are enjoyable and such skills as sitting in the saddle, moving arms and legs independently, using legs to make the pony walk. Simple commands given one aim at a time, that is, 'touch your pony with your feet' – say the words – 'walk on', are most likely to be heard and followed.

In adults, greater joint range and muscle power from exercises on the moving pony allow tasks such as dressing or washing to be performed when previously major help from assistants was necessary.

Instructions must be easy to remember, one task at a time, commands such as:

– walk your pony down the school to a specific marker
– turn your pony
– come back to me.

The helper is of paramount importance in assisting the rider to carry out these tasks and must be consistently aware of the instructor's commands – talking to the rider, not gossiping with friends!

MALADJUSTED CHILDREN

These virtually give no trouble when actually riding as the individual attention of each helper is just what such children need. The therapist, in particular, can be aware of mood changes and avert the undesirable or encourage the new experience, working with the riding instructor in achieving motor skills. The clumsy child also benefits from riding experience through the development of co-ordination, balance and suppleness (Meredith, 1987 *Riding and the Mentally Handicapped* (unpublished); Bicknell, 1981).

To condense the whole philosophy of riding for the disabled into one chapter is impossible. As an introduction to the subject, the chosen disabilities and the general problems cover those most usually presenting at group level. Much has been omitted but it is hoped that this outline will stimulate interest and provide a basis for investigating these subjects in greater detail, and widen research into many other aspects of this rewarding and enriching activity.

REFERENCES

Autrum Jung, A., Lowenstein, W. R., Mackay, D. M. and Tewber, H. L. (1978). *Handbook of Sensory Perception*, vol. 3. Springer-Verlag, New York.

Bicknell, J. (1981). *Goals for the Mentally Handicapped*. Obtainable from Riding for the Disabled Association, National Agricultural Centre, Kenilworth CV8 2LY.

Cotton, E. (1987). Interpreting the motor task (Letter). *Physiotherapy*, 73, 12, 660.

Finnie, N. R. (1974). *Handling the Young Cerebral Palsied Child at Home*, 2nd edition. William Heinemann Medical Books Limited, London.

Gabell, A. and Simons, M. A. (1982). Balance coding. *Physiotherapy*, 68, 9, 286–8.

Kinsman, R., Verity, R. and Waller, J. (1988). A conductive education approach for adults with neurological dysfunction. *Physiotherapy*, 74, 5, 227–30.

Podhajsky, A. (1967). *The Complete Training of Horse and Rider*. Harrap Limited, London.

Shepherd, R. (1987). Movement science and physiotherapy: deriving implications for the clinic. *Proceedings of the WCPT Conference*, WCPT, London.

Sutton, A. and Cottam, P. (1986). *Conductive Education: A System for Overcoming Motor Disorder*. Croom Helm, London.

Watjen, R. L. (1979). *Dressage Riding: A Guide for the Horse and Rider*, 2nd edition, J. A. Allen and Co Limited, London.

Handbook of the Riding for the Disabled Association.
RDA Ring Binder (Green Binder).
Both these titles are regularly updated. They are obtainable from Riding for the Disabled Association, National Agricultural Centre, Kenilworth CV8 2LY.

BIBLIOGRAPHY

Cotton, E. (1975). *Conductive Education and Cerebral Palsy*. Spastics Society, London.

Keim, H. A. (1976). *The Adolescent Spine*. Grune and Stratton Inc, New York.

The Manual of Horsemanship (1981). British Horse Society Pony Club. Obtainable from the British Horse Society, National Agricultural Centre, Kenilworth, Warwickshire CV8 2LY.

Pony Club Instructor's Manual. Obtainable from address above.

Vault Safely by Yvonne Nelson BHSI. Obtainable from the Fortune Centre of Riding Therapy, Avon Tyrell, Christchurch, Dorset BH23 8EE.

Vaulting for the Pony Club by Anne Gittins DipPhysEd. Obtainable from the Pony Club, c/o British Horse Society (address above).

ACKNOWLEDGEMENT

The author thanks Miss A. Smith MCSP at Claremont School, Bristol for her continued interest, help and support.

The record card (Fig. 25/14) was designed by the clinical interest group, Riding for the Disabled, for use by lay helpers after an initial training period.

Chapter 26

Veterinary Physiotherapy

by M. W. BROMILEY MCSP, SRP, RPT(USA)

Treatment described as 'physiotherapy' has been administered to injured animals for many years. These early therapists had no training, many were primarily manipulators, practising a trade handed down from father to son over succeeding generations. All had the advantage of an inherited knowledge of the habits, behavioural patterns and common ailments of the animals they treated. Herbs were much in use as an adjunct to manual skills, as were the 'rubs' applied to muscles, tendons, ligaments and joints. Two world wars and the move from the country to urban living reduced the number of country-bred 'stockmen'. The 'Machine Era' arrived and a new generation of self-styled physiotherapists equipped themselves with ultrasound, muscle stimulators and the like. They had no knowledge of the effect of machines on tissue and as a result many animals suffered unnecessary pain. The machines were claimed to 'cure all'. In most cases they were used without veterinary diagnosis or veterinary permission; the Royal College of Veterinary Surgeons (RCVS) began to query the validity of physiotherapy.

In 1982 the Royal College wrote for guidance to the Chartered Society of Physiotherapy (CSP); from subsequent meetings it became obvious that the RCVS and the majority of their members did not appreciate that the title 'physiotherapist' was unprotected and that many persons using the title were not members of the CSP. In their turn the Chartered Society of Physiotherapists did not know of the existence of the Veterinary Act. This is an act of parliament and is designed to protect animals, not isolate veterinary treatment for the benefit of the profession alone.

VETERINARY SURGEONS ACT

The Veterinary Surgeons Act 1966 provides that (with certain specific exceptions) only veterinary surgeons may carry out acts of veterinary surgery upon animals. 'Veterinary surgery' is so defined by the Act as to include the making of a diagnosis, the carrying out of tests for diagnostic purposes, and both medical and surgical treatment.

Of the exceptions created by the Veterinary Surgery (Exemptions) Order, one permits the treatment of an animal by physiotherapy, *provided* such treatment is given by a person acting under the direction of a veterinarian who has examined the animal and prescribed treatment of the animal by physiotherapy.

In 1984 a Specific Interest Group (SIG) named the Association of Chartered Physiotherapists in Animal Therapy was formed with the agreement of the RCVS. The Royal College issued a directive to their members, recommending that the assistance of qualified physiotherapists be sought if physiotherapy were required for injured animals. Certain parameters were laid down by both the Royal College and the Chartered Society regarding members of the SIG:

All physiotherapists must be paid-up members of the Chartered Society.

The applicant must have had two years post-qualification experience in the human field and have been recommended by two veterinary surgeons after seeing practice with the two veterinary surgeons.

The insurers of the Chartered Society agreed to increase individual liability cover by a further £500,000, provided the physiotherapist was a paid-up member of the SIG. (The cost to be met from the annual subscriptions.) In 1989 the SIG has become a Clinical Interest Group.

PROFESSIONAL STANDARDS AND THE RELATIONSHIP OF THE PHYSIOTHERAPIST TO THE VETERINARY SURGEON AND THE OWNER

It is essential that the physiotherapist retains a professional attitude towards both the veterinary surgeon and their client. Comprehensive notes should be kept and must include the name of the animal, the veterinary diagnosis and the request of the veterinary surgeon for treatment, the number of treatments given, apparatus used, dosage, etc.

A final veterinary report should always be sent to the vet in charge of the case when treatment has finished and it is as well to advise the owner on the follow-up regime that the animal should adopt. Many treatments are ruined by over-enthusiastic owners who do not curtail and control the exercises of the patient when treatment is finishing. Remember, some of the animals can be worth upwards of several million pounds!

A kennel coat is a necessary piece of equipment and if a physiotherapist is working in different yards or kennels it is sensible to keep a coat at each location. These days with the virus prevalent in racing circles and the various illnesses that abound in the dog world, it would be a disaster for the physiotherapist to be the source of transference of infection from one yard to another.

All the normal principles of physiotherapy should be observed: clean equipment, washed down and tested daily, hands washed preferably with disinfectant soap after each animal. If a bridle is taken and used on one horse the bit should be washed in disinfectant before it is put in the mouth of another horse; similarly, equipment in the form of brushes, combs or clippers (all of which may be needed to remove unwanted hair) should always be kept clean and sterile. It is usually best to shave with a razor and then to dispose of the razor. Towels should be kept apart and not used on animals in more than one yard. The appearance of the physiotherapist herself should be neat and tidy. Remember colts can become very upset if any perfume is worn and they are particularly sensitive to perfumed deodorants. Animal skins have a different sensitivity to human and it is better to use veterinary disinfectants at the strength prescribed than to substitute human ones. This also applies to some of the creams and gels such as Movelat. Movelat should *never* be used in a racing yard (for fear that its steroid content be picked up on a dope test) unless the horse is at least three weeks off a run and the vet and the trainer have both been informed. Dope testing is not as stringent as yet in the competitive dog world but no doubt it will come in the foreseeable future.

COMPARATIVE ANATOMY (Figs 26/1, 26/2, 26/3, 26/4)

The World Association of Veterinary Anatomists adopted in 1973 an international nomenclature, the Nomina Anatomica Veterinaria (NAV) based upon Latin. Many of the names in the animal anatomy books will be familiar and some of the anatomical terminology similar, but the planes and ranges of joint movements are different from the human as are the terms of orientation (Fig. 26/5).

To the directional terms applied to the human skeleton are added:

Cranial: The surface of the limb lying relatively near to the head.
Caudal: The surface of the limb lying relatively near to the tail.
Axial: The surface of the digit facing the functional axis of the limb.
Abaxial: The surface of the digit facing away from the functional axis of the limb.

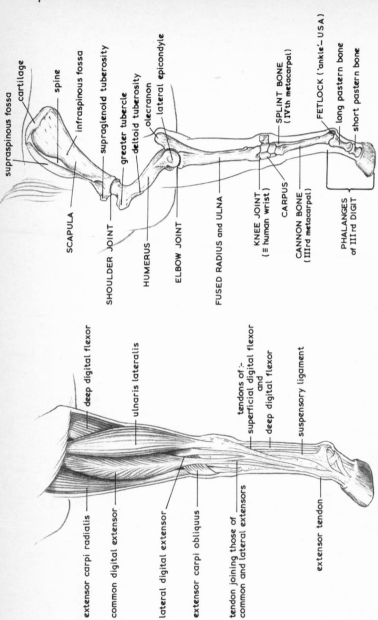

supraspinous fossa
cartilage
spine
infraspinous fossa
supraglenoid tuberosity
greater tubercle
deltoid tuberosity
olecranon
lateral epicondyle
SPLINT BONE (IVth metacarpal)
FETLOCK ('ankle'– USA)
long pastern bone
short pastern bone

SCAPULA
SHOULDER JOINT
HUMERUS
ELBOW JOINT
FUSED RADIUS and ULNA
KNEE JOINT (= human wrist)
CARPUS
CANNON BONE (IIIrd metacarpal)
PHALANGES of IIIrd DIGIT

Fig. 26.2 Bone arrangement of the forelimb of the horse

deep digital flexor
ulnaris lateralis
tendons of :-
superficial digital flexor
and
deep digital flexor
suspensory ligament

extensor carpi radialis
common digital extensor
lateral digital extensor
extensor carpi obliquus
tendon joining those of common and lateral extensors
extensor tendon

Fig. 26.1 Muscle and tendon arrangement in the foreleg of the horse

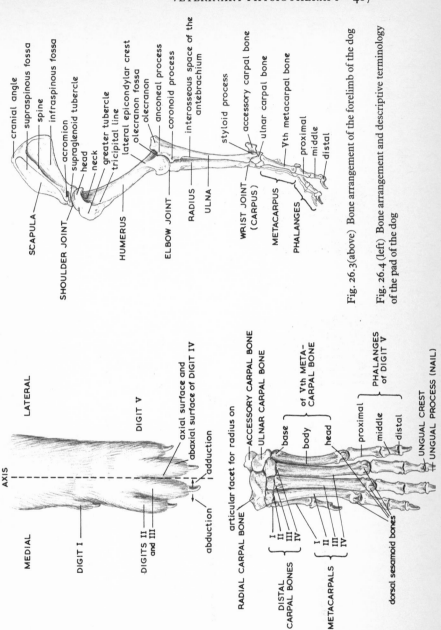

cranial angle
supraspinous fossa
spine
infraspinous fossa
acromion
supraglenoid tubercle
head
neck
greater tubercle
tricipital line
lateral epicondylar crest
olecranon fossa
olecranon
anconeal process
coronoid process
interosseous space of the antebrachium
styloid process
accessory carpal bone
ulnar carpal bone
Vth metacarpal bone
proximal
middle
distal

SCAPULA
SHOULDER JOINT
HUMERUS
ELBOW JOINT
RADIUS
ULNA
WRIST JOINT (CARPUS)
METACARPUS
PHALANGES

Fig. 26.3 (above) Bone arrangement of the forelimb of the dog

Fig. 26.4 (left) Bone arrangement and descriptive terminology of the pad of the dog

AXIS
LATERAL
MEDIAL
DIGIT V
DIGIT I
DIGITS II and III
axial surface and abaxial surface of DIGIT IV
adduction
abduction

articular facet for radius on
RADIAL CARPAL BONE
ACCESSORY CARPAL BONE
ULNAR CARPAL BONE
base
body
head
of Vth META-CARPAL BONE
proximal
middle
distal
PHALANGES of DIGIT V
UNGUAL CREST
UNGUAL PROCESS (NAIL)
DISTAL CARPAL BONES
I
II
III
IV
METACARPALS
I
II
III
IV
dorsal sesamoid bones

Ligament stress and angle of muscle pull vary in each species. The collarbone is missing in some species and the number of vertebrae differ, thus the composition of the brachial and sacral plexuses are not a constant, the number of nerve roots from which they originate changing from species to species. It is important to appreciate all these differences for effective treatment approaches, for example, innervation of muscles and the sensory dermatomes are dependent on the number of nerve roots in the species.

The species are grouped by the veterinary profession into large and small animals.

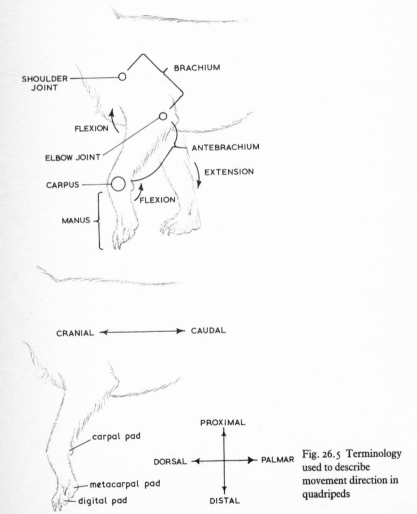

Fig. 26.5 Terminology used to describe movement direction in quadripeds

Large animals

1. Those having a hoof: The horse, donkey, mule, zebra.
2. Those having a cloven hoof: Sheep, cattle, goats and deer which are farmed species. Giraffe inhabit safari parks, as do rhino and hippopotamuses.
3. Those having a pad: The camel and large cats. (They are found in zoos, safari parks and circuses.)

Anatomical variations occur particularly at the distal end of the limbs in the three groups.

The range of spinal movement is minimal in a horse but very extensive in the large cat. The gait pattern and limb sequence varies in each species, thus the angle of G-force experienced as the limb meets the ground also alters. Much can be learned by watching the footfall and the weight distribution while the animal moves.

Small animals

The domestic dog and cat are the most common patients in this group, but zoo work embraces a large number of species including birds of prey. Of the various breeds of dog, the racing greyhound will be foremost among canine patients.

OBSERVATION AND EXAMINATION

Every animal should have been examined by a veterinary surgeon before the case is handed over to the physiotherapist or, in ideal circumstances, a concurrent examination with the vet, physiotherapist and the owner, trainer or handler present, is of most benefit.

It is the job of the veterinary surgeon to eliminate all pathological conditions, particularly in cases where the complaint is 'loss of performance'.

Observation

Accurate observation is of paramount important. This coupled with the ability to recognize an unnatural stance, uneven weight-bearing, a difference in contour, minute differences of the limb movement, the state of the animal's coat, the brightness of the eye, all are aids to discovering the source of the injury and the extent of pain. A close study of normal gait patterns, the overall outline, the normal behavioural stance, foot shape, foot to ground angle, and the normal range of joint movement within a species is essential knowledge for the animal therapist, only then will he or she be able to spot the differences and abnormalities that are associated with injury.

It is advisable to spend time observing the normal variations within a species as well as the different species before trying to locate the abnormal. The dressage horse has a different conformation from the racehorse; the angle of the pastern will vary in each breed; muscle groups develop differently for different tasks; the footfall pattern of the heavy horse has been carefully changed by selective breeding and is considered a fault in the show horse. The racing greyhound is one sided (see p.495); the back of the bassett hound on palpation feels different from the back of a deerhound.

Besides observation of the animals themselves, it is necessary to watch the sport in which the animals partake and to which they hope to return. It is quite impossible to appreciate the muscle strength required by a thoroughbred on the flat or jumping fences in a race unless you have stood at ground level and watched the animal perform. Similarly, it is essential to watch dogs working; police dogs being handled by their trainers; the greyhound both at exercise, slipped and on the racetrack; to see a labrador retrieving; the sheep-dog working with his animals.

If a video recording of an event is available it is of the greatest assistance as it is possible to watch the limb sequence at the time of the accident and to note which part of the animal's body took the most strain and if abnormal joint movements occurred as a result of the accident.

Examination

1 (a) Observation of the animal at rest (Figs 26/6, 26/7, 26/8).
  (b) Being led by handler or groom.
  (c) Horse, lunged or ridden (if injury permits).

2 (a) Passive movement of the joints of the limb involved.
  (b) Test for reflex patterns.

Example: A horse can ventroflex, dorsiflex and side flex the thoraco-lumbar spine. Movements are activated by pressing behind the withers – ventroflexion; behind the girth – dorsiflexion; running the fingers along lateral to the centre of the spine – side flexion away from the pressure.

Extension of the dog's shoulder should produce extension of the wrist (Fig. 26/9).

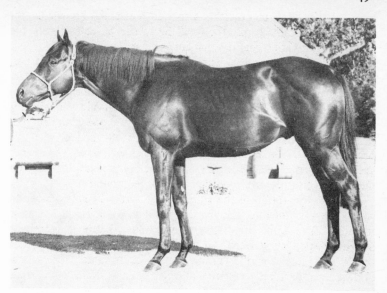

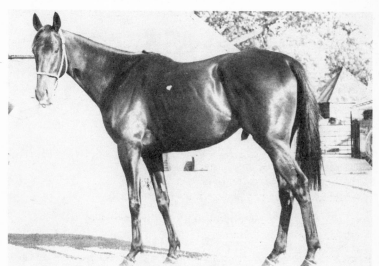

Fig. 26.6 Normal contour of a horse's back

Fig. 26.7 Abnormal contour of a horse's back. *Note* the ridging near the quarters, and the lack of muscle in the neck and quarters

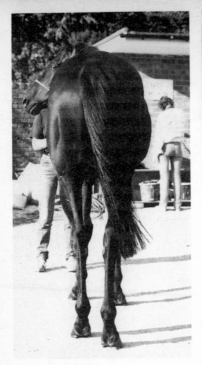
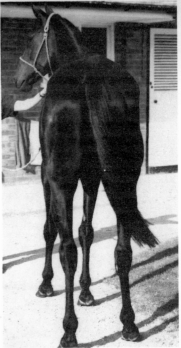

Fig. 26.8 *Left:* Normal contour of a horse's quarters. *Right:* Abnormal contour of a horse's quarters. *Note:* the 'bump' at top of the quarters

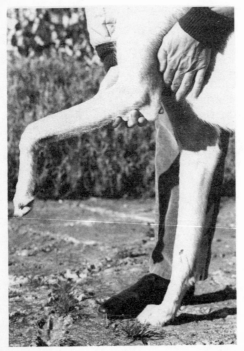

Fig. 26.9 Radial paralysis. The leg should extend fully when stretched forward

3. *Palpation.* The ability to feel with sensitive fingertips for muscle spasm and to palpate deeply to locate pain as a result of muscle or ligament tears is essential. It is wise to observe and palpate the normal animal before attempting to do the same to the injured, and essential to appreciate which muscle or structure is being palpated.

The animal cannot describe where it hurts; effective treatment can only be given if the cause of pain is found, always examine above and below an area found to be sensitive to palpation. The 'stay' system of the horse is such that palpable discomfort may arise as a result of unnatural stance caused by joint or foot discomfort. To understand this phenomenon the following example is described: A horse crippled lame behind was extensively investigated, x-rayed, blood tested; every 'back expert' shook his head after manipulation failed. Examination of the *foot* revealed a carpet tack deeply embedded in the frog – removal gave instant relief!

CAUSES OF INJURY

It is impossible to describe the injuries of all species so only the most common injuries found in the horse and the dog are discussed.

The majority of owners are emotionally involved with their animals and the fact that the injury the animal has suffered may have been caused directly or indirectly as a result of owner error will often make them angry and/or depressed. The physiotherapist should be prepared to deal with both animal and owner.

As with the human, conformation and lack of fitness are two of the predominant factors causing animal injury. To these must be added unnatural behavioural patterns, the result of captivity, and tasks which the animal is asked to perform but for which it was never designed. To these problems in the domesticated animal must be added for the horse, rider error; and the dog, owner error.

Common causes of injury in the horse

Poor shoeing causing an imbalance of gait.
Badly fitted bridles or saddles (the latter the most common cause of back pain).
Being kicked by another horse.
A fall over fences, slipping at speed, or slipping on the road.
Striking one limb with another.
Getting cast. (Stuck upside down when rolling in too small a space.)

Common injuries in horses

Tendon injuries: Rupture, partial or complete, of the flexor tendons of the forelimb. One or both may be involved. Diagnostic ultrasound scanning is becoming an acceptable test for tendon injury.
N.B. There is no structure similar in the human being in any respect to the flexor tendons of the horse.

Joint sprains: All limb joints. The joints of the cervical spine. The sacro-iliac joint. The lumbo-sacral junction.
N.B. The horse has no muscles specifically to move the thoracic or lumbar spine – veterinary anatomists describe the thoracic and lumbar spine as being a rigid structure. There is much controversy regarding the equine spine.

Muscle strains: Triceps, deltoid, pectorals, middle gluteal, hamstrings, quadriceps.
N.B. 'Pulls' are more common than complete tears. Calcification often occurs after a tear in the hamstring group producing a significant diagnostic gait pattern.

Fractures: Most major limb fractures require humane destruction. Micro-fractures of the cannon bone (forelimb) occur in immature animals and recover. Pelvic fractures occur after falls and normally recover given time. Avulsion fractures of the knee and hock are treated by arthroscopy removal.

Wounds: Self-inflicted as a result of the edge of a shoe cutting into an opposing or contralateral limb – 'over-reach' or 'speedy cut'. A fall on the road. Road traffic accidents. Collision with a sharp projection, e.g. barbed wire.

Common causes of injury in the dog

Dog fights.
Road traffic accidents.
Slipping on an unsuitable surface or down stairs.
Jumping too high and twisting in mid air trying to catch a stick or ball.
Being cannoned into by another dog at speed – 'bumped'.
Sudden, unexpected collar restraint by the owner.
N.B. Inherited congenital deformities are increasingly common, e.g. hip dysplasia.

Common injuries in the dog

Joint sprains: The wrist, the hip, the facet joints, the intravertebral joints. (Subluxation of the intravertebral disc is common in most breeds, the long backed being the most at risk.)

Muscle strains: Triceps, deltoid, longissimi dorsi, gracilis.
N.B. All greyhound tracks are *anti-clockwise*, thus all *track greyhounds* in full training are uneven in muscle contour. Coursing greyhounds and all other breeds should have an even muscle outline.

Fractures: Limb fractures, pelvic fractures, shoulder fractures, spinal fractures.
N.B. Unlike the horse, a dog is easy to x-ray; many fractures are reduced and stabilized under open operative procedures and the use of casts for immobilization is common.

Wounds and tears: Cuts of pads and the web of the pad. Wounds due to fights and road accidents. Tears of the claws and dew claws.

MACHINES

If the machines are powered from the mains a muzzle must be worn by the animal.

Massage

In all animals, whether it be with machine or whether it be by hand, massage has a very beneficial effect; not only does the animal relax under the therapist's hands as the pain is removed, but the ability to detect tension within the muscle groups is, from the therapist's point of view, enhanced.

Linda Tellington-Jones (USA) has adopted a method of massage of acupuncture points so effective that she has been able to work with snow leopards in the Moscow zoo, and to calm them, even when they were at their most worried.

To date all massage machines are power operated but some will run off a battery similar to a car battery. The small Pifco type is best for dogs, while, due to the vastness of their muscle bulk, the heavier type Swedish design or the purpose built are ideal for horses.

Electromagnetic machines

Electromagnetic field therapy is very popular with animal owners. There are several machines available: the Blue Boot (USA) – pulsed field, battery operated, designed specifically for sore shins; Magnavet shapes, static field, for soft tissue problems in the limbs; mains operated, alternating field with two pairs of magnets mounted on a rug (Fig. 26/10).

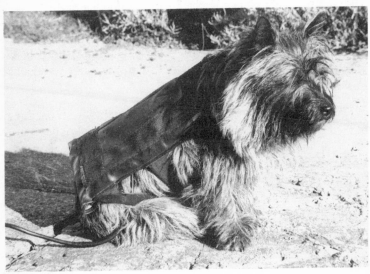

Fig. 26.10 A dog having magnetic field therapy

There is no laboratory work to substantiate the maker's claims of increased circulatory flow and reduction of pain – but a footnote may be of interest. A terrier owned by the author's daughter hurt his back after a fall when ratting. A set of therapeutic magnets was put on the floor by his basket, every day when the machine was switched on he crawled to the magnets and lay on them – he was obviously in less pain after 'treating himself'. As he recovered he ceased to use the magnets.

Animals relax while being treated and there appears to be a reduction of pain.

Field trials backed by radiological evidence at the Equine Research Station at Newmarket have shown no increased rate of fracture healing.

Ultrasound

Some physiotherapists are ultrasound converts, others are not. In the author's experience a battery-powered US machine is one of the most useful therapies in veterinary physiotherapy. Ultrasound has a bad reputation in the veterinary field as most practices own a machine which they 'lend' to their clients.

Prolonged treatments at the incorrect settings (usually at 3 watts to the cm^2) has led to the spontaneous fracture of the cannon bone in several cases. To give an effective treatment the coat of the horse or dog should, if possible, be clipped close. This is not acceptable in the show animal. It is possible to treat limbs under-water. The coat must be rubbed when immersed, because if bubbles are trapped in the hair follicles the beam will be deflected and the treatment will not be effective.

Dosage and treatment time are a matter for common sense. All animals will try to move away if discomfort is felt, if restrained they have the sense to bite or kick should the discomfort continue.

Low level laser therapy

The use of the therapeutic laser is comparatively new; the bulk of the laboratory work has been done by Mester in Budapest using a helium neon (HeNe) laser operating at 632.5mm. Ulcers and wound healing have been improved and bowed tendons, ligaments, muscle and joint injuries in horses have been reported as being improved. At Newmarket the cosmetic appearance of bowed tendons has been shown to be improved but ultrasonic scanning has *not* shown any significant or accelerated recovery of the tendon lesion. Many Chinese workers are applying lasers to acupoints and reporting significant reduction in both acute and chronic pain cases.

Preliminary research on mechanically induced denervation in the rat has demonstrated improved regeneration following HeNe laser therapy. As a therapeutic tool the low level laser appears to enhance tissue repair. Portable battery-operated models are available; contact with the area to be treated is not required, there is no sensation and the machines are silent – ideal for work in correctly selected cases.

Interferential therapy

This is best given using a manual technique. The therapist's hands must be insulated (rubber gloves) or the current will dissipate up the operator's arm. The treatment is only effective if the specific structure at fault is isolated – the greatest disadvantage is the necessity of mains power.

Muscle stimulation (Fig. 26/11)

Weakness of a muscle or muscle groups following injury is the greatest single factor inhibiting the return of the animal athlete to its full pre-injury potential.

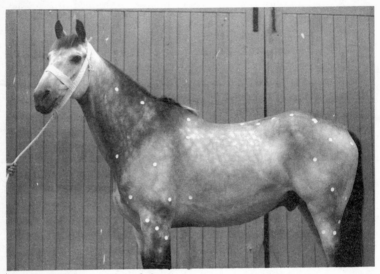

Fig. 26.11 The motor points of a horse

Until recently, stimulation of the injured muscle in the animal was dependent on faradic stimulation (human machines) or the method employed by the late Sir Charles Strong, using a Transeva stimulator. Both were reasonably effective if the animal would tolerate the sensation of the stimuli. Advances in technology have seen the arrival of *neuromuscular stimulators*. These units mimic as accurately as possible the signals of natural nerves. There is minimal skin sensation, even at maximum contraction.

The electronic signals take over the control of muscle metabolism ensuring the preservation of muscle bulk, the ability of the muscle to utilize oxygen and the maintenance of capillary bed density within the muscle. Both slow and fast contracting muscle fibres can be stimulated. These units herald a new era in muscle recovery.

TREATMENT AND REHABILITATION
(Figs 26/12, 26/13)

Once a diagnosis has been made and the physiotherapist has established the nature of the injury, the tissue types involved and the lifestyle to which the animal is required to return, a treatment/rehabilitation programme can be planned. Important points to remember are, firstly, that pain is the main objective finding in the animal; once the pain has been removed, and unfortunately this occurs fairly rapidly with the use of modern machines, the animal has no inbuilt safety factor to stop it over-exerting itself. While pain may have disappeared, as previously stated, this does *not* necessarily mean that the tissue is healed to a degree where it can stand the strain of competition training.

Second, balance in muscle strength is essential to ensure the animal returns to its pre-accident form. For example, a horse with

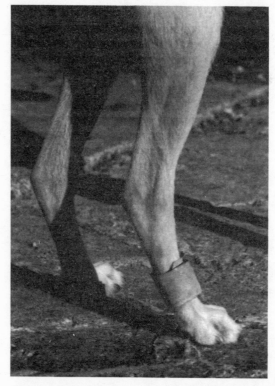

Fig. 26.12 A leg weight attached to a dog

500 VETERINARY PHYSIOTHERAPY

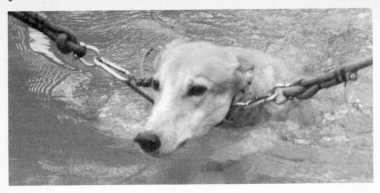

Fig. 26.13 Swimming rehabilitation

weak muscles in one hindquarter may appear to be free of pain and 'working sound' but when under pressure the animal will hang or drift towards the weak side. That is, instead of travelling forward in a straight line, as the weak muscles fatigue, the strong muscles will, with their greater power produce a force that causes the animal to drift slightly sideways, just as a car with one back wheel out of balance, due to a lowered pressure, will cause the car to deviate from a straight line.

As with a human patient the choice of machine must be the responsibility of the therapist in charge of the case. Machines that operate on a rechargeable battery are the most useful as stable yards, kennels, zoos and circuses to name but a few locations, rarely have accessible electrical sockets. It is not the place of this chapter to tell qualified physiotherapists how to use machines, but merely to suggest how machines, followed by a programme of rehabilitation, will help to return an animal to its full fitness potential. Full rehabilitation can be difficult if there is not easy access to either a swimming pool or a treadmill, better still both.

The ideal regime for any animal is, *first*, the machine phase accompanied by passive movements of the joints of the limb or limbs involved. The owner can be taught how to perform these movements and a treatment regime handed to him at the time of the initial examination and first treatment – just as with the spastic child, the parent can be brought in to help the therapist. The *second* phase, machine coupled with swimming (non-weight-bearing), is followed finally by machine and controlled exercise on the treadmill or in a menage; the horse worked in lines with no rider and the dog in an enclosed area such as a menage where it can be encouraged to run in a straight line following a ball.

If the therapist is lucky enough to have her own rehabilitation unit, the swimming pool is of greatest importance, allowing non-weight-bearing exercise for young puppies that are too heavy for their limbs, for horses that have tendon or back problems, in fact for most breeds of domestic animals other than the cat. Swimming coupled with the introduction of work on a treadmill where the exercise can be graded to a certain speed level is of the greatest benefit. The treadmill also assists in the re-education of gait for there is no way an animal can work on a treadmill unless the gait strides are even.

With the zoo animal the treatment programme obviously must vary because the animal is often too dangerous to handle; in these cases the majority of treatments would merely be to relieve pain after a cut or perhaps sprain of a joint and in this situation, particularly with the big cats, the low level laser is very useful.

To those contemplating working with animals, full-time employment is unlikely – the work can be fun, fascinating, frustrating.

BIBLIOGRAPHY

Anatomy

Adams, O.R. (1987). *Lameness in Horses.* Lea and Febiger, Philadelphia.
De Lahunta, A. (1983). *Veterinary Neuro-anatomy and Clinical Neurology.* W.B. Saunders Co, London.
Sisson and Grossman. (1975). *The Anatomy of Domestic Animals.* W.B. Saunders Co, London.
Skerrit and McLelland. (1984). *Functional Anatomy of the Limbs of Domestic Animals.* J. Wright and Sons, Bristol.
Smith, R.N. (1982). *An Anatomy of the Horse.* J. Wright and Sons, Bristol.
Smith, R.N. (1983). *An Anatomy of the Dog.* J. Wright and Sons, Bristol.

Treatment

Bromiley, M.W. (1987). *Equine Injury and Therapy.* Blackwell Scientific Publications Limited, Oxford.
Downer, A.H. (1978). *Physical Therapy for Animals (Selected Techniques).* Charles C. Thomas, Springfield, Ill., USA.
Houlton and Taylor. (1987). *Trauma Management in the Dog and Cat.* J. Wright and Sons, Bristol.
Meagher, J. (1986). *Beating Muscle Injuries for Horses.* USCTA, Boston, USA.
Westermeyer, E. (1979). *The Treatment of Horses by Acupuncture.* Health Science Press, Holsworthy.
Wooley, H. (1988). *Low Power Lasers and their Medical Application.* East Asia Co, London.

Kinesiology

Rooney, J.R. (1981). *The Mechanics of the Horse*. Robert E. Krieger Publishing Co, New York.

Smith, R.N. (1982). *The Locomotor System*. J. Wright and Sons, Bristol.

Smythe, R.H. (1967). *The Horse: Structure and Movement*. J.A. Allen and Co Ltd, London.

Schooling for rehabilitation

Oliveira, N. (1983). *Classical Principles of the Art of Training Horses*. Howley and Russel, Australia.

Richards, P.K. (1983). *The BLOK Training System*. City View Press, Dublin.

Chapter 27

The Elderly

by P. A. FENN CLARK MCSP

Geriatrics, or health care of the elderly, concerns patients of a particular age-group. It is debatable whether work with the elderly is a specialism, so much as a special interest in one of the few remaining fields of generalist practice (Kane, 1988). Age definition, which can range over 40 years in geriatric units, is unsatisfactory (Stevenson, 1981), as 'the elderly', according to the World Health Organization, are aged 60–74; the 'old' 75–90, and 'very old' 90+. Defining geriatrics by chronological age is an arbitrary local decision.

Knowledge about ageing, 'gerontology', was pioneered in the USA; in the UK 'geriatrics' (doctoring of the aged) was, historically, the aspect of ageing which received the most attention. In Great Britain after the Second World War, many old people were to be found in long-stay hospitals for reasons other than their illnesses, and often the only care for the sick was custodial rather than remedial. A few enlightened consultant physicians, having examined and assessed the patients and reorganized these hospitals, founded the British Geriatrics Society in 1947. They based their philosophy on the necessity of accurate diagnosis, on the reversibility of many of the changes commonly seen in their patients, on the possibility of rehabilitation of many of them (with the axiom 'bed is bad') and on the conviction that age should be no bar to receiving the best available medical care (Howell, 1974; Anderson, 1985).

It was soon discovered that many problems of patients in the older age bracket did not stem solely from ill-health, but that health problems were compounded by age-related financial, social, mental, housing, educational and other functional disadvantages. The early geriatricians recruited other professions into the specialty to offer a wider range of agencies and remedies without which medicine alone would fail – so began the concept of the multidisciplinary team. Its rationale is the need to pool professional expertise in order to tackle the patients' multiple problems by an integrated team effort. Each member of the multidisciplinary team works closely not only with the patient and relatives (or carers) but also with the other members of the team to ensure a united service with shared goals.

From the success of crude bed-end exercises devised by Dr Margery Warren, the value of physical rehabilitation was realized. In 1978 the Association of Chartered Physiotherapists in Geriatric Medicine (now the Association of Chartered Physiotherapists with a Special Interest in Elderly People) was founded. This both echoed and foreshadowed the foundation of other special interest groups in the paramedical professions.

In the community the multidisciplinary team is enhanced by home helps, meals-on-wheels services, day centres, incontinence laundry facilities, luncheon and drop-in clubs, various neighbourly initiatives, voluntary organizations and charities. These may have formal and funded links with local social services or health authorities, or be privately organized and endowed by non-statutory bodies such as local churches, retirement organizations and self-help groups. Friends, neighbours and relatives can link with these agencies to form the patients' social network – they may be guided by the formal multidisciplinary team, to reinforce the work of rehabilitation at home.

Physiotherapists working with the elderly need a general understanding of the natural physical and functional changes in the ageing human body, the diseases of the elderly and the differing emphasis in assessment, treatment and rehabilitation which the elderly need. Theoretical and academic knowledge of physiotherapy required is the same as for any other age-group. The skills needed for treatment of the elderly do not differ greatly from those used for any patient: handling, movement, assessment and diagnosis, teaching and treatment with appropriate planning, application and progression of stroke regimes, postoperative protocols, respiratory techniques, etc.

Attitude, though difficult to measure, has been historically deficient in care of the elderly in many professions (Gale and Livesley, 1974). Physiotherapists tend to regard geriatrics as a less than ideal field of practice (Bauer, 1982; Finn, 1986) and to underestimate capabilities of the elderly (Kvitek et al, 1986). Even where there is great skill attitude often remains poor, and is not amenable to direct improvement until the knowledge level is raised, though true competence in practice is only achieved by integrating attitudes and skill with knowledge (Caney, 1983).

Becoming old is a gradual process, but some of the changes start much earlier, and the accumulation of deficits reduces abilities to critical functional thresholds even without particular traumas or pathologies. While medical advances have enabled more people to survive into prolonged retirement many causes of mortality or

longevity remain imponderable. The increasing role of physiotherapists in health education should include education of the elderly
fit in maintaining healthy habits, in adopting safe exercise programmes and in avoiding lethargy.

Let us now consider some of the ways in which the elderly differ
from the rest of the population.

LIFE HISTORY

The elderly, having a longer life history than anyone else's, have
'seen it all'. The physiotherapist can utilize their life-experience to
explain treatments. Familiar primitive actions such as stretching,
taking and holding a deep breath before strenuous effort, rubbing a
sore limb, soothing a fevered brow, learning to write, the lullaby and
cradling of a baby, exemplify certain physiotherapy techniques such
as facilitation, excitation, inhibition, relaxation, irradiation of
neuronal impulses, counter-irritation, palpation.

A person's occupational history is helpful in understanding how
they have become who they are now. Today's elderly have survived
at least one world war, and witnessed the most drastic social, economic, technological and medical advances since the Industrial
Revolution.

SOCIOLOGICAL

The elderly used to be respected and venerated, seen as a valued
source of wisdom and knowledge; children were to be seen and not
heard; and class systems dictated social relationships with elaborate
but widely understood etiquette. All these aspects need to be
remembered when treating or advising an elderly person.

It is particularly important for the elderly that courtesies be
observed. They are sensitive to undue familiarity, and rightly expect
to be addressed by title and surname until they themselves take the
initiative in inviting less formality. They may be reluctant to call
staff by first names and may interpret failure in the niceties of
self-introduction, formal greeting, hand-shaking, as downright
rudeness.

Hierarchical social structures used to ensure authority from
above, obedience and loyal service from below. Standards of living,
education, housing, income, etc. derived largely from social status,
and 'upward mobility' was rarer than nowadays. Professional people
were admired, consulted and respected for their expertise. The
extreme deference to the doctor by some elderly patients stems from

their childhood experience, and they may lose trust in the multi-disciplinary team who openly dispute with or differ from medical opinion. While consultants carry ultimate responsibility for patients, it can disturb the elderly to witness the much freer management style current in today's multidisciplinary teamwork. However, ready acceptance by some elderly patients of professional advice and intervention – 'You know best' – is useful in gaining compliance, though the very old may view the therapist as very young, therefore very inexperienced, therefore incompetent!

Pre-welfare-state 'charity' was the last resort; pride dissuaded many from seeking benefits. Even today, some elderly patients, discounting their National Insurance contributions, try to pay for treatment, or may be reluctant to receive it for fear of bills. They need gentle reassurance.

The attitude of their childhood's society towards hygiene, work, recreational activities, education, religion, ethnic minority groups, law and order, and public morality all affect older patients' attitudes to their own ageing, disability, illness, hospitalization or impending death. By being aware of these views the physiotherapist can do much to avoid any misunderstanding by or with the patients.

TECHNOLOGICAL

Domestic life has changed much in the last 50 years so it is often difficult to imagine some elderly patients' life circumstances. Availability of public utilities (power supplies, water, sewage, telephone, transport) and the now general use of water closets, plumbed hot water and central heating, refrigerators, washing machines, vacuum cleaners, television, even microwave ovens, may be regarded as unnecessary by the aged. Reluctance to use modern technology for overcoming handicap, to accept motorized wheelchairs, stair-lifts, telephone-linked alarm systems, or remote controls is therefore understandable. Sometimes, though, the placebo effect of a miracle of modern science is psychologically beneficial, and a patient may genuinely feel better after his radiograph.

MEDICAL AND SURGICAL

Elderly patients' expectations of admission to hospital are not helped by the conversion of Victorian workhouses into geriatric hospitals. Many, fearing death as the only result, are unwilling to make efforts towards rehabilitation. Confusion of the natural effects of ageing (being old) and the reversible results of disease (being ill) leads to these terms being regarded as synonymous. Unreported illness is more common in the elderly than in younger people (Pathy, 1985). More florid presentations of their more advanced pathology are therefore often seen in geriatric departments (Muir Gray, 1985; Powell and Crombie, 1974). Some disorders, however, manifest more subtly or atypically in the elderly, who will not necessarily feel pain with a heart attack (Day et al, 1987), or show a fever with pneumonia (Berman et al, 1987) and therefore do not perceive themselves as ill and in need of treatment. Decreased mobility due to advanced heart failure or degenerative joint disease is often expected with age; it is seen as irremediable, and therefore accepted without complaint.

Specific symptoms may be difficult to elicit, or terminology may be old-fashioned. Imprecise terms like 'delicate', 'sickly', 'suffering a decline', need careful questioning. A dictionary may be needed for words like 'costive' (constipated), 'dropsy' (dependent oedema), 'ague' (malarial-type fever), 'consumption' (tuberculosis), 'quinsy' (tonsillitis or sore throat) which are part of the patient's vocabulary, but not that of the staff. Many euphemisms are used to describe excretory functions, and staff may be as unaware of their meanings as patients are of the correct names for some parts of the body, let alone their position and function. The Edwardian concept of 'germs' is still useful in explanations to the layman, but it is quite a different matter to describe interferential therapy to a 90-year-old.

THE AGEING BODY

Normal developmental milestones can be pinpointed quite accurately in babies and children, but not so the changes and diminishing abilities of old age.

Theories of ageing

What exact mechanism produces 'ageing' remains an unsolved mystery. A number of factors, physiological and environmental, combine to affect the viability of the human body.

Physiological Longevity is a demonstrably genetically inherited tendency in some families. In *in vitro* experiments cell divisions are self-limiting, cells from the mucosa of young children multiplying through more divisions than those from old people. The maximum appears to be approximately 50 divisions under laboratory conditions, indicating the limited capacity of the body to repair and replace its tissues indefinitely. Likewise, genetically inherited or perinatal defects compromise chances of long life.

Genetic template error leads to decreasingly accurate cell reproduction, and eventual de-differentiation of tissues with consequent impairment of function of specialized organs. As inefficiency multiplies, secondary effects of slowed detoxification and removal of metabolic by-products, reduced tissue nutrition and oxygenation, compromised healing capacity and impaired buffer systems all contribute to ageing. There is a generalized age-related increase in the proportion of white fibrous tissue which is one of the least differentiated body tissues.

The immune system becomes less efficient as the body ages; less prompt both to identify and to overcome invading organisms. This renders the elderly more susceptible to opportunist infections, and they are likely to be more seriously ill in cases where a younger person would recover relatively quickly, hence the importance of 'convalescence' in the recovery of the very old. When immunity becomes functionally impaired, the risk of malignant disease rises, as it does with advancing years.

Natural 'wear and tear' particularly affects tissues which have little or no capacity to reproduce and multiply, for example cardiac muscle, nervous tissue, joint cartilage. The summation and interaction of these insidious and discrete changes produce the gross systemic effects recognized as ageing.

Environmental The body gathers more and more damage from the results of successive diseases, trauma, pollutants, and perhaps inadequate diet or warmth. Until man learned to control his environment, to tame predators, and to ensure food supply and adequate protection from the elements, ageing was an unknown phenomenon. The maximum natural life-span is probably about 100 years, and life expectancy at birth in the developed West is approximately 65–80 years, with a tendency to increase. Factors as yet unknown may influence the patterns and rates of ageing of future generations.

The various systems of the body undergo changes and the significance of these as they affect the physiotherapist will be discussed.

LOCOMOTOR SYSTEM

Bone starts to lose calcium after the age of 25, the rate depending on the amount and vigour of habitual exercise, dietary intake, and increasing in women after the menopause due to hormonal changes.

A 30 per cent de-mineralization may take place before changes are detectable radiologically (Woolf et al, 1987; Goodman, 1985). After a fracture normal bone healing time is not increased if there is osteoporosis although for a previously fit 80-year-old, where there is adequate intact bone, internal fixation is often preferable to prevent the ill-effects of prolonged rest. It is important to prevent further calcium loss from the rest of the skeleton during immobilization. This is best achieved by weight-bearing exercise. Where the fracture site prevents immediate walking every effort should be made to achieve standing, or a non-weight-bearing gait with aids. The mechanism of stressing bone along its longitudinal axis, with accompanying contractions of surrounding muscles, is the most effective way of maintaining blood supply and bone growth, through increasing the intra-medullary pressure (Lewis, 1985).

Maintenance exercises for unaffected limbs and trunk are even more necessary for older people, as the dangers of contracture, stiffness, decubitus lesions and chest complications follow quickly upon disuse atrophy and immobility. Muscle power decreases by up to 3 per cent daily during immobilization on bed rest, and may be reduced by the age of 70 to half what it was at the age of 20. Elderly men are often surprised, even ashamed, at their own lack of strength, and may fail to admit weakness. Tact is needed when muscle testing.

Disuse also decreases the ratio of white fast-twitch to red muscle fibres (Noakes, 1983). This may be due to reduced activity rather than to the ageing process itself, as most old people take less exercise, and even if active are seldom free of the limiting effects of osteoarthrosis. The loss of muscle mass found in the elderly is also affected by its innervation (Nelson et al, 1984; Vandervoort et al, 1986). As irreplaceable anterior horn cells die, the motor end-plates become denervated, and compensatory proliferation of adjacent axon branchings re-inervates some of them. Eventually this compensation cannot keep pace with degeneration, and increasing numbers of muscle fibres become atrophied.

CARDIORESPIRATORY SYSTEM

The respiratory system becomes less flexible. Kyphosis due to osteoporosis of the thoracic spine and ossification of costochondral cartilages reduces mechanical efficiency; hardening of bronchi and bronchioles increases airway resistance, and at microscopic level loss of elastin reduces alveolar extensibility, decreasing total surface area. Diminished vital capacity leads to hypostatic lung changes, increasing susceptibility to pneumonia. These changes mimic obstructive airways disease, even where there is no loss of lung parenchyma. Ciliary motility slows, and the cough reflex becomes sluggish. Coughing becomes less powerful with reduction of intercostal muscle bulk, and the relative usefulness of postural drainage increases compared with other methods of assisting expectoration. Frequent changes of position, and the respiratory effort required to achieve them, are of great importance in respiratory care for the elderly, and careful teaching of diaphragmatic breathing will offset some effects of thoracic rigidity. If inhalers are prescribed the physiotherapist should check their use, and be prepared to select appropriate space inhalers or other dispensers if the patient cannot manage conventional models.

For physiotherapists, cardiac changes are most relevant with regard to exercise capacity. Blood pressure, particularly systolic pressure, increases with age because of raised peripheral resistance due to sclerotic changes in artery and arteriole walls (Dambrink and Weiling, 1987). Heart muscle responds to the increased workload by hypertrophy, but thickening of the myocardium does not produce an increase in stroke volume. Indeed, cardiac reserve decreases, and exercise tolerance in the elderly is best monitored by pulse rate, not allowing an increase of more than 20 or 30 beats per minute from resting rate, or less where there is cardiac pathology or other signs of distress. Cardiomegaly alone is no contra-indication to moderate exercise, but as cardiovascular efficiency is reduced, so is 'sprint' ability, though endurance may be unaffected.

Atherosclerosis is common, although generally considered a disease rather than a natural ageing process, because of its variable incidence in the population, and its step-wise progression. It is also affected by smoking and diet.

In left ventricular failure, patients' mobility may be hampered not only by their cardiac limitation, but also by excessive dependent lower limb oedema. If this is not reduced rapidly, organization and fibrin infiltration will cause permanent swelling and thickening of the tissues. Sequential pressure therapy to reduce this oedema must be applied with caution, as sudden restoration of fluid to the circulation may cause hypervolaemia, raise the blood pressure and further stress the heart. Only one leg should be treated at a time, and the physiotherapist should consult with the physician to ensure that there is adequate kidney function and diuresis.

Due to degenerative changes in the sympathetic nervous system, the heart rate does not readily increase in response to postural change which, with reduced capacity of the veins in the legs to vasoconstrict, often produces postural hypotension. Adequate time must be given for adaptation to an erect stance, and patients may need advice on pacing themselves when rising from bed to avoid fainting or falling.

NEUROLOGICAL FUNCTION

The morphology of brain cells begins to change in the 20s, with successive decrease in numbers throughout the decades, and reduction in brain weight associated with decreased cerebral blood flow. In the absence of specific pathology this does not necessarily reach critical thresholds, even in old age, but a general slowing of mental function is expected. There is conflicting evidence about the effect of ageing on nerve conduction velocity (Payton and Poland, 1983; Nelson et al, 1984) but slowing at neurosynaptic junctions, and loss of dendrites at end-plates, may affect the speed or presence of reflexes. This becomes particularly significant when it starts to affect balance by slowing righting reflexes to the anti-gravity muscles.

The sensory systems

While compensation by other senses can enable an individual to function successfully in the absence or impairment of one of them, gradual deterioration of all the systems will compromise abilities. The elderly take longer to make expected responses (Payton and Poland, 1983) needing time to interpret incoming signals and to process the multiplicity of stimuli.

Telereceptors
Sight: The more sensitive systems are more likely to be affected by nervous system changes. Whereas, for example, in gluteus maximus one motor neurofibril can innervate some 200 muscle fibres, in the eye, the one-to-one ratio of nerve to muscle fibres renders vision more liable to diminution. Visual and spatial perception and discrimination become less accurate. Higher lighting levels are needed to see as well as previously, as loss of retinal rods disturbs dark adaptation. Accommodation to sudden illumination can take 30 seconds or more. Retinal opacity (cataract), reduced lens elasticity, simple glaucoma and senile macular degeneration, while not all necessarily the direct result of ageing, increase in incidence. The physiotherapist must remember this when testing for gait safety in a well-lit department or ward; a floor-level obstacle course may be useful training. The community physiotherapist, aware of the daytime

lighting levels encountered in a patient's home, needs to assess how mobility might be affected at night.

Hearing: Degeneration of hair cell receptors and loss of neurones in the cochlea reduce sensitivity to higher frequencies soon after childhood, leading to deafness in many older people. People can hear vowel sounds after they have lost the ability to pick up the consonants, and are less able to discriminate from unwanted background noise. More time is needed by the deaf elderly to process the meaning of the incoming sounds, and they may use unwittingly acquired lip-reading skills. Deafness is considered so 'normal' that probably only half of the deafness in the population is ever reported, let alone treated.

Exteroceptors

Touch: The sense of touch is not diminished, though in the presence of one stimulus a greater threshold is required for a second stimulus to be noted.

Pain: Superficial pain sensation declines insignificantly; deep pain such as ischaemic pain is diminished, hence the high incidence of 'silent' (painless) myocardial infarctions among the elderly, and the relatively speedy rehabilitation possible in some cases of impacted fracture, uninhibited by pain.

Temperature: Diminution of temperature discrimination is of importance in testing skin sensation before giving heat treatments. The threshold at which temperature change is appreciated rises, and the patient may also think that 'hotter is better'. The benefits of heat as a therapeutic measure for the elderly should not be overlooked, even though extra caution is required. Because of the fragility of the skin of elderly people, greater care should be exercised in giving ice treatments, and the efficiency of the individual's temperature regulation considered.

Proprioceptors

Proprioception declines with age, and can have major results in producing unsteadiness especially if visual function is also impaired and cannot compensate. Blind or partially sighted old people are particularly at risk according to the severity and extent of the loss. If a walking aid is needed, then an increasingly large base is preferable even at the expense of manoeuvrability, i.e. a quadrupod rather than a stick, or a frame with more widely splayed upright struts.

Interoceptors

Visceral and internal appreciation of temperature, pain, pressure and chemical changes diminishes, leading to vagueness in self-reporting. Diagnosis becomes particularly difficult when the symptoms themselves may be vague, as in spinal stenosis (Weinstein, 1988).

AUTONOMIC FUNCTION

Both sympathetic and parasympathetic nervous systems show evidence of degeneration. With reduced efficiency in vasoconstriction, and probable hypothalamic deficit, the aged are especially prone to the effects of cold, capable of appreciating neither temperature loss, nor of the normal physiological responses to it.

Normal febrile response to infection is lowered, so raised heart rate is a much more reliable indicator that the body's defences are being recruited. However, the elderly are more liable to hyperthermia because of reduced sweating. These factors influence the planning of treatment programmes, to include adequate monitored cooling-off time after activities which raise body temperature, and to avoid predisposition to hypothermia.

Bladder function shows evidence of decreased cortical inhibitory activity, with higher resting bladder pressures and reduced bladder capacity, resulting in frequency and urgency which can lead to incontinence.

Although colonic dysfunction has an autonomic component, it is more likely attributable to lack of exercise, low fibre intake or laxative overdose; the most common cause of constipation is ignoring the call of nature.

METABOLIC CHANGES

The major clinical consequence of changes in renal and hepatic function in the elderly is the effect on drug metabolism and excretion. Although not necessarily directly the physiotherapist's concern, all staff in close contact with patients taking medication should note any untoward signs or changes in the patient's state after alterations in prescription, and report them to the physician.

MENTAL FUNCTION

The most widespread normal effect of mental changes is short-term memory loss (benign senescent forgetfulness). Survival skills learned in early years tend to remain relatively intact into extreme age (recognition of harmful stimuli, appropriate response to thirst and hunger, food recognition) but from middle age onwards people commonly complain of not being able to recall names or facts as readily as before, and recently learned material is more difficult to retain.

Ideally the gains of past knowledge and experience offset sensory deprivations and overall performance of the elderly fit is not compromised until some insult to the body, disease or trauma, supervenes.

The mentally ill elderly fall into four main categories:

1. Elderly people with physical illnesses which also cause mental symptoms

Properly, these patients should not be classed as psychiatric. Acute confusional states very often have physical causes: sudden onset of mental symptoms preceding or accompanying onset of physical manifestations, for example the bronchopneumonia sufferer who first presents wandering out of doors in nightclothes. Such cases are reversible, given the correct treatment of the physical causes.

Chronic brain syndromes are intractable due to long-term progressive, irreversible organic brain damage.

Some Physical Causes of Confusion in the Elderly

Incipient or sub-acute infection: such as urinary or respiratory tract infection.

Change of location: for example a recent move from home to hospital or vice versa, or into institutional care. Sometimes confusion is only apparent when the patient is away from the familiar surroundings which have enabled continued function by force of habit.

Withdrawal of alcohol: after considerable drinking confusion may not develop until the second or third day after withdrawal. Thiamine deficiency in the chronic alcoholic produces longer-standing confusion which, if not reversible, may be arrestable.

Constipation (Ellard, 1988): As previously stated this may be caused by delaying response to the call of nature if mobility is impaired and help is needed to get to the toilet. It may be improved by taking adequate exercise.

Adverse or heightened reaction: to medication; allergy or toxicity.

Pain: Even when not complaining of pain, the confusion it causes may cloud abilities to analyse and describe it.

Sensory deprivation: diminished sight, hearing or perception.

Hypothermia or hyperthermia: Hypothermic patients should be left as undisturbed as possible until their core temperature has been normal for at least 24 hours, even if this means temporarily postponing chest treatment. Hyperthermic patients, especially those with circulatory or cardiac disorders, should not receive any treatment liable to raise their body temperature further, as in sudden spells of hot weather they are at higher than normal risk (Bull and Morton, 1975).

Dehydration.

Malnutrition: leading to internal chemical imbalance, deficiency in essential body salts, proteins and vitamins.

Electrolyte imbalance: or raised urea and creatinine.

Cerebral impairment: by low pressure hydrocephalus, intracranial neoplasm, tertiary syphilis, or slow subdural haemorrhage.

Physiotherapy should be appropriate to the physical illness, with caution regarding impaired understanding; a simple, direct approach will be the most effective (Andreae and Moon, 1983).

2. Long-standing patients who have been mentally ill throughout their lives, and have grown into old age with their illness

These patients will be found both in hospital and community. In the past, patients whose severe mental disturbance led to behaviour which society found unacceptable were virtually banished to mental asylums. These were huge long-stay institutions, isolated in remote country areas, and their forgotten inmates became permanently separated from normal life. Now that policy has changed to integrated community care, with closure of many vast mental hospitals, it will become more common to meet such patients in domestic settings, staffed houses, smaller residential care establishments, or general hospitals.

Until then, as the elderly often show multiple problems, the incidence of physical disorders in elderly chronic mental patients is expected to rise. It is the physiotherapist who is in a position to diagnose and refer patients with intercurrent physical disease.

3. The elderly functionally ill

These are patients who are subject to the disabling effects of reversible affective disorders, with no intrinsic structural damage to brain tissue. There may be predisposing physical factors to their mental state, for example long-term joint pain can produce severe depression, even suicide. Physiotherapists have a role in reducing such arthritic pain, advising on management and providing walking aids.

A depressed patient tends to hypokinesia which, in the elderly, leads to stiffness, muscle atrophy, further disinclination to move and progressive reduction in stamina. Exercise classes and individual movement programmes can help to reduce these effects and, during recovery, the change of scenery achieved by leaving the ward or home to attend physiotherapy can be beneficial.

4. The elderly with senile mental disease

Alzheimer's disease produces slow degeneration of the brain cortex, with smoothing and flattening of the sulci and gyri; there are plaque formations with microscopically detectable cell changes, although post-mortem studies do not correlate uniformly with the degree of impairment suffered (Kellett, 1988; Wilcock, 1988). The disease is progressive and remorseless, with a prognosis of increasing disability until death about 7 to 10 years after date of onset. Patients often remain remarkably physically healthy and mobile until the terminal stage, when pneumonia is a common cause of death.

Arteriosclerotic dementia is characterized by its step-wise progression, often exacerbated by transient ischaemic attacks, and other effects of circulatory deficit. Its course and prognosis vary according to severity of vascular changes. Neurological problems often accompany the mental signs, rendering rehabilitation less feasible in later stages, when management and education of carers in mobility, transfers and hygiene become predominant.

Hospitalization is often the only option in the most immobile dependent stages. Ideally, liaison beds jointly administered by consultants and staffed by nurses qualified in both psychiatry and medicine for the elderly should be available, as many aspects of care require more bodily help than registered mental nurses are qualified to give. Problems of incontinence, poor mobility, helping and handling, feeding and so on, which are amenable to physical management, are of particular concern to the physiotherapist, who has a role in educating other staff in a psychogeriatric hospital or department (Oddy, 1987).

APPROACH TO THE TREATMENT OF THE ELDERLY PATIENT

Not all the gross changes that may be expected with age are within the physiotherapist's ability to help. However, any may impinge upon the patient's quality of functional movement, and therefore on the approach to treatment and management. Interests of the different professions in the multidisciplinary team do overlap and all members should be familiar with the others' roles, and ready to refer/discuss problems appropriately as they arise. Professional jealousy and boundary defensiveness have no part in good team practice (Isaacs, 1981). It would be ridiculous to withhold from each other the skills and knowledge we should impart to a patient/carer, and it is important that statutory carers are well equipped (Young, 1988).

The distinctive characteristic of physiotherapy with the elderly is the comprehensiveness of the initial assessment. Unlike some specialties, where the presenting symptomatic problem is the major focus, the whole patient should be assessed; specific dysfunctions, pain, immobility, debility, impaired sensation or motivation, spasticity, incomprehension, non-compliance and so on, are seen in relation not only to each other and to the ability of the whole person, but also in relation to the contributions of other team members.

Whether the patient is treated as an outpatient or in a day hospital, a ward, his/her home or in an institution, it is essential to link the information about movement and function to life at home. A joint home assessment with the occupational therapist is much to be recommended.

Gathering the data

Because of a long history (either due to progressive deterioration of chronic degenerative diseases or merely to the length of the patient's life) there may well be more relevant history. A synopsis can usually be sought by talking with the spouse, or anyone regularly in close contact with the patient. Any relevant records, hospital notes or clinical summaries should be read.

Multidisciplinary consultation in ward meetings, rounds and case conferences are useful for sharing information; the general practitioner's knowledge about the patient can be invaluable. Any previous physiotherapy notes should be consulted.

The interview

As earlier indicated the normal courtesies should not be overlooked. The patient should be comfortable and able to see and hear the physiotherapist as well as possible. Language should be adapted to the patient's understanding, with answers being used as the clue to comprehension. Don't talk down to the patient.

Open-ended questions, like 'Tell me about what you find difficult' are most likely to elicit useful information. If the patient sees non-complaining or underrating their own symptoms as a virtue, it is often more fruitful to ask if anywhere hurts or aches, than to use the word 'pain'.

Adequate time and accurate note-taking are vital. The examination may have to extend over some days, but differences in self-reporting from day to day should not be discounted. The emphasis that the patient places on what is reported and whether the personal pattern is random or predictable will enable the physiotherapist to work out priorities in deciding treatment.

The patient may:

- Put the most painful thing first/last.
- Put the most worrying thing first/last.
- Report only what he/she thinks the physiotherapist wants to hear.
- Report only things he/she feels the physiotherapist can remedy.
- Try not to shock the hearer.
- Give undue significance to something quite minor – this should prompt the physiotherapist to probe 'why'.
- Report things that cause dysfunction or pain or other symptoms.

The physiotherapist should also assess whether the self-reporting is congruous with the obvious problems and diagnosis, and should note the quality of the history, memory and ideas. Independent witnesses of the patient's abilities, and discrepancies between their accounts will highlight fluctuations in performance or motivation.

The examination

The patient is examined systematically, often using a scheme or check list so that nothing is overlooked. Gradually a picture of any functional disabilities in daily life is revealed. If physical or emotional pain is caused, it is important not to leave the patient feeling worse than before the physiotherapist came. The gross examination may reveal problems, thus enabling the physiotherapist to focus the examination more closely on abnormal or difficult movements or activities.

The main difference between the examination by the physiotherapist and that by other members of the multidisciplinary team will be the examination of movement, its speed, co-ordination, quality, associated reactions, power, stamina, range and function, degree and causes of difficulty. This applies to every movement, whether of the thorax in respiration, or getting up out of bed, or of a single painful digit which may have been overlooked by other staff during a major crisis of, say, a fractured neck of femur.

Problem list

The problem list is ideally made *with* the patient and/or the main relative or carer. Problems not within the ambit of physiotherapy should be noted for referral to the appropriate member of the team, and the patient/carer told about the referral.

The patient may be too acutely ill to understand or co-operate in the drawing-up of a treatment programme. The physiotherapist should treat the unconscious or aggressively confused person according to the observable needs at the time, and wait for the patient to recover enough reason and comprehension to co-operate with an organized plan.

It is sometimes necessary to distinguish between what really is problematic, rather than what appears to be: a patient born blind may be perfectly capable of coping with this disability. If the patient has a low self-esteem or a tendency to magnify difficulties, an objective positive review of what *is* possible may be more useful than concentrating on 'problems'.

Time may be needed to discuss disabilities which cannot be remedied. Other problems may be amenable to physiotherapy but if there are too many to attend to all of them, priorities should be set with the patient/carer, and realistic, measurable goals agreed.

Aims of intervention

Treatment aims must be realistic, or both patient and physiotherapist will become disillusioned and discouraged. While it may not be possible to make an accurate prediction of the degree of overall recovery from what may seem a catastrophic event such as a cerebrovascular accident or a coronary thrombosis, it will cheer the patient to have some intermediate goals by which to mark progress, and these should be expressed in a way that patient and carers understand. The overall aim of the physiotherapist that the patient should achieve unsupported sitting-to-standing balance should be expressed to the patient/carer as ability to sit up on the edge of the bed. When this is achieved, the next aim can be set: to be able to lean forward without toppling sideways or without becoming breathless, and so on.

The physiotherapist will have time schedules for these goals, but will not necessarily share these with the patient/carer. Whether the goals are met at all will be a measure of effectiveness. Whether they are met within the time expected will be a measure of efficiency. The outcomes of different treatment methods should be compared so that the most efficient and effective regimes are used in future. No treatment modality should be ruled out solely on the grounds of the patient's age.

The physiotherapist is not responsible only for individual treatments, but should plan who best will implement the whole treatment regime outside physiotherapy attendances, be it patient, carer, physiotherapist, helper, nurse (Werner, 1985), and should also act as educator, adviser, supplier of certain mobility aids and appliances, monitor of abilities (especially in progressive conditions) and referer to other agencies.

At each attendance there is a less extensive, informal re-assessment of the patient's overall state, changes in symptoms and the functional progress maintained, made or lost, the effectiveness of learned ways of coping, and new or intercurrent factors.

THE ROLE OF THE PHYSIOTHERAPIST

Physiotherapists working with the elderly may not only *treat* the patient, although in hospitals this will often be the obvious rôle (with all the other members of the multidisciplinary team available within their own defined specialties); they must also remember their obligations to act responsibly for the good of the patient even though this may involve activities which are not strictly physiotherapy (Purtilo, 1986). While it may not seem to be 'physiotherapy' to accompany an old woman with a walking frame to the toilet, the physiotherapist will be well placed to make an assessment of the balance, stamina, speed, agility, independence, motivation and competence of the patient.

During treatment sessions she may also hear many confidences and details relevant to the patient's total rehabilitation, and find herself acting as an informal counsellor (Saunders and Maxwell, 1988). While confidentiality is a very important part of this relationship, it must be made clear that any information thus received is information received by the *whole team* through one of its members.

It would be wrong to hide from the team a secret confidence, for example, that the patient always uses trips to the toilet to flush away the pills that she was supposed to have swallowed at the last drug round.

Community physiotherapists will find their rôle widened to include many aspects of health education, preventive work and informal education and advice. Regular appearances at day centres or old people's homes provide excellent opportunities to review the activities of the residents, to be seen as a resource for staff training, and to note problems which may need attention. Even where there is no formal commitment to provide exercise classes, the physiotherapist may find local volunteers or staff only too willing to be guided as to the kind of exercises suitable for their elderly folk. Group exercise classes or movement with music and even dancing are useful and effective ways of involving the reluctant or under-stimulated (Kennard, 1983) although the value of such exercises in improving performance may vary (Molloy et al, 1988).

The number of elderly people in the (UK) population is rising and the birth rate is falling, so there is an increasing proportion of elderly with a decreasing number of younger carers (Central Statistical Office, 1987). This will result in less physiotherapists to treat more older patients, and every resource must be recruited. The work of physiotherapy helpers in care of the elderly already demonstrates the enormous potential of less skilled personnel. Physiotherapists should take every opportunity to pass on their handling and helping skills to those who care for elderly people, and to educate themselves and the general population in preparing for as healthy and mobile old age as possible.

REFERENCES

Anderson, F. (1985). An historical overview of geriatric medicine: definition and aims. In *Principles and Practice of Geriatric Medicine* (ed. Pathy, M. S. J.). John Wiley Limited, Chichester.

Andreae, M. C. and Moon, M. H. (1983). A physiotherapist's approach to psychogeriatrics. *New Zealand Journal of Physiotherapy*, 11, 3, 13–15.

Bauer, D. (1982). Fact or fiction: the 'four-uns' of geriatrics. *Fisioterapie*, 38, 4, 84–6.

Berman, P., Hogan, D. B. and Fox, R. A. (1987). The atypical presentation of infection in old age. *Age and Ageing*, 16, 4, 201.

Bull, C. M. and Morton, J. (1975). Seasonal and short-term relationships of temperature with deaths from myocardial infarction and cerebral infarction. *Age and Ageing*, 4, 1, 19.

Caney, D. (1983). Competence – can it be assessed? *Physiotherapy*, 69, 8, 302.

Central Statistical Office (1987). *Key Data*. HMSO, London.

Dambrink, J. H. A. and Weiling, W. (1987). Circulatory response to postural change in healthy male subjects in relation to age. *Clinical Science*, **72**, 335–41.

Day, J. J., Bayer, A. J., Pathy, M. S. J. and Chadha, J. S. (1987). Acute myocardial infarction: diagnostic difficulties and outcome in advanced old age. *Age and Ageing*, **16**, 4, 239.

Ellard, J. (1988). Growing old: what it is and what it is not. *Geriatric Medicine*, **18**, 6, 71.

Finn, A. H. (1986). Attitudes of physiotherapists towards geriatric care. *Physiotherapy*, **72**, 3, 129.

Gale, J. and Livesley, B. (1974). Attitudes towards geriatrics. A report of the King's survey. *Age and Ageing*, **3**, 1, 49.

Goodman, C. E. (1985). Nutrition and exercise regime that reverses bone loss. *Geriatric Medicine*, **15**, 11, 14.

Howell, T. (1974). Origins of the British Geriatric Society. *Age and Ageing*, **2**, 3, 69.

Isaacs, B. (1981). Ageing and the doctor. In *The Impact of Ageing* (ed. Hobman, D.), pp. 155 *et seq.* Croom Helm, Beckenham.

Kane, R. L. (1988). Beyond caring: the challenge to geriatrics. *Journal of the American Geriatric Society*, **36**, 467–72.

Kellett, J. M. (1988). Dementia evaluation shows half Alzheimer's diagnoses are MID. *Geriatric Medicine*, **18**, 10, 13.

Kennard, K. (1983). A touch of music for physiotherapists. *Physiotherapy*, **69**, 4, 114.

Kvitek, S. D. B., Shaver, B. J., Blood, H. and Shepard, K. F. (1986). Age bias: physical therapists and older patients. *Journal of Gerontology*, **41**, 6, 706–9.

Lewis, C. B. (1985). Modifying treatment programmes in the elderly. *Clinical Management in Physical Therapy*, **5**, 6, 14–17.

Molloy, D. W., Delaquerriere, R. and Grilly, R. G. (1988). The effects of a three-month exercise programme on neurophysiological function in elderly institutionalized: a randomized controlled trial. *Age and Ageing*, **17**, 5, 303.

Muir Gray, J. (1985). Social and community aspects of ageing. In *Principles and Practice of Geriatric Medicine* (ed. Pathy, M. S. J.), p. 17. John Wiley Limited, Chichester.

Nelson, R. M., Soderberg, G. L. and Urbscheit, N. L. (1984). Alteration of motor-unit discharge characteristics in aged humans. *Physical Therapy*, **64**, 1, 29–34.

Noakes, T. D. (1983). Physical activity and ageing. *Fisioterapie*, **38**, 4, 88–92.

Oddy, R. (1987). Promoting mobility in patients with dementia: some suggested strategies for physiotherapists. *Physiotherapy Practice*, **3**, 18–27.

Pathy, M. S. J. (ed.) (1985). *Principles and Practice of Geriatric Medicine*, p. 3. John Wiley Limited, Chichester.

Payton, O. D. and Poland, J. L. (1983). Ageing process implications for clinical practice. *Physical Therapy*, **63**, 1, 41–7.

Powell, C. and Crombie, A. (1974). The Kilsyth questionnaire: a method of screening elderly people at home. *Age and Ageing*, **3**, 1, 23.

Purtilo, R. (1986). Professional responsibility in physiotherapy. *Physiotherapy*, **72**, 12, 579.

Saunders, C. and Maxwell, M. (1988). The case for counselling in physiotherapy. *Physiotherapy*, **74**, 11, 592.

Stevenson, O. (1981). Caring and dependency. In *The Impact of Ageing* (ed. Hobman, D.), p. 128. Croom Helm, Beckenham.

Vandervoort, A. A., Hayes, K. C. and Bélanger, A. Y. (1986). Strength and endurance of skeletal muscle in the elderly. *Physiotherapy Canada*, **38**, 3, 167–73.

Werner, S. (1985). Suggestions for a training programme for home helpers for the aged and disabled. *Fisioterapie*, **41**, 4, 115–17.

Wilcock, G. K. (1988). Recent research into dementia. *Age and Ageing*, **17**, 2, 73.

Woolf, A. D., McMurdo, M. E. T. and MacLennan, W. L. (1987). Answering a vexed question: how to treat osteoporosis? *Geriatric Medicine*, **17**, 2, 61.

Young, P. (1988). Home-care assistants: a new multifunctional role. *Geriatric Medicine*, **18**, 8, 13.

BIBLIOGRAPHY

Andrews, K. (1987). *Rehabilitation of the Older Adult*. Edward Arnold, London.

Andrews, K. and Brocklehurst, J. (1987). *British Geriatric Medicine in the 1980s*. King Edward's Hospital Fund for London.

Hawker, M. (ed.) (1983). *The Older Patient and the Role of the Physiotherapist*. Faber and Faber, London.

Jackson, O. (ed.) (1983). *Physical Therapy of the Geriatric Patient*. Churchill Livingstone, Edinburgh.

Jackson, O. (ed.) (1987). *Therapeutic Considerations for the Elderly*. Churchill Livingstone, Edinburgh.

Mitchell, L. (1988). *The Magic of Movement – A Tonic for Older People*. Age Concern, London.

Squires, A. (ed.) (1988). *Rehabilitation of the Older Patient*. Croom Helm, Beckenham.

Wagstaff, P. and Coakley, D. (ed.) (1988). *Physiotherapy and the Elderly Patient*. Croom Helm, Beckenham.

Key Points for Good Practice (1985). Published by, and obtainable from, the Association of Chartered Physiotherapists with a Special Interest in Elderly People, c/o The Chartered Society of Physiotherapy, London WC1R 4ED.

ACKNOWLEDGEMENTS

The author thanks the following for their help in the preparation of this chapter:

Miss Lydia Potter, Assistant Librarian, Normanby College, King's College Hospital, London SE5 9RS.
Mrs R. G. Fenn Clark.

Chapter 28

The Dying

by P. A. DOWNIE FCSP

In 1988 St Christopher's Hospice, London, celebrated its 21st anniversary of splendid work for dying patients. When it opened in 1967 it heralded the start of what has now been called 'a new hospice movement'. In medieval times a hospice was a half-way house, a resting place, for the pilgrim as he made his way to some great holy shrine. Such a place was likely to be within a religious house, and through the centuries hospices became shelters not only for the pilgrim but also for the sick, the destitute and the dying. Many religious communities maintained this role until quite recently – the Hostel of God (now Trinity Hospice) was run by the Society of Saint Margaret until the late 1970s – and St Joseph's Hospice in Hackney is still in the care of the Irish Sisters of Charity (Downie, 1973, 1974a).

After 1967 the hospice movement burgeoned and today (1989) there are well over 150 hospices, palliative care units, continuing care units, worldwide. Most of them care for adult patients, but Helen House in Oxford cares specifically for children. With the increasing numbers of AIDS patients a new need for specialist care for those in the terminal stages of the disease has become apparent, and the first hospice in the UK especially for such people has opened at the Mildmay Hospital, London.

In the USA care for the dying has been virtually non-existent until latterly, with the exception of the Calvary Hospital in the Bronx district of New York. This has stood like a beacon since the 1890s, always in the care of the Roman Catholic church and currently administered by the Sisters of the Little Company of Jesus. For many years they have included a physiotherapist as a key member of their team (Downie, 1974b). However, hospices are now being established and much interest in the care of the dying has been fostered. From the USA has come a great deal of literature on the subject of thanatology (study of death), bereavement, reactions to dying, counselling, etc.

Currently in the UK it is almost certain that a physiotherapist, and an occupational therapist, will be found as part of the team. There is little doubt that they have a definite part to play in the overall care of the dying (Chatterton, 1988).

DEATH AND DYING

We are often reminded that death is a taboo subject although with the increased number of special units one might feel that this attitude should have changed. Elizabeth Kubler Ross in the USA helped in the understanding of dying patients' feelings, as well as in the realization of the stages in bereavement; the work of Cicely Saunders towards the understanding and alleviation of pain has revolutionized the basic needs of many patients. Much of Kubler Ross's work can be classed as common sense and this is the prime requirement of the philosophy of approach to the dying patient. While the stages which she describes (Kubler Ross, 1970) are usually discussed in the context of bereavement it is interesting to see how they fit in with the reactions which a person suffers when faced with disagreeable truths, e.g. the patient who is told that he has multiple sclerosis, the mother who is told her baby has spina bifida, the young man who has to be told that his leg needs amputation after an accident. These stages can be summarized as follows: denial of the fact, followed by anger and then the stage of bargaining; depression follows and finally comes the stage of acceptance. Not every patient or family will react in the same way, nor will they all go through each of the stages. If one understands that these reactions are normal it will help the physiotherapist when she comes to treat what to her may be considered 'a difficult patient'.

Care of the dying cannot be neatly slotted into a definite period of time; the actual process of dying may be sudden or it may be a progressive decline, of failing faculties and functions. It is about the latter group that most of the practical comments will be made, since it is these patients who require the encouragement and reassurance to accept their weaknesses and to live. It is of these that the question 'Should the patient be told of his approaching death?', will be asked. In general the answer is probably 'Yes', in as much as they are able to bear it. There is no need to be cold and dogmatic; rather sow the seed and then wait and see what follows. Certainly this telling should be done early in the care of patients so that they are able to assimilate the truth and be helped to come to an understanding. Patients suffering from progressive disease, and particularly those who may have been treated with cytoxic drugs, become less and less able to respond to the demands of brain and body and consequently they look always to the familiar things.

The role of the physiotherapist

Many therapists are reluctant to acknowledge the part that they can play in the overall care of the dying. They are often frightened, not only of the questions which such patients might ask them, but also of their own reactions to what may be a distressing occasion.

What then should be the approach of such individuals? I suggest that basically it must be one of calmness, of reassurance, and of matter-of-factness. There is no place for sentimental slush; but this does *not* mean being hard and unsympathetic. Rather does it mean showing understanding and care, and, above all, being realistic. The Latin word *caritas* (love) covers this meaning so well – not the shallow meaning of physical love, but the deep compassionate understanding of a person's whole being.

Physiotherapy is not prescribed because a patient is dying, but is a continuing part of treatment that was started when the patient was more well. When I use the word physiotherapy I am thinking in the wide term of rehabilitation and total patient care. Some patients with a progressive disease, such as multiple sclerosis, motor neurone disease or severe arthritis, may have been in long-term hospitals for many years and received regular physiotherapy. To withdraw from treating such patients when they rapidly deteriorate would be most unkind, for this is the moment of truth when they require all the help that can be given. When one is privileged to partake in the work of any of the specialist homes for the dying, it becomes patently clear that the goal for each patient must be to live each day as it comes; for the physiotherapist this means adjusting the treatment each day.

Both doctor and physiotherapist, and, indeed, any member of the health care team, need to understand and appreciate the purpose behind treatment for the progressively ill or dying patient. Above all they need to accept that such care is as important as the care which they would bestow upon a young man who receives injuries in an industrial accident. Physiotherapy for the dying should not be regarded as a waste of time. Death is neither a disaster nor a failure of medicine, but a natural event which terminates people's existence. Physiotherapy that helps the patient to accept his dying and eases his physical discomfort should be prescribed without hesitation.

Complicated treatments are not advocated, but with perception and adroitness it is possible to help many patients up to the point of death. There is no doubt that physiotherapy and occupational therapy have much to offer patients who are reaching the end of their lives. Active encouragement to continue to live each day will help the patient to a better adjustment of approaching death, and the mere fact that somebody is interested in a dying patient's whim or fancy can be therapeutic. For the paralysed and bedridden patient, passive and active assisted movements of limbs will help the circulation and ease uncomfortable joints. Massage has the dual advantage of physical help as well as providing an opportunity for the patient to talk. It needs to be continually repeated that the prerequisite in care of the dying is the ability to give time and to be able to listen and support. The role of the physiotherapist is essentially in this area.

Doctors do not prescribe physiotherapy because a patient is dying but if there is a mutual understanding between doctor and physiotherapist then he may well ask her to treat a dying patient so that he may be enabled to die more peacefully. Into this category comes the progressively ill patient who develops pneumonia – 'the old man's friend' as Osler described it. Often, simple physiotherapeutic measures can relieve distress, and then it is justified; heroics in such cases are to be abhorred.

Relatives also need support. If the dying patient is being nursed at home, the visiting physiotherapist can help by showing the relatives how to offer unobtrusive help, how to move painful limbs and how to support where necessary as the patient potters round the room. This help with involvement in care will alleviate the feelings of inadequacy and despair which you so often encounter in families who are trying to cope and do not know how.

Dying patients latch on to unexpected things and people. The physiotherapist must be prepared for this and act accordingly. The author remembers a 60-year-old man who had been diagnosed as having a carcinoma of the bronchus for which no treatment was advised. He was admitted with an acute superimposed chest infection for which physiotherapy was requested. When seen he was acutely distressed and ill. Gentle breathing exercises and vibrations to the chest wall were instituted and with continuous oxygen he gradually relaxed and was able to co-operate. Over two or three days he improved, the infection cleared and he was mobilized to the point of going home. Suddenly his condition deteriorated and at the patient's request the physiotherapist was sent for – in his own gasping words to the ward sister he said: 'She's the only one who's done anything for me.' When I reached him it was abundantly obvious that he was dying with no physical treatment being possible or justified; all I could do was to remain with his wife by the bedside. Care and compassion to the point of death must be accepted when one accepts the treatment of a patient with a progressive illness.

I have questioned whether physiotherapy should be prescribed when a patient is dying, but equally I ask the question, when is a patient dying? I remember a lady, aged 45, with disseminated carcinoma from a primary breast tumour. She developed 'pneumonia', and because the family could not cope was admitted to a nursing home for care and comfort. Twelve months later she was still in the nursing home being kept comfortable on opiates. It was decided to seek another opinion and she was re-assessed. Following this she was transferred for rehabilitation with a view to trying at home. She was weaned off drugs, mobilized, and a month later returned home where she remained for 18 months before dying.

Physiotherapy can also be used in helping nurses to handle patients with greater ease and comfort. Often the patient with advanced malignant disease may have bone metastases and nurses are afraid of handling limbs for fear they may fracture. Nothing transmits itself more readily than fear and if a nurse is afraid of handling such limbs, the patient will soon become aware of this. Firm gentle handling is necessary and often the presence of a physiotherapist, used to moving injured limbs, can give the required confidence to both nurse and patient alike.

The yardstick of all care of the dying is to improve the quality of life remaining in the individual patient; it may entail keeping one patient drowsy and thus unaware of pain, while allowing another patient to live more actively and even more dangerously than might normally have been considered (Graeme, 1975). A physiotherapist involved with care for a dying person needs to be able to appreciate the purpose of life as a whole; she must never be surprised by strange requests; she must certainly not attempt to impose her own ideas upon the patient; and her approach must be positive yet sympathetic.

PHILOSOPHICAL QUESTIONS

Questions will be raised as to the reality of treating the dying: the physiotherapist may say, 'I have to treat dying patients and I cannot see the point – they won't recover and I could use the time more profitably'. Who are we to accept the truth of such a question? I would suggest that it is not for any one of us to say that a patient will not recover – very remarkable things do happen and I think it is right that we continue modified treatments, particularly for those patients whom we have known for a long time.

'What do I say if a patient asks me if she/he is dying?' At first sight, how difficult but most patients do not want an answer – that question is often the cry of desperation to be allowed to talk their way through their thoughts. Don't ignore it and don't run away. Rather sit down and listen, or, give some massage and listen, and turn the question to 'why are you asking me that' or 'what makes you think this?' You will almost certainly find at the end that you have said almost nothing or you have been given time to provide the practical help required. Don't lie to such patients; if you don't know the answer, say so with complete frankness, *but* offer either to find out the answer or at least to find someone else who can help. In all these situations remember the hospital chaplain – he is there to help *you* as well as the patients.

'What do I do if I am asked to treat a dying patient for the very first time?' Here is another often asked question – particularly by students and newly qualified physiotherapists. Invariably it is asked in the context of the patient with disseminated cancer or some other progressive chronic disease, who develops a pneumonia. To any who postulate this question, I always say that if by treating such patients they will die more peacefully, then treat them; when in doubt in your own mind, ask yourself if you would allow your own parents to be treated – if you can honestly answer yes, then treat them. BUT, if you are unhappy about giving such treatments then you must say so. No one will think the less of you for so doing.

Euthanasia

In recent times there has again been much talk about the desirability to legalize the practice of euthanasia. Over the years many respected and responsible people have spoken for it; there have been, in the last 50 years, three bills presented to Parliament – all have failed. Any professional who has dealings with the chronically sick or dying patient may find herself caught up in this debate. For this reason the following paragraphs are offered.

Despite all the writings of people like Dame Cicely Saunders, Robert Twycross, Sylvia Lack and others, there are many who still equate dying with pain and so the question of euthanasia is raised. It is as well for physiotherapists to be aware of this, to understand the implications, and to be prepared to speak out fearlessly against it. Nowadays pain control, both physical and mental, is better understood; pain is more able to be treated adequately and should not therefore present problems. The positive answer to euthanasia is education of this aspect, and reassurance to the public that such treatment is possible.

The word euthanasia is derived from a Greek word meaning 'peaceful death', but the modern connotation implies the deliberate ending of a person's life. In 1973 the late Cardinal Heenan stated the Christian teaching on the care of the incurably ill as follows:

It is not for me to give medical and legal arguments against euthanasia. Nor shall I discuss the social implication of killing sick people whether with or without their consent. I do not intend to deal with those for whom men are high-grade animals without responsibility to any law not made by man. It is my task to give briefly the Christian teaching on treatment of the incurably sick.

(1) The first principle is that Almighty God as the author of life is also the Lord of life. God alone is Creator. Parents are called pro-creators. That is our way of saying that they are not absolute in their authority over the life they bring into the world. This is a fundamental truth accepted by all civilized societies until our own day.

(2) The second principle is that no private person has the right to destroy life whether his own or another's.

(3) Thirdly, there are legitimate differences of opinion among believers regarding the rights of the State over life. In general terms these concern killing in war and in peace. Not all agree that the State can authorize the killing (a) of aggressors by force of arms and (b) of criminals by execution. Some Christians hold that killing is legitimate in a just war or in self-defence. Pacifists regard no price as too high to pay for peace. They deny the right and duty of the State to maintain military defences. Some Christians, who are not necessarily pacifists, hold that the capital punishment of criminals is immoral.

(4) Direct killing of the incurably sick, disabled or insane is never justified.

(5) The Catholic church condemns the direct killing of the living fetus although saving the life of the mother may indirectly involve the death of the fetus.

(6) It is not permissible to withhold nourishment or normal medical aids with the object of hastening a patient's death.

It is not for the theologian to define in detail what is meant by normal medical aids. The kiss-of-life or mechanical resuscitation of a patient suffering from shock would now be regarded as normal. The prolonged use of machines to maintain the action of heart or lungs though commonplace would be regarded as extra-ordinary means of preserving life. In certain circumstances such means might and perhaps ought to be discontinued on ethical grounds.

The patient and the doctor have different responsibilities. It may be the duty of the doctor and relatives to provide the opportunity of treatment to save or prolong life. It may be their duty in the old phrase 'to allow nature to take its course'. It is not the duty of the patient to accept treatment which will purchase a further lease of life at the cost of great suffering or discomfort. Thus it would be unethical for the surgeon merely for the sake of research to persuade a patient to submit to an operation which might save the patient from death only to survive in misery.

For the Christian there are many fates worse than death. Often death is the last friend rather than the last enemy. In the *Canterbury Tales* Chaucer says, 'Death is an end of every worldly sore.' Shelley also pays tribute to death: 'How wonderful is Death, Death and his brother sleep!' Death is not a misfortune to be warded off at all costs. The death of God's friends is precious in His sight because it is a homecoming. That is why we need not hesitate to alleviate pain merely from fear of bringing nearer the hour of death. It is good ethics to ensure the comfort of the dying. It disposes of the chief argument in support of euthanasia.

The moral sense and compassion of doctors and nurses must decide what is for the patient's good. It is not euthanasia to refuse to use extra-ordinary methods to conquer a critical condition in a patient already suffering from a chronic terminal illness. To help patients to die in peace and dignity is part of the art of nursing and medicine.

These are the general principles. If we depart from them either to co-operate in suicide or to execute incurables we trespass on God's province and run the risk of destroying the whole moral law. With the decline of religion people have already begun to confuse legality with morality. Abortion and homosexual practices are regarded by many as morally acceptable because they are now permitted by law. If euthanasia were to become legal no sick or old person would be safe. The law of God is also the law of reason.

These are clear facts which should help all physiotherapists to understand better the very real difficulties which can arise in caring for the dying. It is an issue which cannot be evaded and one with which all right-thinking professionals should be concerned. It is probably true to say that it is not death itself which people fear, it is the process of dying and the very real fear of being subjected to unpleasant treatments with no real purpose save that of satisfying medical science. If this latter fear can be confidently resolved, and the patient and his family convinced and reassured that he will neither be allowed to suffer pain, nor be regarded as useless and a nuisance, then the question of euthanasia should not even be contemplated.

DAY CARE

With the growth of hospices a feature which has developed is that of providing day care for an increasing number of patients. Some units were concerned as to how their patients managed when they were discharged from the unit after an admission for symptom control management, etc.; some units were equally concerned at the number of patients who needed their expert advice but could not be admitted because of lack of beds. For both purposes a day centre seemed the obvious answer: discharged patients could be followed-up regularly – weekly, twice-weekly or as required; new patients could be assessed and then seen as necessary. For the latter this also meant that they were able to get to know the hospice staff so that if or when admission was necessary it would be to an environment that they already knew (Wilkes, 1982).

Most of the day centres now in being regard having their own transport arrangements as an essential requirement. Usually this is provided by a rota of volunteers who will ferry the patients as necessary. The staff will include, apart from doctors and nurses, a physiotherapist, an occupational therapist, chiropodist, social worker, voluntary helpers, access to a chaplain and, almost certainly, the services of a hairdresser (Wilkes et al, 1978).

Liaison is maintained with the patient's GP as well as with the district nurse and community services who may already be visiting at home. Stress is laid on supporting relatives and carers: the fact that a patient is able to come regularly to the unit can be reassuring to a carer who may otherwise not be able to have any time to him/herself.

THE DYING CHILD

By its very definition the death of a child or adolescent is inevitably premature. From the time the parents respond to the earliest signs of life in their, as yet unborn, child so they start to invest in hopes for his/her future. Names start to be explored; personality and potential for this new person begins to emerge.

Death of a child may occur in a number of circumstances: miscarriage, stillbirth and sudden infant death may occur within the families that the therapist is working with. She may have little to contribute in a direct way but a sensitivity to the pain that the family is experiencing and an awareness of local support available may be a very real way of helping such a family to reassemble its life.

Death may occur suddenly as the result of acute illness, accident or trauma. The therapist may be involved within the intensive care unit – she can make a contribution to the ease, dignity and comfort of the last part of a child's life and join with the whole team in supporting the family.

Death of a child may be anticipated. A number of childhood illnesses and disabilities are progressive or degenerative in nature, e.g. fibrocystic disease, muscular dystrophies and atrophies. Through the early part of the child's life there may be new achievement as maturation progresses more rapidly than the degeneration. Then comes a level period followed by a tangible deterioration. The therapist may well have worked with the child and his family throughout each of these phases. She may have established a considerable rapport with each member of the family. She too has to acknowledge the changed circumstances. It may be very difficult for the family to accept this changing situation. The therapist can no longer work for rehabilitation, but has a contribution to make to the child and his family. To escape from this tangle requires honesty, communication and, if possible, the support of a broad-based team bringing counselling skills to all who are involved. Each individual has his/her own needs. The child, his mother, father, siblings and friends are all individuals, and it is important to allow each family member to work through their own feelings both as an individual and as part of the family.

Children approach death in different ways related to their age, maturation, life experiences, personality and family attitudes and beliefs. Some children will have experienced the death of a grandparent, a neighbour or a pet – these events will help to establish that death is irreversible.

As an awareness of the approach of their own death grows so many children and young people will need to explore questions such as, 'Am I dying?' 'What will happen to me?' The therapist working with youngsters in this circumstance can use her established rapport to help the child voice his anxieties and fears and use other team members with the skills to help him through this difficult stage of life. She can help the child feel comfortable with needing to talk about these things.

No two people approach the death of someone close in exactly the same way. The parents of a dying child have many feelings in common but also their own separate understandings and perceptions. It is important that each is given the opportunity to explore their needs as individuals as well as receiving support as a couple. They may have questions about when, how or where the child will die. Will they recognize the signs of significant change? What will they be able to do? How will they respond? What will they tell the other children? If the child is being nursed at home they may want to know who to call and when and how.

Brothers and sisters of dying children have needs themselves. These will vary according to the age of the sibling. As far as possible they should be involved in the care of their brother/sister and be aware as to what is going on. It is easier to help them through the facts of their brother's/sister's last days of life than to allow them to develop fantasies.

For the family of a disabled child the death will bring with it changes to their life – much of their daily routine will have been directed at meeting the child's needs, visiting hospitals, going to therapy and attending support groups and school. With the death of their child comes the loss of these support networks within which is invested a considerable memory of the child and those who knew him/her. Some families may need to maintain contact with these known supports for variable periods until they have established new ones. Bereavement counselling may lead to one such new contact; if therapists become involved in such counselling they will need to recognize what is normal grief from that which may be pathological. For the latter the therapist will need to know where to seek further help.

True care for the dying patient does not involve sophisticated treatments; it demands care, understanding and compassion of the very highest standards. Unashamedly, I have stressed this throughout the chapter. At the same time the ability to 'switch off' is equally important, and this is why it is so important for all involved with caring for the dying to think 'positively'. Death should be seen as a natural part of life, and *not* as a disaster.

Note: This chapter has not attempted to touch upon the problems of patients in intensive care units – it has concentrated on the patient who is dying from long-term illness. It is written to encourage the physiotherapist not to be frightened, put off or embarrassed at the thought of treating a dying person. They are still human beings with all the faults and frailties which we know so well; they require help, and if as physiotherapists we can provide this, then we must do so.

REFERENCES

Chatterton, P. (1988). Physiotherapy for the terminally ill. *Physiotherapy*, **74**, 1, 42–6.

Downie, P.A. (1973). Havens of peace. *Nursing Times*, August 16, 1068–70.

Downie, P.A. (1974a). Hostel of God. *Nursing Mirror*, October 10, 66–8.

Downie, P.A. (1974b). A personal commentary on the care of the dying on the North American continent. *Nursing Mirror*, October 10, 68–70.

Graeme, P.D. (1975). Support for the dying patient and his family. In *Cancer, the Patient and the Family*, John Sherratt and Sons, Altrincham.

Kubler-Ross, E. (1970). *On Death and Dying*. Tavistock Publications, London.

Wilkes, E., Crowther, G.O. and Greaves, C.W.K.H. (1978). A different kind of day hospital – the patient with pre-terminal cancer and chronic disease. *British Medical Journal*, **2**, 1053–6.

Wilkes, E. (1982). The day unit. In *The Dying Patient* (ed. Wilkes, E.), pp. 300–305. MTP Press, Lancaster.

BIBLIOGRAPHY

Albanus (1978). To die or not to die. *Therapy*, May 5.

Buckman, R. (1988). *I Don't Know What to Say. How to Help and Support Someone Who is Dying*. Macmillan, London.

Corr, C. A. and Corr, D. M. (eds) (1983). *Hospice Care: Principles and Practice*. Faber and Faber, London. Published in the USA by Springer Publishing Co Inc, New York.

Hinton, J. (1972). *Dying*, 2nd edition. Penguin Books, Harmondsworth.

Lamerton, R. (1980). *Care of the Dying*. Penguin Books, Harmondsworth.

Kubler-Ross, E. (1983). *On Children and Death*. Macmillan Publishing Co, New York.

Lewis, C.S. (1961). *A Grief Observed*. Faber and Faber, London.

On Dying Well: An Anglican Contribution to the Debate on Euthanasia (1975).

Parkes, C.M. (1986). *Bereavement*, 2nd edition. Penguin Books, Harmondsworth.

Wells, R. (1988). *Helping Children Cope with Grief*. Sheldon Press, London.

Wilkes, E. (ed.) (1982). *The Dying Patient: The Medical Management of Incurable and Terminal Illness*. MTP Press, Lancaster.

ACKNOWLEDGEMENTS

The author thanks the following for advice, help and constructive criticism:

Mrs A. Scott-Malden MCSP, physiotherapist at the Priscilla Bacon Lodge, Norwich.

Miss C. Bungay MCSP and Miss M. John BSC, MSC (senior clinical psychologist, Department of Child Health, St George's Hospital, London) who wrote the short section on the dying child.

The late Cardinal John Heenan gave permission in a personal letter to the author for the use of his statement on euthanasia.

Further Reading

In addition to the references and bibliography at the end of most of the chapters, the following is a select list of titles which touch on the wider aspects of some of the subjects within the book. They are divided into *Books* and *Papers*. Where books are listed the current editions are shown, but most textbooks are regularly updated and the reader should check whether there has been a new edition. This can be ascertained by asking the librarian at the hospital or postgraduate centre library, or by checking in Whittaker's *Books in Print* (now on microfiche) which is to be found in the reference section of all public libraries.

Books

Anderson, R. and Bury, M. (eds) (1988). *Living With Chronic Illness. The Experience of Patients and their Families*. Unwin Hyman, London.

Baum, M. (1988). *Breast Cancer*, 2nd edition. Oxford University Press, Oxford.

Bond, M. (1986). *Stress and Self-awareness. A Guide for Nurses*. Heinemann Medical Books, London.

Brearley, G. and Birchley, P. (1986). *Introducing Counselling Skills and Techniques. With Particular Application for the Paramedical Professions*. Faber and Faber, London.

Clarke, D. C. (1986). *Mentally Handicapped People, Living and Learning*, revised edition. Baillière Tindall, London.

Davidson's Principles and Practice of Medicine. A Textbook for Students and Doctors, 15th edition. (1987). Churchill Livingstone, Edinburgh.

Downie, R. S. and Calman, K. C. (1987). *Healthy Respect: Ethics in Health Care*. Faber and Faber, London.

Doyle, D. (1987). *Domiciliary Terminal Care. A Handbook for Doctors and Nurses*. Churchill Livingstone, Edinburgh.

Evans, T. R. (ed.) (1986). *ABC of Resuscitation*. British Medical Association, London.

Gillis, L. (1988). *Human Behaviour in Illness. Psychology and Interpersonal Relationships*, 4th edition. Faber and Faber, London.

Hattersley, J., Hosking, G. P., Morrow, D. and Myers, M. (1987). *People with Mental Handicap. Perspectives of Intellectual Disability*. Faber and Faber, London.

Hollins, S. and Grimer, M. (1988). *Going Somewhere. People with Mental Handicaps and their Pastoral Care*. SPCK, London.

Kennedy, I. (1983). *The Unmasking of Medicine*. Granada Books, London.

Ludman, H. (1988). *ABC of Ear, Nose and Throat*, 2nd edition. British Medical Association, London.

Malin, N. (ed.) (1988). *Reassessing Community Care. With Particular Reference to Provision for People with Mental Handicap and for People with Mental Illness.* Croom Helm, London.

Medicine in Old Age, 2nd edition. (1988). British Medical Association, London.

Oakhill, A. (ed.) (1988). *The Supportive Care of the Child with Cancer.* John Wright, London.

Piff, C. (1985). *Let's Face It.* Gollancz, London.

Reid, J., Rubin, P. and Whiting, B. (1985). *Lecture Notes on Clinical Pharmacology*, 2nd edition. Blackwell Scientific Publications Limited, Oxford.

Riseborough, P. and Walter, M. (1988). *Management in Health Care: the Allied Professions.* John Wright, London.

Rogers, H. J. and Spector, R. C. (1986). *Aids to Pharmacology*, 2nd edition. Churchill Livingstone, Edinburgh.

Standacher, C. (1988). *Beyond Grief.* Souvenir Press, London.

Turner, P. and Volans, G. (1988). *Drugs Handbook, 1988–89.* Macmillan Press, London.

Warburg, T. L. (1988). *A Voice at Twilight.* Owen, London.

Whitehead, S. (1988). *Illustrated Operation Notes. A Guide for Students to General Surgical Procedures.* Edward Arnold, London.

Wilson, F. and Park, W. G. (1980). *Basic Resuscitation and Primary Care.* MTP Press, Lancaster.

Wright, P. and Treacher, A. (eds) (1982). *The Problem of Medical Knowledge: Examining the Social Construction of Medicine.* Edinburgh University Press, Edinburgh.

Wyngaarden, J. B. and Smith, L. H. (eds) (1985). *The Cecil Textbook of Medicine*, 17th edition, W. B. Saunders Co, Philadelphia.

Papers

Brudvig, T. J. (1988). Therapeutic horseback riding on a military base: one PT's experience. *Clinical Management of Physiotherapy*, 8, 3, 30–2.

Chernin, E. (1988). The 'Harvard System': a mystery dispelled. *British Medical Journal*, 297, 106–3.

Cunha, U. V. (1988). Differential diagnosis of gait disorders in the elderly. *Geriatrics*, 43, 8, 33–8.

Dordel, H. J. (1988). Mobility training following brain trauma: results of intensive individual treatment. *International Journal of Rehabilitation Results*, 10, 4 (supp.), 279–90.

Durance, J. P. and O'Shea, B. J. (1988). Upper limb amputees – a clinical profile. *International Disability Studies*, 10, 2, 68–72.

Gilchrist, W. J., Newman, R. J., Hamblen, D. L. and Williams, B. O. (1988). Prospective randomized study of an orthopaedic geriatric in-patient service. *British Medical Journal*, 297, 1116–18.

Goodhart, C. B. (1988). Embryo experiments. *British Medical Journal*, 297, 782–3.

Henalla, S. M., Kirwan, P., Castleden, C. M., Hutchins, C. J. and Breeson, A. J. (1988). The effect of pelvic floor exercises in the treatment of genuine urinary stress incontinence in women at two hospitals. *British Journal of Obstetrics and Gynaecology*, 95, 6, 602–6.

Kennie, D. C., Reid, J., Richardson, I. R., Kiamari, A. A. and Kelt, C. (1988). Effectiveness of geriatric rehabilitative care after fractures of the proximal femur in elderly women: a randomized clinical trial. *British Medical Journal*, 297, 1083–6.

Kloth, L. C. and Feeder, J. A. (1988). Acceleration of wound healing with high voltage, monophasic pulsed current. *Physical Therapy*, 68, 4, 503–8.

Malchow, D. and Clark, J. D. (1987). Interviewing the amputee. A step toward rehabilitation. *Orthotics and Prosthetics*, 41, 3, 50–9.

Mental Handicap: Three special issues on Mental Handicap will be located in *Physiotherapy* (1985). 71, 3, 99–123; 71, 4, 170–5; 71, 5, 216–24.

Physiotherapy in Psychiatry: A special issue will be located in *Physiotherapy*, 71, 6, 257–68.

Useful Organizations

Of necessity this is only a select list of organizations and agencies which can offer help, advice and counselling. Mostly they relate to the conditions mentioned in this book, and they have been divided into two sections, general and children. A useful guide book for extensive information about many organizations is the *Directory for the Disabled* edited by A. Darnborough and D. Kinrade and published by Woodhead-Faulkner, Cambridge CB2 3PF. It is regularly updated.

General

The organizations are listed alphabetically.

Age Concern
Bernard Sunley House, Pitcairn Road
Mitcham, Surrey CR4 3LL   01–640 5431

Alzheimer's Disease Society
Bank Buildings, Fulham Broadway
London SW6 1EP   01–381 3177

Association of Carers
1st Floor, 21–23 New Road
Chatham, Kent ME4 4QJ   0634 813981

British Association of Cancer United
Patients (BACUP)
121–123 Charterhouse Street
London EC1M 6AA   01–608 1661

British Burns Association
British Research Group
c/o Birmingham Accident Hospital
Birmingham B15 1NA   021–643 7041

British Diabetic Association
10 Queen Anne Street
London W1M 0BD   01–323 1531

British Geriatrics Society
1 St Andrew's Place, Regents Park
London NW1 4LB   01–935 4004

British Institute of Mental Handicap
Wolverhampton Road
Kidderminster
Worcs DY10 3PP   0562 850251

Colostomy Welfare Group
38–9 Eccleston Square (2nd Floor)
London SW1V 1PB   01–828 5175

Disabled Drivers' Association
Ashwellthorpe
Norfolk NR16 1EX   050841 449

Disabled Living Foundation
380–384 Harrow Road
London W9 2HU   01–289 6111

Disfigurement Guidance Centre
52 Crossgate
Cupar, Fife KY15 5HS   03374 281

HEADWAY
National Head Injuries Association
200 Mansfield Road
Nottingham NG1 3HX   0602 622382

Hysterectomy Support Group
11 Henryson Road
London SE4 1HL   01–690 5987

Ileostomy Association of Great Britain
and Ireland
Amblehurst House
Chobham, Woking
Surrey GU24 8PZ   09905 8277

Intractable Pain Society of Great Britain
and Northern Ireland
9 Bedford Square
London WC1B 3RA   01–631 1650

Let's Face It
10 Wood End
Crowthorne
Berkshire RG11 6DQ   0344 774405

Marie Curie Cancer Care
28 Belgrave Square
London SW1X 8QG   01–235 3325

Mastectomy and Breast Care Association
of Great Britain
26 Harrison Street (off Grays Inn Road)
London WC1H 8JG   01–837 0908

MIND
National Association for Mental Health
22 Harley Street
London W1N 2ED   01–637 0741

National Association for Colitis and
Crohn's Disease
98A London Road, St Albans
Herts AL1 1NX

National Association of Laryngectomee
Clubs
38 Eccleston Square
London SW1V 1PB   01–834 2704

National Association of Limbless
Disabled
31 The Mall, Ealing
London W5 2PX   01–579 1758

National Eczema Society
5 Tavistock Place
London WC1H 9SR   01–388 4097

National Schizophrenia Fellowship
79 Victoria Road
Surbiton, Surrey KT6 4NS   01–390 3651

National Society for Phenylketonuria
c/o Worth Cottage, Lower Scholes
Pickles Hill
Keighley BD22 0RR   0535 44865

Prader-Willi Syndrome Association
c/o 30 Follett Drive
Abbots Langley
Herts WD5 0LO   0923 674543

The Psoriasis Association
7 Milton Street
Northampton NN2 7JG   0604 711129

Rape Crisis Centre
PO Box 69, London WC1X 9NJ
(Local lists available)

Riding for the Disabled Association
National Agricultural Centre (Avenue R)
Kenilworth
Warwickshire CV8 2LY   0203 56107

Royal Association for Disability and
Rehabilitation (RADAR)
25 Mortimer Street
London W1N 8AB   01–637 5400

Tay Sachs and Allied Diseases
Association
c/o 17 Sydney Road, Barkingside
Ilford, Essex IG6 2ED   01–550 8989

Terence Higgins Trust
BM AIDS
London WC1N 3XX
Helpline   01–242 1010

Women's National Cancer Control
Campaign
1 South Audley Street
London W1Y 5DQ   01–499 7532

The Vitiligo Group
PO Box 919
London SE21 8AW

Children

A useful booklet giving details of many organizations, as well as information about allowances and how to claim them, may be obtained from the Voluntary Council for Handicapped Children, National Children's Bureau, 8 Wakley Street, London EC1V 7QE. It is called *Help Starts Here.*

Association for Spina Bifida and
Hydrocephalus (ASBAH)
22 Upper Woburn Place
London WC1H OEP   01–388 1382

British Epilepsy Association
Ansley House, 40 Hanover Square
Leeds
West Yorkshire LS3 1BE   0532 439393

Compassionate Friends
6 Denmark Street
Bristol BS1 5DQ   0272 292778
(this is an organization for bereaved parents)

Contact-a-Family
16 Strutton Ground
London SW1P 2HP   01–222 2695

Cystic Fibrosis Research Trust
5 Blyth Road
Bromley, Kent BR1 3RS   01–464 7211

Down's Syndrome Association
12–13 Clapham Common, South Side
London SW4 7AA   01–720 0008

Handicapped Adventure Playground
Association
Fulham Palace Playground
Bishop's Avenue
London SW6 6EA   01–731 4443

Muscular Dystrophy Group of Great
Britain
Nattrass House, 35 Macaulay Road
London SW4 OQP   01–720 8055

National Association for the Welfare of
Children in Hospital (NAWCH)
7 Exton Street
London SE1 8UE   01–261 1738

National Childbirth Trust
9 Queensborough Terrace
London W2 3TB   01–221 3833

National Society for Mentally
Handicapped Children (MENCAP)
117–123 Golden Lane
London EC1Y ORF   01–253 9433

Pre-school Playgroups Association
61 Kings Cross Road
London WC1   01–833 0991

Spastics Society
12 Park Crescent
London W1N 4EQ   01–636 5020

Toy Libraries Association
Seabrook House, Wyllyotts Manor
Darkes Lane
Potters Bar EN6 5HL   0707 44571

Professional groups

The following are Specific Clinical Interest Groups of the Chartered Society of Physiotherapy. Anyone interested in joining a group should write to the secretary of the relevant group, c/o the Chartered Society of Physiotherapy, 14 Bedford Row, London WC1R 4ED.

Association of Paediatric Chartered Physiotherapists
Association of Chartered Physiotherapists in Animal Therapy
Riding for the Disabled
Association of Chartered Physiotherapists in Obstetrics and Gynaecology
Association of Chartered Physiotherapists in Psychiatry
Association of Chartered Physiotherapists in Mental Handicap
Association of Chartered Physiotherapists with a Special Interest in Elderly People

Index